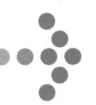

ACSM's
Guidelines for
Exercise Testing
and Prescription
SEVENTH EDITION

SENIOR EDITOR
Mitchell H. Whaley, PhD, FACSM
Professor and Chair
School of Physical Education, Sport and Exercise Science
Ball State University
Muncie, Indiana

ASSOCIATE EDITOR—CLINICAL
Peter H. Brubaker, PhD, FACSM
Associate Professor and Executive Director
Healthy Exercise and Lifestyle Programs
Department of Health and Exercise Science
Wake Forest University
Winston-Salem, North Carolina

ASSOCIATE EDITOR—FITNESS
Robert M. Otto, PhD, FACSM
Professor and Director
Human Performance Laboratory
Department of Health, Physical Education, and
Human Performance Sciences
Adelphi University
Garden City, New York

AUTHORS
Lawrence Armstrong, PhD, FACSM
Gary J. Balady, MD
Michael J. Berry, PhD, FACSM
Shala E. Davis, PhD, FACSM
Brenda M. Davy, PhD, RD, LC
Kevin P. Davy, PhD, FACSM
Barry A. Franklin, PhD, FACSM
Neil F. Gordon, MD, PhD, MPH, FACSM

I-Min Lee, MD, FACSM
Timothy McConnell, PhD, FACSM
Jonathan N. Myers, PhD, FACSM
Frank X. Pizza, PhD,
Thomas W. Rowland, MD, FACSM
Kerry Stewart, EdD, FACSM
Paul D. Thompson, MD, FACSM
Janet P. Wallace, PhD, FACSM

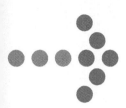

ACSM's
GUIDELINES FOR
EXERCISE TESTING
AND PRESCRIPTION

SEVENTH EDITION

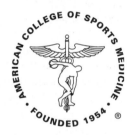

**AMERICAN COLLEGE
OF SPORTS MEDICINE**

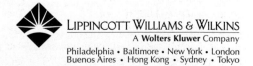

LIPPINCOTT WILLIAMS & WILKINS
A **Wolters Kluwer** Company
Philadelphia · Baltimore · New York · London
Buenos Aires · Hong Kong · Sydney · Tokyo

Executive Acquisitions Editor: Peter J. Darcy
Managing Editor: Linda S. Napora
Marketing Manager: Christen D. Murphy
Production Editor: Jennifer Ajello
Designer: Risa Clow
Illustrator: Kimberly M. Battista
Compositor: Seven Worldwide
Printer: RR Donnelley & Sons – Crawfordsville
ACSM's Publications Committee Chair: Jeffrey L. Roitman, Ed.D, FACSM
ACSM Group Publisher: D. Mark Robertson

351 West Camden Street
Baltimore, Maryland 21201-2436 USA

530 Walnut Street
Philadelphia, Pennsylvania 19106-3621 USA

Printed in the United States of America

First Edition, 1975
Second Edition, 1980

Third Edition, 1986
Fourth Edition, 1991

Fifth Edition, 1995
Sixth Edition, 2000

Library of Congress Cataloging-in-Publication Data

American College of Sports Medicine.
   ACSM's guidelines for exercise testing and prescription / American College of Sports
Medicine ; [senior editor, Mitchell H. Whaley; associate editor—clinical, Peter H.
Brubaker, associate editor—fitness, Robert M. Otto; authors, Lawrence Armstrong...et
al.].—7th ed.
    p.; cm
  Includes bibliographical references and index.
  ISBN 13: 978-0-7817-4590-1
  ISBN 10: 0-7817-4590-X
  1. Exercise therapy. 2. Exercise tests. I. Title: Guidelines for exercise testing and
prescription. II. Whaley, Mitchell H., 1955- III. Brubaker, Peter H., 1961- IV. Otto,
Robert M. V. Armstrong, Lawrence E., 1949- VI. Title.
  [DNLM: 1. Exertion. 2. Exercise Test—standards. 3. Exercise Therapy—standards. WE
103 A514a 2005]
  RM725.A48 2005
  615,8'2—dc22

2004057756

To purchase additional copies of this book call our customer service department at **(800) 638-
3030** or fax orders to **(301) 824-7390.** International customers should call **(301) 714-2324.**

Visit Lippincott Williams & Wilkins on the Internet: http://www.lww.com. Lippincott
Williams & Wilkins customer service representatives are available from 8:30 am to 6:00 pm, EST,
Monday through Friday, for telephone access.

For more information concerning American College of Sports Medicine certification and suggested preparatory materials, call **(800) 486-5643** or visit the American College of Sports
Medicine Website at **www.acsm.org.**

06 07
3 4 5 6 7 8 9 10

This text is humbly dedicated to the more than 18,000 professionals who have attained certification and/or registration from the American College of Sports Medicine since 1975. It is from the daily efforts of this prestigious group—mostly working in the trenches—that many advances in health and fitness, and clinical exercise practice routines/regimens are first tried, and then refined, and finally become guidelines. *We are indebted to all of you, and most thankful for your collective desire to advance the fields of exercise testing and prescription.*

Sir Isaac Newton said, "If I have seen further . . . it is by standing upon the shoulders of giants." Traditionally, *ACSM's Guidelines for Exercise Testing and Prescription* has been written and reviewed by representatives of the Committee on Certification and Registry Boards (formerly known as the Certification and Education Committee and the Preventive and Rehabilitative Exercise Committee) of the American College of Sports Medicine. Several individuals on the committee and others from the college contributed to each edition. The primary responsibility for writing and editing each edition was assumed by the following individuals:

First Edition, 1975
Karl G. Stoedefalke, PhD, Co Chair
John A. Faulkner, PhD, Co-Chair
Samuel M. Fox, MD
Henry S. Miller, Jr., MD
Bruno Balke, MD

Second Edition, 1980
R. Anne Abbott, PhD, Chair
Karl G. Stoedefalke, PhD
N. Blythe Runsdorf, PhD
John A. Faulkner, PhD

Third Edition, 1986
Steven N. Blair, PED, Chair
Larry W. Gibbons, MD
Patricia Painter, PhD
Russell R. Pate, PhD
C. Barr Taylor, MD
Josephine Will, MS

Fourth Edition, 1991
Russell R. Pate, PhD, Chair
Steven N. Blair, PED
J. Larry Durstine, PhD
Duane O. Eddy, PhD
Peter Hanson, MD
Patricia Painter, PhD
L. Kent Smith, MD
Larry A. Wolfe, PhD

Fifth Edition, 1995
W. Larry Kenney, PhD,
Senior Editor
Reed H. Humphrey, PhD, PT,
Associate Editor Clinical
Cedric X. Bryant, PhD, Associate
Editor Fitness
Donald A. Mahler, MD
Victor F. Froelicher, MD
Nancy Houston Miller, RN
Tracy D. York, MS

Sixth Edition, 2000
Barry A. Franklin, PhD, Senior Editor
Mitchell H. Whaley, PhD, Associate
Editor Clinical
Edward T. Howley, PhD, Associate
Editor Fitness
Authors:
Gary J. Balady, MD
Kathy A. Berra, MSN, ANP
Lawrence A. Golding, PhD
Neil F. Gordon, MD, PhD, MPH
Donald A. Mahler, MD
Jonathan N. Myers, PhD
Lois M. Sheldahl, PhD
Special Contributors:
Martin Grais, MD
David L. Herbert, Esq
William G. Herbert, PhD
David P. Swain, PhD
Sheri L. Tokarczyk. MS, PA-C
Andrew J. Young, PhD

Preface

This seventh edition of *ACSM's Guidelines for Exercise Testing and Prescription* represents the next step in the evolution of this text first published by the American College of Sports Medicine in 1975. What started in 1975 as 48 pages of *guidelines* related to 1) admitting adults into exercise programs, 2) exercise testing administration, and 3) exercise prescription, has evolved into one of the single most widely read and referenced texts of its kind in the world (more than 100,000 copies of the sixth edition have been sold since 2000). The primary purpose of this revised edition was to present the most current information in a usable form for health/fitness and clinical exercise professionals, physicians, nurses, physician assistants, physical and occupational therapists, dietitians, and health care administrators. This edition continues the emphasis on preventing illness through physical activity/exercise in apparently healthy persons and those with risk factors, as well as prescribing exercise for patients with diagnosed chronic disease. Furthermore, these guidelines acknowledge the efficacy of self-guided physical activity regimens for many individuals, and recommendations for such are provided at various places throughout the book.

There are several additional ACSM texts that complement and expand on the *Guidelines*. For more detailed treatment of topics covered in the *Guidelines*, the reader is directed to its companion publication, the *ACSM's Resource Manual for Guidelines for Exercise Testing and Prescription,* fifth edition. Additional information on selected chronic diseases and/or conditions, particularly those not covered in the *Guidelines,* may be found in two ACSM texts: *ACSM's Exercise Management for Persons with Chronic Diseases and Disabilities*, and *ACSM's Resources for Clinical Exercise Physiology*. When combined with the *Guidelines*, these resources represent the fundamental knowledge that must be mastered by candidates seeking ACSM credentials in preventive and rehabilitative exercise programming. Finally, the *ACSM Fitness Book* serves a vital role for the general public by providing self-guided fitness assessments and an easy-to-use progressive exercise program for adults with few to no chronic disease risk factors.

The ACSM also recognizes the importance of exercise-related guidelines and position statements published by other professional organizations (e.g., American Heart Association, American Association for Cardiovascular and Pulmonary Rehabilitation, American Thoracic Society, American College of Obstetrics and Gynecology), and relevant content and references from such documents are included within these *Guidelines*. Needless to say, all exercise program professionals should stay abreast of revisions to these other dynamic documents.

Substantive revisions have been made to most chapters of the seventh edition for the purpose of incorporating: 1) the most current public health and clinical information; 2), state-of-the-art, research-based recommendations; and 3) accumulated feedback from readers of previous editions of the *Guidelines*. The quantitative data thresholds, clinical laboratory cutoffs considered "abnormal," and normative fitness data found throughout the fifth and sixth editions have been carried forward and updated where appropriate. An exercise *intensity* classification table and a new table of health benefits from the *dose-response* perspective are included in Chapter 1. A new preparticipation screening algorithm is found in Chapter 2, along with a modification of the ACSM/AHA screening questionnaire. The algorithm and questionnaire, along with revised program supervision guidelines found in Chapter 7, are more closely linked to the ACSM risk stratification categories found in Chapter 2. Furthermore, the seventh edition contains guidelines for a broader spectrum of chronic conditions than found in previous editions, with the intent of presenting a lean set of essential testing and programming modifications while outsourcing additional supporting material to the *Resource Manual*. In addition, a continued effort was made to incorporate figures and boxes to highlight key points in the text, set off information that merited special attention with colored screening, and more clearly designate subheadings in a descending order of importance.

Beyond the revisions to the content of this text, we hope those who use *Guidelines* will consider the flow of information throughout the book as it was our intent to provide a continuum of coverage of topics that would serve both health/fitness and clinical exercise professionals. To this end, please note that Section I contains important information on benefits/risks of exercise (Chapter 1) and preparticipation screening (Chapter 2) that are relevant to all who deliver, or supervise those who deliver, exercise testing and prescription services. Section II begins with preexercise assessment and interpretation guidelines (Chapter 3) that should be read by both the health/fitness and clinical professional. The health/fitness professional may then proceed to Chapter 4 for additional assessment and interpretation guidelines more relevant to the low-risk adult, whereas the clinician may want to proceed to Chapters 5 and 6, which provide clinical exercise testing and interpretation guidelines more applicable to the moderate- to high-risk adult. Section III, Exercise Prescription, begins with a foundational chapter (Chapter 7) that is relevant for all who design and supervise exercise programs, regardless of the target population. A condensed version of the behavioral concepts presented in the sixth edition (Chapter 12) has been incorporated into the fundamental prescription principles in Chapter 7. A broader discussion of behavioral concepts is contained within the newest edition of the *ACSM Resource Manual*. Subsequent chapters in Section III provide guidelines regarding *modifications* of the fundamental testing, and prescriptive and programming principles for patients with selected chronic conditions, as well as for children and elderly people. The reader should have a solid grasp of the principles presented in Chapter 7 before progressing to Chapters 8 through 10.

The seventh edition has been prepared by a volunteer writing team with representative expertise in health/fitness and clinical exercise physiology, cardiology, epidemiology, pediatrics, and pulmonology. Our acknowledgments begin with Virginia Hall-Moore, who provided exemplary administrative support to the editorial team throughout the planning, writing, and editing phases of this project. Special thanks also go to Associate Editors, Peter H. Brubaker, PhD, FACSM, and Robert M. Otto, PhD, FACSM, for their author recruitment, chapter contributions, editorial expertise, and unwavering commitment to the project. Furthermore, we express our appreciation to Cathy Stewart (former National

Director of Certification at ACSM) and Leonard A. Kaminsky, PhD, FACSM (Senior Editor of the fifth edition of *ACSM's Resource Manual for Guidelines for Exercise Testing and Prescription*) for their involvement and critical contributions and feedback during each of our editorial meetings as we prepared this text. We also express our sincere gratitude to Linda Napora, our managing editor, for her encouragement and expertise, and her never-ending patience with our odyssey through the publication process. And finally, as was stated in the dedication, we want to acknowledge the huge contributions made by authors of previous editions of the *Guidelines*; it can truly be said that this edition continues to rely heavily on their wisdom regarding exercise testing and prescription principles.

This text has undergone an extensive review by external and internal experts; the latter include many members of the American College of Sports Medicine, and specifically, members of the ACSM Committee on Certification and Registry Boards. The College and authors wish to express their appreciation to those individuals who contributed ideas, comments, critical reviews, and editorial assistance.

Mitchell H. Whaley, PhD, FACSM
Senior Editor

NOTA BENE

The views and information contained in the seventh edition of *ACSM's Guidelines for Exercise Testing and Prescription* are provided as *guidelines* as opposed to *standards of practice*. This distinction is an important one, because specific legal connotations may be attached to such terminology. The distinction also is critical inasmuch as it gives the exercise professional the freedom to deviate from these guidelines when necessary and appropriate in the course of exercising independent and prudent judgment. *ACSM's Guidelines for Exercise Testing and Prescription* presents a framework whereby the professional may certainly—and in some cases has the obligation to—tailor to individual client or patient needs and alter to meet institutional or legislated requirements.

Contributors

Authors

Lawrence E. Armstrong, PhD, FACSM
Professor, Department of
Kinesiology
Human Performance Laboratory
University of Connecticut
Storrs, Connecticut

Gary J. Balady, MD
Co-Director, Noninvasive
Cardiac Labs
Boston Medical Center
Professor of Medicine
Boston University School of
Medicine
Boston, Massachusetts

Michael J. Berry, PhD, FACSM
Professor, Department of Health and
Exercise Science
Wake Forest University
Winston-Salem, North Carolina

Shala E. Davis, PhD, FACSM
Associate Professor, Department of
Movement Studies and Exercise
Science
East Stroudsburg University
East Stroudsburg, Pennsylvania

Brenda M. Davy, PhD, RD, LD
Assistant Professor, Department of
Human Nutrition, Foods and
Exercise
Virginia Polytechnic Institute and
State University
Blacksburg, Virginia

Kevin P. Davy, PhD, FACSM
Associate Professor, Department of
Human Nutrition, Foods and
Exercise
Virginia Polytechnic Institute and
State University
Blacksburg, Virginia

Barry A. Franklin, PhD, FACSM
Director, Cardiac Rehabilitation and
Exercise Laboratories
Beaumont Rehab and Health Center
William Beaumont Hospital
Royal Oak, Michigan
Professor of Physiology
Wayne State University
Detroit, Michigan

**Neil F. Gordon MD, PhD, M.PH.,
FACSM**
President, Intervention Center
for Heart Disease Prevention
St. Joseph's/Candler Health System
Savannah, Georgia

I-Min Lee, MD, ScD
Associate Professor, Department
of Medicine
Harvard Medical School
Associate Epidemiologist,
Department of Preventive Medicine
Brigham and Women's Hospital
Boston, Massachusetts

Timothy R. McConnell, PhD, FACSM
Assistant Professor
Coordinator, Graduate Student
Department of Science and Athletics
Bloomsburg University
Bloomsburg, Pennsylvania

Jonathan N. Myers, PhD, FACSM
Clinical Assistant Professor of
Medicine
Department of Cardiology
Stanford University
Palo Alto VA Health Care System
Palo Alto, California

Francis X. Pizza, PhD
Professor
Department of Kinesiology
The University of Toledo
Toledo, Ohio

Thomas W. Rowland, MD, FACSM
Professor, Department of Pediatrics
Tufts University School of Medicine
Boston, Massachusetts
Director, Pediatric Cardiology
Bay State Medical Center
Springfield, Massachusetts

Kerry Stewart, EdD, FACSM
Associate Professor of Medicine
Division of Cardiology
Director, Johns Hopkins Heart
Health
Johns Hopkins Bayview Medical
Center
Baltimore, Maryland

Paul D. Thompson, MD, FACSM
Director, Preventive Cardiology
Hartford Hospital
Hartford, Connecticut

Janet P. Wallace, PhD, FACSM
Professor and Director of Adult
Fitness
Department of Kinesiology
Indiana University
Bloomington, Indiana

Contents

Section IV Appendices

Abbreviations

AACVPR	American Association of Cardiovascular and Pulmonary Rehabilitation	CAD	coronary artery disease
		CDC	Centers for Disease Control and Prevention
ABI	ankle/brachial systolic pressure index	CHF	congestive heart failure
		CHO	carbohydrate
ACE	angiotensin-converting enzyme	CI	cardiac index
		COPD	chronic obstructive pulmonary disease
ACGIH	American Conference of Governmental Industrial Hygienists	CPAP	continuous positive airway pressure
ACOG	American College of Obstetricians and Gynecologists	CPR	cardiopulmonary resuscitation
		CPK	creatine phosphokinase
ACP	American College of Physicians	CRQ	Chronic Respiratory Questionnaire
ACSM	American College of Sports Medicine	DBP	diastolic blood pressure
		DOMS	delayed onset muscle soreness
ADL	activities of daily living		
AHA	American Heart Association	ECG	electrocardiogram (electrocardiographic)
AICD	automatic implantable cardioverter defibrillator	EF	ejection fraction
		EIB	exercise-induced bronchoconstriction
AIHA	American Industrial Hygiene Association	EIH	exercise-induced hypotension
AMA	American Medical Association	ERV	expiratory reserve volume
AMS	acute mountain sickness	ES	Exercise Specialist®
AST	aspartate aminotrans-ferase	FC	functional capacity
		$FEV_{1.0}$	forced expiratory volume in one second
AV	atrioventricular		
BIA	bioelectrical impedance analysis	FFM	fat-free mass
		F_{IO_2}	fraction of inspired oxygen
BLS	basic life support		
BMI	body mass index	F_{ICO_2}	fraction of inspired carbon dioxide
BP	blood pressure		
BR	breathing reserve	FN	false negative
BUN	blood urea nitrogen	FP	false positive
C	ceiling (heat stress) limit	FRV	functional residual volume
CABG(S)	coronary artery bypass graft (surgery)	FVC	forced vital capacity

GXT	graded exercise test	P_aO_2	partial pressure of arterial oxygen
HAPE	high-altitude pulmonary edema	PAC	premature atrial contraction
HDL	high-density lipoprotein	PAR-Q	Physical Activity Readiness Questionnaire
HFD	Health/Fitness Director®		
HFI	Health/Fitness Instructor$_{SM}$	PD	Program Director$_{SM}$
HR	heart rate	PE_{max}	maximal expiratory pressure
HR_{max}	maximal heart rate	PI_{max}	maximal inspiratory pressure
HRR	heart rate reserve		
HR_{rest}	resting heart rate	PNF	proprioceptive neuro-muscular facilitation
IC	inspiratory capacity		
ICD	implantable cardioverter defibrillator	Po_2	partial pressure of oxygen
IDDM	insulin-dependent diabetes mellitus	PTCA	percutaneous translumi-nal coronary angioplasty
KSAs	knowledge, skills, and abilities	PVC	premature ventricular contraction
LAD	left axis deviation	PVD	peripheral vascular disease
LBBB	left bundle-branch block		
LDH	lactate dehydrogenase	RER	respiratory exchange ratio
LDL	low-density lipoprotein		
L-G-L	Lown-Ganong-Levine	RAD	right axis deviation
LLN	lower limit of normal	RAL	recommended alert limit
LV	left ventricle (left ventricular)	RBBB	right bundle-branch block
MCHC	mean corpuscular hemo-globin concentration	rep	repetition
		RIMT	resistive inspiratory muscle training
MET	metabolic equivalent	1-RM	one repetition maximum
MI	myocardial infarction	RPE	rating of perceived exertion
MUGA	multigated acquisition (scan)		
MVC	maximal voluntary contraction	RQ	respiratory quotient
		RV	residual volume
MVV	maximal voluntary ventilation	RVG	radionuclide ventriculog-raphy
NCEP	National Cholesterol Education Program	RVH	right ventricular hypertrophy
NIDDM	non–insulin-dependent diabetes mellitus	S_aO_2	percent saturation of arterial oxygen
NIH	National Institutes of Health	SBP	systolic blood pressure
NIOSH	National Institute for Occupational Safety and Health	SEE	standard error of estimate
		SPECT	single photon emission computed tomography
NYHA	New York Heart Association		

SVT	supraventricular tachycardia	VMT	ventilatory muscle training
THR	target heart rate	$\dot{V}O_2$	volume of oxygen consumed per minute
TLC	total lung capacity		
TN	true negative	$\dot{V}O_{2max}$	maximal oxygen uptake
TP	true positive	$\dot{V}O_{2peak}$	peak oxygen uptake
TPR	total peripheral resistance	$\dot{V}O_2R$	oxygen uptake reserve
		$\%\dot{V}O_2R$	percentage of oxygen uptake reserve
TV	tidal volume		
VC	vital capacity	VT	ventilatory threshold
$\dot{V}CO_2$	volume of carbon dioxide per minute	WBGT	wet-bulb globe temperature
$\dot{V}_E$	expired ventilation per minute	WHR	waist-to-hip ratio
		W-P-W	Wolff-Parkinson-White
$\dot{V}_{Emax}$	maximal exercise ventilation	YMCA	Young Men's Christian Association
$\dot{V}_I$	inspired ventilation per minute	YWCA	Young Women's Christian Association

Portland Community College Library

971-722-4935
www.pcc.edu/library

Borrowed Items 4/27/2016 19:01
XXXXX3928

Item Title	Due Date
33019005868246	5/18/2016
Complete conditioning for soccer	
33019006562541	5/18/2016
ACSM's guidelines for exercise testing and prescription	
33019007675227	5/18/2016
Weight training	
33019007768147	5/18/2016
High-Intensity 300	
33019007772495	5/18/2016
Training for speed, agility, and quickness	

Thank you for using the self-check out machine

Health Appraisal, Risk Assessment, and Safety of Exercise

Benefits and Risks Associated With Physical Activity

This chapter provides operational definitions for terminology used throughout the book related to physical activity and fitness, and then provides a review of: 1) the current public health recommendations for physical activity, 2) the health and fitness benefits associated with regular physical activity and/or exercise, and 3) the risks associated with exercise. The chapter concludes with a brief description of recommendations for reducing the incidence and severity of exercise-related complications in primary and secondary prevention programs.

Physical Activity and Fitness Terminology

It is important to summarize several key terms defined elsewhere[1,2] that are used throughout the text. *Physical activity* is defined as bodily movement that is produced by the contraction of skeletal muscle and that substantially increases energy expenditure. *Exercise*, a type of physical activity, is defined as planned, structured, and repetitive bodily movement done to improve or maintain one or more components of physical fitness. *Physical fitness* is a multidimensional concept that has been defined as a set of attributes that people possess or achieve that relates to the ability to perform physical activity[1], and is comprised of skill-related, health-related, and physiologic components[2]. Skill-related components of physical fitness include agility, balance, coordination, speed, power, and reaction time, and are associated mostly with sport and motor skills performance. Health-related physical fitness is associated with the ability to perform daily activities with vigor, and the possession of traits and capacities that are associated with a low risk of premature development of hypokinetic diseases (e.g., those associated with physical inactivity). Health-related components of fitness include cardiovascular endurance, muscular strength and endurance, flexibility, and body composition. Physiologic fitness differs from health-related fitness in that it includes nonperformance components that relate to biological systems influenced by habitual activity. Physiologic fitness includes:

- Metabolic fitness: The status of metabolic systems and variables predictive of the risk for diabetes and cardiovascular disease
- Morphologic fitness: The status of body compositional factors such as body circumference, body fat content, and regional body fat distribution
- Bone integrity: The status of bone mineral density

Both health-related and physiologic fitness measures are closely allied with health promotion and disease prevention and can be modified through regular physical activity and exercise.

Professionals should recognize that both the quality and quantity of physical activity recommendations described in later chapters of this text relate to exercise recommendations and should not be viewed as inconsistent or contrary to existing physical activity recommendations for the general public[3-6].

In addition to definitions for physical activity, exercise, and physical fitness, there is a recognized need to standardize the use of terms related to physical activity intensity[3,7]. This issue has been problematic in that adjectives such as *light, low, moderate, vigorous,* and *hard* have been associated with a wide range of physiologic equivalents, such as metabolic equivalents (METs) or percentages of maximal oxygen uptake. Likewise, several of the aforementioned terms have been used to describe quantities of physical activity expressed in kilocalories expended per session or per week. To aid in the standard use of terminology describing physical activity intensity, the authors of the Surgeon General's report[3] provided a classification scheme, which has been modified several times[7,8] and is summarized in Table 1-1. The table contains an ordinal set of adjectives that are arbitrarily anchored to a set of physiologic intensity ranges. In addition, the physiologic intensity ranges have been expressed in both relative and absolute terms. *Relative intensity* is defined using a percentage of an individual's maximal oxygen uptake reserve or heart rate reserve, whereas *absolute intensity* has been defined using METs with values for each intensity category provided across a range of functional capacities.

The following points should be considered when interpreting the information within Table 1-1:

- The linking of adjectives to physiologic ranges (e.g., light $\approx$20%–39% $\dot{V}O_2R$) is based on participation in activities ranging from 20 to 60 minutes, which represents the recommended session duration within most exercise prescriptions.

Table 1-1. Classification of Physical Activity Intensity

	Relative Intensity		Absolute Intensity Ranges (METs) Across Fitness Levels			
Intensity	$\dot{V}O_2R$ (%) HRR (%)	Maximal HR (%)	12 MET $\dot{V}O_{2max}$	10 MET $\dot{V}O_{2max}$	8 MET $\dot{V}O_{2max}$	6 MET $\dot{V}O_{2max}$
Very light	<20	<50	<3.2	<2.8	<2.4	<2.0
Light	20–39	50–63	3.2–5.3	2.8–4.5	2.4–3.7	2.0–3.0
Moderate	40–59	64–76	5.4–7.5	4.6–6.3	3.8–5.1	3.1–4.0
Hard (vigorous)	60–84	77–93	7.6–10.2	6.4–8.6	5.2–6.9	4.1–5.2
Very hard	≥85	≥94	≥10.3	≥8.7	≥7.0	≥5.3
Maximal	100	100	12	10	8	6

Adapted from United States Department of Health and Human Services. Physical activity and health: A report of the Surgeon General, 1996; American College of Sports Medicine. Position Stand: The recommended quantity and quality of exercise for developing and maintaining cardiorespiratory and muscular fitness, and flexibility in healthy adults. Med Sci Sports Exerc 1998;30:975–991; Howley ET. Type of activity: resistance, aerobic and leisure versus occupational physical activity. Med Sci Sports Exerc 2001;33:S364–S369.

Abbreviations: METs, metabolic equivalent units (1 MET = 3.5 mL·kg^{-1}·min^{-1}); $\dot{V}O_2R$, oxygen uptake reserve; HRR, heart rate reserve.

- The theoretic basis for the table is the link between the *adjective* and the *relative physiologic range*, with the remainder of the columns containing data to illustrate the concept that a given MET value (e.g., 4 METs) represents varying *relative* intensities across the range of fitness levels typically found within healthy adults (e.g., 6–12 METs).
- Maximal aerobic capacity typically declines across the life span[7]; therefore, a given MET value (e.g., 4 METs) typically represents a higher *relative* intensity for older compared with younger individuals. However, it should be recognized that physically active older individuals may have fitness levels at or above that of sedentary younger adults.
- Although the varying MET range associated with *moderate* physical activity found within Table 1-1 differs from the absolute range found in earlier versions of this text (i.e., 3–6 METs independent of fitness level or age)[4,9], it should be noted that the ranges are quite consistent for individuals with functional capacities less than or equal to 10 METs. Therefore, brisk walking at 3 to 4 mph still represents *moderate*-intensity physical activity for most healthy adults.

Public Health Perspective for Current Recommendations

An important mission of the American College of Sports Medicine (ACSM) is to promote increased physical activity and fitness to the public. In order to advance this mission, exercise program professionals must be familiar with existing public health statements that relate to physical activity and must stay abreast of the evolving scientific literature related to current and future physical activity recommendations. Current recommendations[3,5] have expanded the traditional emphasis on formal *exercise* prescriptions to include a broader public health perspective on *physical activity*. The intent of these reports is twofold: 1) to increase both professional and public awareness of the health benefits associated with daily physical activity, and 2) to draw attention to the amounts and intensities of physical activity necessary to achieve these benefits, which are lower than those thought necessary to achieve the traditional physiologic training effect associated with exercise[7]. A major theme within these public health reports[3-5] is that more traditional exercise recommendations[7] have overlooked the numerous health benefits associated with regular participation in intermittent, moderate-intensity physical activity (e.g., <20 minutes per session and <50% of maximal aerobic power). In fact, it was recognized that health benefits can be obtained from a range of activities, with longer total duration required for less intense activities, and shorter total duration required for more intense activities.

Two key factors—feasibility and efficacy—were important in the development of the recommendations that emphasized moderate-intensity physical activity, which can be accumulated to achieve health benefits. The end result represented an attempt to balance feasibility and efficacy in developing public health recommendations for physical activity. Because Americans are highly sedentary (the 1998 estimates indicating that almost 40% of adults do not engage in any leisure-time physical activity)[10], persuading sedentary individuals to become physically active is more likely to be successful when the target level of physical activity is moderate, rather than the traditional higher-intensity level. Thus, there was an attempt to define the lowest, most effective level of physical activity that could provide health benefits.

Two conclusions from the Surgeon General's Report, *Physical Activity and Health*[3], remain prudent general guidelines for physical activity and public health:

- "Significant health benefits can be obtained by including a moderate amount of physical activity (e.g., 30 minutes of brisk walking or raking leaves, 15 minutes of running, or 45 minutes of playing volleyball) on most, if not all, days of the week. Through a modest increase in daily activity, most Americans can improve their health and quality of life."
- "Additional health benefits can be gained through greater amounts of physical activity. People who can maintain a regular regimen of activity that is of longer duration or of more vigorous intensity are likely to derive greater benefit."

An important component of the current recommendations[3-5] that has not been emphasized sufficiently is the dose-response relationship between physical activity and health. In other words, some activity is better than none, and more activity (up to a point) is better than less. Although the optimal dose of physical activity has yet to be defined, the well-established relationship between physical activity and various health benefits clearly supports the need for professionals to encourage the public to engage in at least moderate amounts and intensities of daily physical activity. The health benefits of increasing physical activity within the general population are potentially enormous because of both the high prevalence of sedentary lifestyle[10] and the impact of increased physical activity on lowering disease risk[11].

DIVERGENT PHYSICAL ACTIVITY RECOMMENDATIONS

Although the Surgeon General's recommendation of 30 minutes of light to moderate activity on most days of the week is a well-established public health recommendation, more recent reports have made recommendations for greater volumes of physical activity[6,12,13]. Are the recommendations found within these reports in conflict with those found within the Surgeon General's report? For the most part, the answer is no. The clear focus of these recent reports was *energy balance,* and their recommendations identified the higher volume of physical activity necessary to prevent weight gain and reduce weight regain following weight reduction. In 2001, ACSM updated its Position Stand on weight loss and prevention of weight gain for adults[12], and concluded that overweight adults should increase their activity to approximately 45 minutes of exercise per day (i.e., 200–300 minutes/week) to facilitate weight loss and prevent weight regain. The following year, in a report on guidelines for healthy eating, the Institute of Medicine (IOM) recommended 60 minutes a day of moderate-intensity physical activity to prevent weight gain and accrue additional weight-independent health benefits. And finally, in 2003, the International Association for the Study of Obesity (IASO) concluded that 45 to 60 minutes of moderate physical activity per day is required to prevent the transition to overweight and obesity in adults, and that prevention of weight regain may require 60 to 90 minutes of moderate activity per day. Taken collectively, these reports emphasize the additional volume of physical activity, above the 30 minutes cited within the Surgeon General's report, that is likely necessary to: 1) prevent the onset of obesity, 2) effect weight loss in overweight adults, and 3) prevent weight regain in formerly obese adults. However, these reports also acknowledge the myriad health benefits associated with 30 minutes a day of moderate-intensity physical activity. This consensus is clearly supported by recent studies in men and women of different races, showing risk reductions of some 20% to 50% in coronary heart disease and cardiovascular disease incidence rates with moderate-intensity physical activity, which can be accumulated in short bouts, compared with sedentary behavior[14–18]. The recommendations also agree that there is a dose-response relationship, with greater benefits occurring at higher duration and/or intensity of physical activity.

Benefits of Regular Physical Activity and/or Exercise

A large body of laboratory- and population-based studies has documented the many health and fitness benefits associated with physical activity and endurance exercise training, such as improved physiologic, metabolic, and psychologic parameters, as well as decreased risk of many chronic diseases and premature mortality (Box 1-1)[3,19]. Physical activity and exercise clearly prevent occurrences of cardiac events; reduce the incidence of stroke, hypertension, type 2 diabetes mellitus, colon and breast cancers, osteoporotic fractures, gallbladder disease, obesity, depression, and anxiety, and delay mortality[3,19–25]. Additionally, several studies have examined the impact of change in physical activity or fitness in relation to developing coronary heart disease or dying prematurely[26–32]. These data indicate that individuals who change from a sedentary lifestyle to being physically active, or who change from being physically unfit to physically fit, experience lower rates of disease and premature mortality compared with those who continue to remain sedentary or unfit. This holds true from middle age to older age (forties to eighties), indicating that it is never too late to become physically active to achieve health benefits[27].

DOSE-RESPONSE RELATIONSHIP

In recent years, there has been much interest in the nature and shape of the dose-response curve between physical activity and health[19]. Although physical activity clearly has been documented to reduce the risk of the diseases listed previously (see Box 1-1), the data are far less clear regarding the minimal dose of physical activity that is required, as well as what further risk reductions occur with additional amounts (duration and/or intensity) of physical activity. Besides the scientific value of these data, such information is also pertinent for public health recommendations in order to balance the feasibility of the recommendations proposed with their efficacy in preventing various diseases or health conditions. Therefore, further research is needed to more clearly define the minimal dose of physical activity associated with prevention of various diseases and health conditions and to clarify the shape of the dose-response curve. It is also likely that the minimum dose and shape of the dose-response curve differs for various health conditions. For example, in the discussion of public health recommendations, it seems that greater amounts of

BOX 1-1	Benefits of Regular Physical Activity and/or Exercise*

Improvement in Cardiovascular and Respiratory Function
- Increased maximal oxygen uptake resulting from both central and peripheral adaptations
- Decreased minute ventilation at a given absolute submaximal intensity
- Decreased myocardial oxygen cost for a given absolute submaximal intensity
- Decreased heart rate and blood pressure at a given submaximal intensity
- Increased capillary density in skeletal muscle
- Increased exercise threshold for the accumulation of lactate in the blood
- Increased exercise threshold for the onset of disease signs or symptoms (e.g., angina pectoris, ischemic ST-segment depression, claudication)

Reduction in coronary artery disease risk factors
- Reduced resting systolic/diastolic pressures
- Increased serum high-density lipoprotein cholesterol and decreased serum triglycerides
- Reduced total body fat, reduced intraabdominal fat
- Reduced insulin needs, improved glucose tolerance
- Reduced blood platelet adhesiveness and aggregation

Decreased morbidity and mortality
- Primary prevention (i.e., interventions to prevent the initial occurrence)
  - Higher activity and/or fitness levels are associated with lower death rates from coronary artery disease
  - Higher activity and/or fitness levels are associated with lower incidence rates for combined cardiovascular diseases, coronary artery disease, stroke, type 2 diabetes, osteoporotic fractures, cancer of the colon and breast, and gallbladder disease
- Secondary prevention (i.e., interventions after a cardiac event [to prevent another])
  - Based on meta-analyses (pooled data across studies), cardiovascular and all-cause mortality are reduced in postmyocardial infarction patients who participate in cardiac rehabilitation exercise training, especially as a component of multifactorial risk factor reduction
  - Randomized controlled trials of cardiac rehabilitation exercise training involving postmyocardial infarction patients do not support a reduction in the rate of nonfatal reinfarction ▶

> ▶ **Box 1-1, continued**

Other postulated benefits

- Decreased anxiety and depression
- Enhanced physical function and independent living in older persons
- Enhanced feelings of well being
- Enhanced performance of work, recreational, and sport activities

*Adapted from references 3, 19: United States Department of Health and Human Services. Physical activity and health: a report of the Surgeon General, 1996; Kesaniemi YK, Danforth E Jr, Jensen MD, et al. Dose-response issues concerning physical activity and health: an evidence-based symposium. Med Sci Sports Exerc 2001;33:S351–358.

physical activity are required to prevent unhealthy weight gain compared with the amount needed to reduce the risk of cardiovascular disease.

Whereas Box 1-1 contains a list of health related benefits attributed to a more active lifestyle, Table 1-2 summarizes the available data on the inverse dose-response relationship between physical activity and selected health outcomes[19]. The categories use an evidence-based approach developed by the National Institutes of Health[33], which places greater emphasis on data from large, randomized clinical trials. Although randomized trails are considered the gold standard for clinical research, it is often impractical to conduct such studies. For example, studies of physical activity and the primary prevention of coronary heart disease would require many subjects (thousands to tens of thousands) followed for several years. It would be impossible to maintain good compliance with physical activity over this time, and in addition would be prohibitively expensive. To emphasize this point, it is to be noted that cigarette smoking is clearly believed to cause lung cancer, even though no randomized clinical trials on this topic have ever been conducted. Table 1-2 summarizes results from a large body of observational studies, which indicate an inverse dose-response relationship between physical activity and a variety of health conditions. The clearest of these relationships is for all-cause mortality, cardiovascular disease, and coronary heart disease. A smaller body of evidence also indicates likely inverse dose-response relations for weight and fat distribution, type 2 diabetes mellitus, colon cancer, quality of life, and independent living in older persons. Finally, a small body of data, including data from randomized clinical trials, suggests the lack of an inverse dose-response for blood pressure and depression and anxiety. More research is needed on certain health conditions to define the dose-response relationship for physical activity.

When the knowledge of the additional health and fitness benefits associated with greater quantities and intensities of physical activity and/or exercise is combined with the fact that the list of chronic diseases favorably affected by exercise continues to grow, there remains a clear need for medically and scientifically sound primary and secondary prevention programs. These exercise programs should be designed and supervised by qualified professionals who possess training in exercise testing and prescription (see Appendix F for academic and experience prerequisites for ACSM certification).

Table 1-2. Evidence for Dose-Response Relationship Between Physical Activity and Health Outcome*

Variable	Evidence for Inverse Dose-Response Relationship	Category of Evidence
All-cause mortality	Yes	C
Cardiovascular and coronary heart disease	Yes	C
Blood pressure and hypertension	No†	B
Blood lipids and lipoproteins	Insufficient data	
Coagulation and hemostatic factors	Insufficient data	
Overweight, obesity, and fat distribution	Yes	C
Type 2 diabetes mellitus	Yes‡	C
Colon cancer	Yes	C
Low back pain, osteoarthritis, and osteoporosis	Insufficient data	
Quality of life and independent living in older persons	Yes	C
Depression and anxiety	No†	B

*From Kesaniemi YK, Danforth E Jr, Jensen MD, et al. Dose-response issues concerning physical activity and health: an evidence-based symposium. Med Sci Sports Exerc 2001;33:S351–358.

†No indicates a lack of evidence for a "dose-response" for the relationship between the health outcome and physical activity; it does not indicate the absence of a favorable relationship.

‡Inverse dose-response for primary prevention, but not for improvement in blood glucose control in patients with diabetes.

Category definitions:
- *Category A:* Evidence is from endpoints of well-designed randomized clinical trials (RCTs) (or trials that depart only minimally from randomization) that provide a consistent pattern of findings in the population for which the recommendation is made. It requires substantial numbers of studies involving substantial number of participants.
- *Category B:* Evidence is from endpoints of intervention studies that include only a limited number of RCTs, post hoc or subgroup analysis of RCT, or meta-analysis of RCTs. In general, Category B pertains when few randomized trials exist, they are small in size, and the trial results are somewhat inconsistent, or the trials were undertaken in a population that differs from the target population of the recommendation.
- *Category C:* Evidence is from outcomes of uncontrolled or nonrandomized trials or observational studies.
- *Category D:* Expert judgment is based on the panel's synthesis of evidence from experimental research described in the literature and/or derived from the consensus of panel members based on clinical experience or knowledge that does not meet the listed criteria. This category is used only in cases where the provision of some guidance was deemed valuable but an adequately compelling clinical literature addressing the subject of the recommendation was deemed insufficient to justify placement in one of the other categories (A through C).

Risks Associated With Exercise

Habitual physical activity reduces the incidence of atherosclerotic cardiovascular disease. Nevertheless, vigorous physical exertion also acutely and transiently increases the risk of sudden cardiac death[34,35] and acute myocardial infarction[36,37]. It is important to remember that exercise only provokes cardiovascular events in individuals with preexisting heart disease, whether diagnosed or occult. Exercise does not provoke cardiac events in individuals with normal cardiovascular systems. Consequently, the risk of exercise for any population depends on its prevalence of cardiac disease.

SUDDEN DEATH AMONG YOUNG INDIVIDUALS

Among individuals younger than 35, the risk of sudden cardiac death during exercise is low because the prevalence of occult disease is low. The absolute incidence of death during or within an hour of sports participation among United States high school and college athletes has been estimated as one death per year for every 133,000 men and 769,000 women, respectively[38]. These numbers overestimate the incidence of *cardiac* events because only 100 of the 136 deaths with identifiable causes of death in this report were caused by cardiac disease. The reason for lower rates of exercise-related cardiac death among women is unclear, but is characteristic of most studies on this topic.

Congenital cardiac abnormalities and nonatherosclerotic, acquired myocardial disease are the primary cause of exercise-related cardiac deaths in younger individuals. Atherosclerotic coronary artery disease is rare (Table 1-3)[38–40]. In the United States, the most common cause of exercise-related sudden cardiac death is hypertrophic cardiomyopathy[38,40,41]. This is not true for other populations. For example, arrhythmogenic right ventricular cardiomyopathy is the most frequent cause of exercise-related sudden cardiac death in Italy[42]. Such observations suggest that the causes of exercise-related sudden death differ by both the age of the subjects and the population examined.

Table 1-3. Cardiac Causes of Death in High School and College Athletes* (*N* = 100)

Disorder	Men	Women
Hypertrophic cardiomyopathy†	50	1
Probable hypertrophic cardiomyopathy	5	0
Coronary artery anomalies‡	11	2
Myocarditis	7	—
Aortic stenosis	6	—
Cardiomyopathy	6	—
Atherosclerotic coronary disease	2	1
Aortic rupture	2	—
Subaortic stenosis	2	—
Coronary aneurysm	—	1
Mitral prolapse	1	—
Right ventricular cardiomyopathy	—	1
Cerebral arteriovenous malformation	—	1
Subarachnoid hemorrhage	—	1

*Adapted from Van Camp SP, Bloor CM, Mueller FO, et al. Nontraumatic sports death in high school and college athletes. Med Sci Sports Exerc 1995;27:641–647.

†Three also had coronary anomalies; one had Wolff-Parkinson-White syndrome.

‡Includes anomalous left coronary artery (LCA) from right sinus of Valsalva (*N* = 4); intramural left anterior descending (LAD) (*N* = 4); anomalous LCA from pulmonary artery (*N* = 2); anomalous right coronary artery (RCA) from left sinus (*N* = 2); hypoplastic RCA (*N* = 2); and ostial ridge of the LCA (*N* = 2). Three subjects with coronary anomalies also had hypertrophic cardiomyopathy and are tabulated with that group.

EXERCISE EVENTS IN THOSE WITH SICKLE CELL TRAIT

In contrast to the overall low incidence of exercise-related deaths in young subjects, individuals with sickle cell trait have a remarkably higher incidence of exertion-related death. Sickle cell trait is much more common in the African-American than the White population. Kark et al.[43] examined deaths during basic training in 2 million U.S. military recruits between 1977 and 1981. All of the sudden, "unexplained" deaths were related to physical exertion and attributed to cardiac events, heat illness, or exertional rhabdomyolysis. It is not possible to decipher exactly how many of the exercise-related deaths were related to cardiac causes. Nevertheless, the relative risk of sudden unexplained death among African-Americans with sickle cell trait was 27 times higher than in those without it. The absolute death rate in African-Americans with sickle cell trait during 8 to 11 weeks of basic training can be estimated as one death for every 3,105 recruits, with an annual rate of one death for every 478 to 660 recruits. This is remarkably higher than the annual rate of exercise deaths among other populations of military age. Athletic trainers and others who supervise young athletes during vigorous exertion should be aware of this potential problem in African-American athletes.

EXERCISE-RELATED CARDIAC EVENTS IN ADULTS

The risks of exercise in adults are considerably higher than in younger subjects because of the increased prevalence of atherosclerotic cardiovascular disease. The most widely cited studies, performed in Rhode Island[44] and Seattle[35], estimated an incidence of sudden cardiac death during vigorous exertion in healthy adults as only one death per year for every 15,000 to 18,000 individuals. This is a low incidence of cardiovascular events, but both studies demonstrated that the rate of sudden cardiac death during or immediately after vigorous exertion was higher than that during more leisurely activities. Exercise also acutely increases the risk of acute, nonfatal myocardial infarction[36,37]. Interestingly, both the incidences of exertion-related sudden cardiac death[35] and acute myocardial infarction[36,37] are higher in individuals who exercise infrequently.

The mechanism of sudden cardiac death and acute myocardial infarction in previously asymptomatic adults is probably acute coronary plaque rupture leading to coronary thrombosis. Atherosclerosis decreases the flexibility of the coronary arteries. The increased frequency of cardiac contraction and the increased excursion of the coronary arteries during exercise produce increased bending and flexing of these arteries. This increased flexing can produce cracking in the atherosclerotic plaque, which leads to platelet aggregation and subsequent acute coronary thrombosis. Such atherosclerotic plaque disruption with acute thrombotic occlusion has been documented by angiography in individuals with exercise-induced cardiac events[45–47].

RISKS OF CARDIAC EVENTS DURING EXERCISE TESTING

As noted, the risk of exercise varies with the prevalence of underlying coronary artery disease in the population. Consequently, the risk of exercise stress testing also varies with the populations studied. Exercise stress testing performed in previously healthy individuals has a low rate of cardiovascular events, whereas exercise testing in high-risk patients has a higher risk. The overall risk of exercise testing in a mixed subject population is approximately six cardiac events (e.g., myocardial infarction, ventricular fibrillation, other important dysrhythmia or death) per 10,000 tests (Table 1-4). These results include exercise testing that is supervised by nonphysicians[48].

RISKS OF CARDIAC EVENTS DURING CARDIAC REHABILITATION

Individuals with diagnosed coronary artery disease are at the highest risk of experiencing a cardiac event during exercise, and it has been estimated that vigorous exercise increases the risk of a cardiac event 100 times in this population[49]. Nevertheless, studies of cardiac events during cardiac rehabilitation document that the risk of vigorous exercise in such supervised populations is extremely low (Table 1-5). Obviously, these data cannot be extrapolated to vigorous exercise in cardiac patients who are not supervised because such patients are not monitored, nor are facilities for cardiac resuscitation readily available. However, a review of seven randomized and four nonrandomized trials of home-based cardiac rehabilitation indicated that there was no increase in cardiovascular complications of this approach versus formal center-based exercise programs[25].

As discussed, acute plaque disruption is the likely cause of most cardiac events in previously asymptomatic individuals. In contrast, both acute plaque rupture and ventricular dysrhythmias arising from previously infarcted myocardium contribute to cardiac events in patients with diagnosed coronary heart disease.

PREVENTION OF EXERCISE-RELATED CARDIAC EVENTS

The development and evaluation of strategies to reduce the risk of vigorous exercise have been negatively impacted by a low incidence of events. Interventions cannot be proposed and tested because an enormous number of subjects would have to participate to document effectiveness. Consequently, recommendations for strategies to reduce cardiac events are based primarily on common sense and expert opinion. Furthermore, the paucity of exercise-related cardiac events makes it difficult to quantify the benefit of any routine screening procedures. Some experts recommend extensive preparticipation screening of young subjects prior to sports participation using electrocardiography[50] or echocardiography[51]. However, this approach is controversial and not presently recommended by all organizations. An expert panel from The American Heart Association recommends a preparticipation physical examination of young athletes, but does not recommend routine electrocardiography or echocardiography[52]. Some experts and organizations recommend routine exercise stress testing prior to initiating vigorous exercise programs in adults with risk factors. This approach also is controversial and not endorsed by all expert panels. The ACSM recommends exercise stress testing prior to vigorous exercise for "moderate" or "high-risk individuals" including men over 45 and women over 55 years of age, individuals with more than one coronary disease risk factor, and those with known coronary disease (see Chapter 2). Most authorities agree with these recommendations for those with established coronary artery disease (CAD). In contrast, the American College of Cardiology and the American Heart Association Guidelines for Exercise Testing considered the use-

Table 1-4. Cardiac Complications During Exercise Testing*

Reference	Year	Site	No. Tests	MI	VF	Death	Hospitalization	Comment
Rochmis[56]	1971	73 U.S. centers	170,000	NA	NA	1	3	34% of tests were symptom limited; 50% of deaths in 8 hr; 50% over next 4 days
Irving[57]	1977	15 Seattle facilities	10,700	NA	4.67	0	NR	
McHenry[55]	1977	Hospital	12,000	0	0	0	0	
Atterhog[58]	1979	20 Swedish centers	50,000	0.8	0.8	6.4	5.2	
Stuart[59]	1980	1,375 U.S. centers	518,448	3.58	4.78	0.5	NR	"VF" includes other dysrhythmias requiring treatment
Gibbons[60]	1989	Cooper Clinic	71,914	0.56	0.29	0	NR	Only 4% of men and 2% of women had CAD
Knight[48]	1995	Geisinger Cardiology Service	28,133	1.42	1.77	0	NR	25% were inpatient tests supervised by non-MDs

*Events are per 10,000 tests.

Abbreviations: MI, myocardial infarction; VF, ventricular fibrillation; CAD, coronary artery disease; MD, medical doctor; NA, not applicable; NR, not reported.

Table 1-5. Number of Participants for One Cardiac Event in Cardiac Rehabilitation Programs*

Reference	Cardiac Arrest	MI	Fatalities	MI and Arrest
Van Camp[61]	111,996	293,990	783,972	81,101
Digenio[62]	120,000	—	160,000	120,000
Vongvanich[63]	89,501	268,503	268,503	67,126
Franklin[64]	146,127	97,418	292,254	58,451
Average	116,906	219,970	752,364	81,669

*Adapted from Franklin BA, Bonzheim K, Gordon S, et al. Safety of medically supervised outpatient cardiac rehabilitation exercise therapy: a 16-year follow-up. Chest 1998;114:902–906.

Abbreviation: MI, myocardial infarction.

fulness of routine exercise testing prior to vigorous exercise in asymptomatic persons as less well established by evidence or opinion (Class IIB)[53,54]. Such divergence of opinion leaves the decision about the necessity of a preparticipation exercise test in healthy subjects largely to the clinician.

Procedures for reducing the risks of vigorous exercise during exercise training, exercise stress testing, and cardiac rehabilitation have not been evaluated rigorously. Nevertheless, several simple measures seem prudent. Individuals with known cardiovascular disease should receive medical clearance prior to vigorous exercise training. Individuals who seek to start an exercise program should be queried as to their reasons for initiating exercise, because some patients with new symptoms of cardiovascular disease initiate exercise programs in an attempt to reassure themselves that they are well. It is also important that practitioners supervising vigorous exercise programs or testing have training in cardiac life support and established procedures for dealing with emergencies. These procedures should be reviewed and practiced at least several times yearly (see Appendix B). Also, because the incidences of exercise-related sudden cardiac death and acute myocardial infarction are more frequent in physically unfit subjects, individuals initiating exercise programs should be encouraged to start slowly and progress gradually. It is also important that exercising adults know the prodromal symptoms of CAD. Some victims of exercise-related cardiac events underestimated the importance of their symptoms prior to death[44]. Finally, if young or older individuals develop exercise-induced symptoms such as chest discomfort, unexpected dyspnea, or syncope, they should be fully evaluated by a physician prior to returning to vigorous activity.

REFERENCES

1. Caspersen CJ, Powell KE, Christenson GM. Physical activity, exercise, and physical fitness: definitions and distinctions for health-related research. Public Health Rep 1985;100:126–131.
2. President's Council on Physical Fitness. Definitions: health, fitness, and physical activity. Research Digest, 2000.
3. United States Department of Health and Human Services. Physical activity and health: a report of the Surgeon General, 1996.
4. Pate RR, Pratt M, Blair SN, et al. Physical activity and public health. A recommendation from the Centers for Disease Control and Prevention and the American College of Sports Medicine. JAMA 1995;273:402–407.

5. National Institutes of Health. Physical activity and cardiovascular health. NIH Consensus Development Panel on Physical Activity and Cardiovascular Health. JAMA 1996;276:241–246.
6. Food and Nutrition Board, Institute of Medicine. Dietary reference intakes for energy, carbohydrates, fiber, fat, protein and amino acids (macronutrients). Washington, DC: National Academy Press, 2002.
7. American College of Sports Medicine. Position Stand: The recommended quantity and quality of exercise for developing and maintaining cardiorespiratory and muscular fitness, and flexibility in healthy adults. Med Sci Sports Exerc 1998;30:975–991.
8. Howley ET. Type of activity: resistance, aerobic and leisure versus occupational physical activity. Med Sci Sports Exerc 2001;33:S364–S369.
9. Franklin BA, Whaley MH, Howley E. ACSM's Guidelines for Exercise Testing and Prescription. 6th ed. Baltimore: Lippincott Williams & Wilkins, 2000.
10. Schoenborn CA, Barnes PM. Leisure-time physical activity among adults: Advanced Statistics from Vital and Health Statistics No. 325; April 7, 2002. United States, 1997–1998. 2002.
11. Hahn RA, Teutsch SM, Rothenberg RB, et al. Excess death from nine chronic diseases in the United States, 1986. JAMA 1990;264:2654–2659.
12. American College of Sports Medicine. Position Stand: Appropriate intervention strategies for weight loss and prevention of weight regain for adults. Med Sci Sports Exerc 2001;33:2145–2156.
13. Saris W, Blair SN, van Baak M, et al. How much physical activity is enough to prevent unhealthy weight gain? Outcome of the IASO 1st Stock Conference and consensus statement. Obesity Rev 2003;4:101–114.
14. Manson JE, Greenland P, LaCroix AZ, et al. Walking compared with vigorous exercise for the prevention of cardiovascular events in women. N Engl J Med 2002;347:716–725.
15. Lee IM, Sesso HD, Paffenbarger RS Jr. Physical activity and coronary heart disease risk in men: does the duration of exercise episodes predict risk? Circulation 2000;102:981–986.
16. Lee IM, Rexrode KM, Cook NR, et al. Physical activity and coronary heart disease in women: is "no pain, no gain" passe? JAMA 2001;285:1447–1454.
17. Sesso HD, Paffenbarger RS Jr, Lee IM. Physical activity and coronary heart disease in men: The Harvard Alumni Health Study. Circulation 2000;102:975–980.
18. Tanasescu M, Leitzmann MF, Rimm EB, et al. Exercise type and intensity in relation to coronary heart disease in men. JAMA 2002;288:1994–2000.
19. Kesaniemi YK, Danforth E Jr, Jensen MD, et al. Dose-response issues concerning physical activity and health: an evidence-based symposium. Med Sci Sports Exerc 2001;33:S351–358.
20. Jolliffe JA, Rees K, Taylor RS, et al. Evidence-based rehabilitation of coronary heart disease (Cochran Review). In: The Cochran Library, Issue 3, 2002. Oxford Update Software. Cochran Library, 2002.
21. Lee IM, Oguma Y. Physical Activity. 3rd ed. In: Schottenfeld D, Fraumeni JFJ, eds. San Francisco: Oxford University Press, in press.
22. Feskanich D, Willett W, Colditz G. Walking and leisure-time activity and risk of hip fracture in postmenopausal women. JAMA 2002;288:2300–2306.
23. Leitzmann MF, Rimm EB, Willett WC, et al. Recreational physical activity and the risk of cholecystectomy in women. N Engl J Med 1999;341:777–784.
24. Sahi T, Paffenbarger RS Jr, Hsieh CC, et al. Body mass index, cigarette smoking, and other characteristics as predictors of self-reported, physician-diagnosed gallbladder disease in male college alumni. Am J Epidemiol 1998;147:644–651.
25. Wenger NK, Froelicher ES, Smith LK, et al. Cardiac rehabilitation. Clinical Practice Guideline No. 17. Rockville, MD: U.S. Department of Health and Human Services, Public Health, Agency for Health Care Policy and Research and National Heart, Lung, and Blood Institute, 1995.
26. Hein HO, Suadicani P, Sorensen H, et al. Changes in physical activity level and risk of ischaemic heart disease. A six-year follow-up in the Copenhagen male study. Scand J Med Sci Sports 1994; 4:57–64.
27. Paffenbarger RS Jr, Hyde RT, Wing AL, et al. The association of changes in physical-activity level and other lifestyle characteristics with mortality among men. N Engl J Med 1993;328:538–545.
28. Blair SN, Kohl HW 3rd, Barlow CE, et al. Changes in physical fitness and all-cause mortality. A prospective study of healthy and unhealthy men. JAMA 1995;273:1093–1098.
29. Wannamethee SG, Shaper AG, Walker M. Changes in physical activity, mortality, and incidence of coronary heart disease in older men. Lancet 1998;351:1603–1608.
30. Erikssen G, Liestol K, Bjornholt J, et al. Changes in physical fitness and changes in mortality. Lancet 1998;352:759–762.

31. Bijnen FC, Feskens EJ, Caspersen CJ, et al. Baseline and previous physical activity in relation to mortality in elderly men: the Zutphen Elderly Study. Am J Epidemiol 1999;150:1289–1296.

32. Manson JE, Hu FB, Rich-Edwards JW, et al. A prospective study of walking as compared with vigorous exercise in the prevention of coronary heart disease in women. N Engl J Med 1999;341:650–658.

33. Expert Panel on Detection Evaluation and Treatment of Overweight and Obesity in Adults. National Institutes of Health. Clinical guidelines on the identification, evaluation, and treatment of overweight and obesity in adults: the evidence report. Arch Intern Med 1998;158:1855–1867.

34. Thompson PD, Funk EJ, Carleton RA, et al. Incidence of death during jogging in Rhode Island from 1975 through 1980. JAMA 1982;247:2535–2538.

35. Siscovick DS, Weiss NS, Fletcher RH, et al. The incidence of primary cardiac arrest during vigorous exercise. N Engl J Med 1984;311:874–877.

36. Mittleman MA, Maclure M, Tofler GH, et al. Triggering of acute myocardial infarction by heavy physical exertion. Protection against triggering by regular exertion. Determinants of Myocardial Infarction Onset Study Investigators. N Engl J Med 1993;329:1677–1683.

37. Giri S, Thompson PD, Kiernan FJ, et al. Clinical and angiographic characteristics of exertion-related acute myocardial infarction. JAMA 1999;282:1731–1736.

38. Van Camp SP, Bloor CM, Mueller FO, et al. Nontraumatic sports death in high school and college athletes. Med Sci Sports Exerc 1995;27:641–647.

39. Maron BJ, Roberts WC, McAllister HA, et al. Sudden death in young athletes. Circulation 1980; 62:218–229.

40. Burke AP, Farb A, Virmani R, et al. Sports-related and non-sports-related sudden cardiac death in young adults. Am Heart J 1991;121:568–575.

41. Maron BJ, Shirani J, Poliac LC, et al. Sudden death in young competitive athletes. Clinical, demographic, and pathological profiles. JAMA 1996;276:199–204.

42. Thiene G, Nava A, Corrado D, et al. Right ventricular cardiomyopathy and sudden death in young people. N Engl J Med 1988;318:129–133.

43. Kark JA, Posey DM, Schumacher HR, et al. Sickle-cell trait as a risk factor for sudden death in physical training. N Engl J Med 1987;317:781–787.

44. Thompson PD, Stern MP, Williams P, et al. Death during jogging or running. A study of 18 cases. JAMA 1979;242:1265–1267.

45. Black A, Black MM, Gensini G. Exertion and acute coronary artery injury. Angiology 1975;26: 759–783.

46. Ciampricotti R, Deckers JW, Taverne R, et al. Characteristics of conditioned and sedentary men with acute coronary syndromes. Am J Cardiol 1994;73:219–222.

47. Hammoudeh AJ, Haft JI. Coronary-plaque rupture in acute coronary syndromes triggered by snow shoveling. N Engl J Med 1996;335:2001.

48. Knight JA, Laubach CA Jr, Butcher RJ, et al. Supervision of clinical exercise testing by exercise physiologists. Am J Cardiol 1995;75:390–391.

49. Cobb LA, Weaver WD. Exercise: a risk for sudden death in patients with coronary heart disease. J Am Coll Cardiol 1986;7:215–219.

50. Kragel AH, Roberts WC. Sudden death and cardiomegaly unassociated with coronary, valvular, congenital or specific myocardial disease. Am J Cardiol 1988;61:659–660.

51. Corrado D, Basso C, Schiavon M, et al. Screening for hypertrophic cardiomyopathy in young athletes. N Engl J Med 1998;339:364–369.

52. Maron BJ, Thompson PD, Puffer JC, et al. Cardiovascular preparticipation screening of competitive athletes. A statement for health professionals from the Sudden Death Committee (clinical cardiology) and Congenital Cardiac Defects Committee (cardiovascular disease in the young), American Heart Association. Circulation 1996;94:850–856.

53. Gibbons RJ, Balady GJ, Beasley JW, et al. ACC/AHA guidelines for exercise testing: executive summary. A report of the American College of Cardiology/American Heart Association Task Force on Practice Guidelines (Committee on Exercise Testing). Circulation 1997;96:345–354.

54. Gibbons RJ, Balady GJ, Bricker J, et al. ACC/AHA 2002 guideline update for exercise testing: a report of the American College of Cardiology/American Heart Association Task Force on Practice Guidelines (Committee on Exercise Testing). 2002. American College of Cardiology web site www.acc.org/clinical/guidelines/exercise/dirIndex.htm

55. McHenry PL. Risks of graded exercise testing. Am J Cardiol 1977;39:935–937.

56. Rochmis P, Blackburn H. Exercise tests. A survey of procedures, safety, and litigation experience in approximately 170,000 tests. JAMA 1971;217:1061–1066.

57. Irving JB, Bruce RA, DeRouen TA. Variations in and significance of systolic pressure during maximal exercise (treadmill) testing. Am J Cardiol 1977;39:841–888.
58. Atterhog JH, Jonsson B, Samuelsson R. Exercise testing: a prospective study of complication rates. Am Heart J 1979;98:572–579.
59. Stuart RJ Jr, Ellestad MH. National survey of exercise stress testing facilities. Chest 1980;77:94–97.
60. Gibbons L, Blair SN, Kohl HW, et al. The safety of maximal exercise testing. Circulation 1989;80: 846–852.
61. Van Camp SP, Peterson RA. Cardiovascular complications of outpatient cardiac rehabilitation programs. JAMA 1986;256:1160–1163.
62. Digenio AG, Sim JG, Dowdeswell RJ, et al. Exercise-related cardiac arrest in cardiac rehabilitation. The Johannesburg experience. S Afr Med J 1991;79:188–191.
63. Vongvanich P, Paul-Labrador MJ, Merz CN. Safety of medically supervised exercise in a cardiac rehabilitation center. Am J Cardiol 1996;77:1383–1385.
64. Franklin BA, Bonzheim K, Gordon S, et al. Safety of medically supervised outpatient cardiac rehabilitation exercise therapy: a 16-year follow-up. Chest 1998;114:902–906

Preparticipation Health Screening and Risk Stratification

This chapter presents guidelines related to preparticipation health screening and risk stratification for individuals initiating a self-guided physical activity regimen or those entering primary or secondary prevention exercise programs. To this end, the American College of Sports Medicine (ACSM) recognizes other published guidelines by the American Heart Association (AHA) and the American Association of Cardiovascular and Pulmonary Rehabilitation (AACVPR)[1–5]. Exercise program professionals should review these other documents, as well as revisions to them, when establishing program-specific policies for preparticipation health screening and medical clearance.

To aid in the development of a safe and effective exercise prescription and optimize safety during exercise testing, it is important to screen potential participants for risk factors and/or symptoms of various cardiovascular, pulmonary, and metabolic diseases, as well as conditions (e.g., pregnancy, orthopedic injury) that may be aggravated by exercise. The purposes of the preparticipation health screening include the following:

- Identification and exclusion of individuals with medical contraindications to exercise
- Identification of individuals at increased risk for disease because of age, symptoms, and/or risk factors who should undergo a medical evaluation and exercise testing before starting an exercise program
- Identification of persons with clinically significant disease who should participate in a medically supervised exercise program
- Identification of individuals with other special needs

Preparticipation Screening Algorithm

Preparticipation screening procedures should be valid, cost effective, and time efficient. Procedures range from *self-administered* questionnaires to sophisticated diagnostic tests. Exercise program professionals should establish preparticipat screening procedures appropriate for their clients or a facility's target population. To provide guidance on the appropriate depth and breadth of preparticipation health screening, ACSM offers the algorithm presented in Table 2-1. The algorithm defines three *levels* of screening with the intent of presenting a logical sequence of assessment and decision making. It is generally accepted that many sedentary individuals can safely begin a light- to moderate-intensity (see

Table 2-1. ACSM Pre-Participation Screening Algorithm

	Screening Recommended Prior to Self-Guided[a] Physical Activity	Screening Recommended Prior to Professionally-Guided[b] Exercise Testing/Prescription		
Level-1 — Risk Stratification & Medical Clearance (Chapter 2)	1. Complete ACSM/AHA Questionnaire or PAR-Q (Figures 2-1 & 2-2) 2. Determine need for medical clearance and obtain if recommended 3. Proceed to Level 2	1. Identify presence of major CAD risk factors (Table 2-2) and major signs/symptoms suggestive of cardiovascular, pulmonary or metabolic disease (Table 2-3). This process could include the use of the ACSM/AHA Questionnaire (Figure 2-1)(2). This process may also include a more elaborate, facility-specific medical/health history questionnaire. 2. Determine ACSM risk category from Table 2-4 for use in Levels 2 and 3. 3. Determine need for medical clearance prior to testing and/or participation and obtain if recommended based on ACSM risk category 4. Proceed to Level 2 and follow recommendations based on ACSM risk category		
Level-2 — Additional Pre-Participation Assessment (Chapters 3-4)	• Initiate general physical activity recommendations as outlined by the United States Surgeon General[6] • For a specific self-guided exercise assessment and examples of both aerobic and resistance training regimens see Chapters 4-6 of the ACSM Fitness Book[10]. • Individuals identified as needing medical clearance in Level 1 may benefit from participation in a professionally-guided pre-exercise assessment and prescription.	**Low Risk** • Perform informed consent for testing (sample Figure 3-1) and/or training[c] • Complete appropriate assessment procedures outlined in Chapters 3-4 • Medical history, physical examination, laboratory tests, body composition, etc	**Moderate Risk** Perform informed consent for testing (sample Figure 3-1) and/or training[c]	**High Risk** Perform informed consent for testing (sample Figure 3-1) and/or training[c] ↑ *Both the depth and breadth of pre-exercise test assessment should increase as a function of risk category. Refer to Chapters 3 & 4 for advanced assessment procedures.*
Level-3 — Exercise Test Considerations (Chapters 4-5)		• Further medical examination and exercise testing not necessary[d] prior to initiation of exercise training • Medical supervision for submaximal or maximal exercise testing not necessary	• Medical examination and exercise testing recommended prior to initiation of vigorous exercise training • Medical supervision[e] recommended for maximal exercise testing	• Medical examination and exercise testing recommended prior to initiation of moderate or vigorous exercise training • Medical supervision[e] recommended for maximal or submaximal exercise testing

Moderate exercise intensity = 40-59% $\dot{V}O_2R$; Vigorous exercise intensity = > 60% $\dot{V}O_2R$ (See Table 1-1)

a Physical activity regimen that is initiated and guided by the individual with little or no input or supervision from an exercise program professional.

b Professionally-guided implies that the fitness/clinical assessment is conducted by - and exercise program designed and supervised by - appropriately trained personnel that possess academic training and practical/clinical knowledge, skills and abilities commensurate with the credentials defined in Appendix F, or the ACSM Program Director® or Health/Fitness Director®.

c Published samples of appropriate consent forms for participation in preventive and rehabilitative exercise programs are found in references 3 & 9.

d The designation of not necessary reflects the notion that a medical examination, exercise test, and medical supervision of exercise testing would not be essential in the pre-activity screening; however, they should not be viewed as inappropriate.

e When medical supervision of exercise testing is "recommended," the physician should be in proximity and readily available should there be an emergent need.

Table 1–1) physical activity regimen without the need for extensive medical screening [2,6–8]; therefore, Level 1 screening may be all that is necessary for most individuals seeking to adopt a more active lifestyle. However, it should be noted that many exercise programs incorporate all three levels described in Table 2-1 into their procedures regardless of the outcome from each level. This should not be viewed as inappropriate, because information gained in subsequent screening steps can enhance the safety and effectiveness of the exercise prescription. Furthermore, the preparticipation screening recommendations in Table 2-1 relate to both self- and professionally guided exercise regimens; therefore, physicians and other allied health professionals counseling clients or patients to adopt a more active lifestyle should provide appropriate screening as part of the physical activity counseling process. Finally, regardless of the scope of preparticipation screening employed, information should be interpreted by qualified professionals and results should be documented [2].

RISK STRATIFICATION AND MEDICAL CLEARANCE

The initial screening step in Table 2-1 is designed to yield information regarding risk stratification and the need for medical clearance prior to beginning or significantly increasing physical activity. This process requires identification of the presence of:

- Coronary artery disease (CAD) risk factors (Table 2-2)
- Signs or symptoms of cardiovascular, pulmonary and/or metabolic disease (Table 2-3)
- Known cardiovascular, pulmonary, and/or metabolic disease

As an initial, minimal step, it is recommended that prospective exercisers complete a *self-administered* questionnaire that serves to alert those with elevated risk to consult their physician (or other appropriate health care provider) prior to participation [2,9,10]. As *self-administered* surveys, such forms can be incorporated into: 1) physical activity promotional materials designed for the general public, 2) routine paperwork completed within the scope of a physician office visit, or 3) entry procedures at health/fitness or clinical exercise program facilities. The modified AHA/ACSM Health/Fitness Facility Preparticipation Screening Questionnaire (Fig. 2-1) and the Physical Activity Readiness Questionnaire (PAR-Q; Fig. 2-2) [11] represent examples of self-administered surveys recommended for use at Level 1 screening for individuals seeking either self- or professionally guided regimens. When medical clearance is recommended from the questionnaire results, participants should be advised to obtain such clearance prior to participation. Individuals recommended for medical clearance may further benefit from initial participation in a professionally guided program. Although both surveys are effective in identifying individuals who would benefit from medical consultation prior to participation, the AHA/ACSM questionnaire provides greater detail regarding cardiovascular disease risk factors and symptoms, and it identifies a broader scope of chronic diseases that might be aggravated by exercise. Thus, the AHA/ACSM questionnaire is more useful for identifying ACSM risk strata (Table 2-4). Although the use of either questionnaire is acceptable at Level 1 screening, many health/

(text continues on page 27)

Table 2-2. Coronary Artery Disease Risk Factor Thresholds for Use With ACSM Risk Stratification

Positive Risk Factors	Defining Criteria
1. Family history	Myocardial infarction, coronary revascularization, or sudden death before 55 years of age in father or other male first-degree relative, or before 65 years of age in mother or other female first-degree relative
2. Cigarette smoking	Current cigarette smoker or those who quit within the previous 6 months
3. Hypertension	Systolic blood pressure ≥140 mm Hg or diastolic ≥90 mm Hg, confirmed by measurements on at least two separate occasions, or on antihypertensive medication
4. Dyslipidemia	Low-density lipoprotein (LDL) cholesterol ≥130 mg·dL^{-1} (3.4 mmol·L^{-1}) or high-density lipoprotein (HDL) cholesterol <40 mg·dL^{-1} (1.03 mmol·L^{-1}), or on lipid-lowering medication. If total serum cholesterol is all that is available use ≥200 mg·dL^{-1} (5.2 mmol·L^{-1}) rather than low-density lipoprotein (LDL) ≥130 mg·dL^{-1}
5. Impaired fasting glucose	Fasting blood glucose ≥100 mg·dL^{-1} (5.6 mmol·L^{-1}) confirmed by measurements on at least two separate occasion
6. Obesity†	Body mass index ≥30 kg·m^{-2} or Waist girth >102 cm for men and >88 cm for women or Waist/hip ratio: ≥0.95 for men and ≥0.86 for women
7. Sedentary lifestyle	Persons not participating in a regular exercise program or not meeting the minimal physical activity recommendations‡ from the U.S. Surgeon General's Report

Negative Risk Factor	Defining Criteria
1. High-serum HDL cholesterol§	≥60 mg·dL^{-1} (1.6 mmol·L^{-1})

Hypertension threshold based on National High Blood Pressure Education Program. The Seventh Report of the Joint National Committee on Prevention, Detection, Evaluation, and Treatment of High Blood Pressure (JNC7). 2003. 03-5233.

Lipid thresholds based on National Cholesterol Education Program. Third Report of the National Cholesterol Education Program (NCEP) Expert Panel on Detection, Evaluation, and Treatment of High Blood Cholesterol in Adults (Adult Treatment Panel III). NIH Publication No. 02-5215, 2002.

Impaired FG threshold based on Expert Committee on the Diagnosis and Classification of Diabetes Mellitus. Follow-up report on the diagnosis of diabetes mellitus. Diabetes Care 2003;26:3160–3167.

Obesity thresholds based on Expert Panel on Detection Evaluation and Treatment of Overweight and Obesity in Adults. National Institutes of Health. Clinical guidelines on the identification, evaluation, and treatment of overweight and obesity in adults—the evidence report. Arch Int Med 1998;158:1855–1867.

Sedentary lifestyle thresholds based on United States Department of Health and Human Services. Physical activity and health: a report of the Surgeon General. 1996.

†Professional opinions vary regarding the most appropriate markers and thresholds for obesity and therefore, allied health professionals should use clinical judgment when evaluating this risk factor.

‡Accumulating 30 minutes or more of moderate physical activity on most days of the week

§Notes: It is common to sum risk factors in making clinical judgments. If HDL is high, subtract one risk factor from the sum of positive risk factors, because high HDL decreases CAD risk.

Table 2-3. Major Signs or Symptoms Suggestive of Cardiovascular, Pulmonary, or Metabolic Disease*†

Sign or Symptom	Clarification/Significance
Pain, discomfort (or other anginal equivalent) in the chest, neck, jaw, arms, or other areas that may result from ischemia	One of the cardinal manifestations of cardiac disease, in particular coronary artery disease Key features *favoring an ischemic origin* include: • *Character:* Constricting, squeezing, burning, "heaviness" or "heavy feeling" • *Location:* Substernal, across midthorax, anteriorly; in both arms, shoulders; in neck, cheeks, teeth; in forearms, fingers in interscapular region • *Provoking factors:* Exercise or exertion, excitement, other forms of stress, cold weather, occurrence after meals Key features *against an ischemic origin* include: • *Character:* Dull ache; "knifelike," sharp, stabbing; "jabs" aggravated by respiration • *Location:* In left submammary area; in left hemithorax • *Provoking factors:* After completion of exercise, provoked by a specific body motion
Shortness of breath at rest or with mild exertion	Dyspnea (defined as an abnormally uncomfortable awareness of breathing) is one of the principal symptoms of cardiac and pulmonary disease. It commonly occurs during strenuous exertion in healthy, well-trained persons and during moderate exertion in healthy, untrained persons. However, it should be regarded as abnormal; when it occurs at a level of exertion that is not expected to evoke this symptom in a given individual. Abnormal exertional dyspnea suggests the presence of cardiopulmonary disorders, in particular left ventricular dysfunction or chronic obstructive pulmonary disease.
Dizziness or syncope	Syncope (defined as a loss of consciousness) is most commonly caused by a reduced perfusion of the brain. Dizziness and, in particular, syncope *during* exercise may result from cardiac disorders that prevent the normal rise (or an actual fall) in cardiac output. Such cardiac disorders are potentially life-threatening and include severe coronary artery disease, hypertrophic cardiomyopathy, aortic stenosis, and malignant ventricular dysrhythmias. Although dizziness or syncope shortly *after* cessation of exercise should not be ignored, these symptoms may occur even in healthy persons as a result of a reduction in venous return to the heart.
Orthopnea or paroxysmal nocturnal dyspnea	Orthopnea refers to dyspnea occurring at rest in the recumbent position that is relieved promptly by sitting upright or standing. Paroxysmal nocturnal dyspnea refers to dyspnea, beginning usually 2 to 5 hours after the onset of sleep, which may be relieved by sitting on the side of the bed or getting out of bed. Both are symptoms of left ventricular dysfunction. Although nocturnal dyspnea may occur in persons with chronic obstructive pulmonary disease, it differs in that it is usually relieved after the person relieves himself or herself of secretions rather than specifically by sitting up.

continued

Table 2-3. Major Signs or Symptoms Suggestive of Cardiovascular, Pulmonary, or Metabolic Disease*† (continued)

Sign or Symptom	Clarification/Significance
Ankle edema	Bilateral ankle edema that is most evident at night is a characteristic sign of heart failure or bilateral chronic venous insufficiency. Unilateral edema of a limb often results from venous thrombosis or lymphatic blockage in the limb. Generalized edema (known as anasarca) occurs in persons with the nephrotic syndrome, severe heart failure, or hepatic cirrhosis.
Palpitations or tachycardia	Palpitations (defined as an unpleasant awareness of the forceful or rapid beating of the heart) may be induced by various disorders of cardiac rhythm. These include tachycardia, bradycardia of sudden onset, ectopic beats, compensatory pauses, and accentuated stroke volume resulting from valvular regurgitation. Palpitations also often result from anxiety states and high cardiac output (or hyperkinetic) states, such as anemia, fever, thyrotoxicosis, arteriovenous fistula, and the so-called idiopathic hyperkinetic heart syndrome.
Intermittent claudication	Intermittent claudication refers to the pain that occurs in a muscle with an inadequate blood supply (usually as a result of atherosclerosis) that is stressed by exercise. The pain does not occur with standing or sitting, is reproducible from day to day, is more severe when walking upstairs or up a hill, and is often described as a cramp, which disappears within 1 or 2 minutes after stopping exercise. Coronary artery disease is more prevalent in persons with intermittent claudication. Diabetics are at increased risk for this condition.
Known heart murmur	Although some may be innocent, heart murmurs may indicate valvular or other cardiovascular disease. From an exercise safety standpoint, it is especially important to exclude hypertrophic cardiomyopathy and aortic stenosis as underlying causes because these are among the more common causes of exertion-related sudden cardiac death.
Unusual fatigue or shortness of breath with usual activities	Although there may be benign origins for these symptoms, they also may signal the onset of, or change in the status of cardiovascular, pulmonary, or metabolic disease.

*Modified from Gordon S, Mitchell BS. Health appraisal in the non-medical setting. In: Durstine JL, King AC, Painter PL, eds. ACSM's resource manual for guidelines for exercise testing and prescription. Philadelphia: Lea & Febiger, 1993:219–228.

†These signs or symptoms must be interpreted within the clinical context in which they appear because they are not all specific for cardiovascular, pulmonary, or metabolic disease.

FIGURE 2-1. AHA/ACSM Health/Fitness Facility Preparticipation Screening Questionnaire*

Assess your health status by marking all *true* statements

History
You have had:
_____ a heart attack
_____ heart surgery
_____ cardiac catheterization
_____ coronary angioplasty (PTCA)
_____ pacemaker/implantable cardiac
defibrillator/rhythm disturbance
_____ heart valve disease
_____ heart failure
_____ heart transplantation
_____ congenital heart disease

*If you marked any of these statements in this section, consult your physician or other appropriate health care provider before engaging in exercise. You may need to use a facility with a **medically qualified staff.***

Symptoms
_____ You experience chest discomfort with exertion.
_____ You experience unreasonable breathlessness.
_____ You experience dizziness, fainting, or blackouts.
_____ You take heart medications.

Other health issues
_____ You have diabetes.
_____ You have asthma or other lung disease.
_____ You have burning or cramping sensation in your lower legs when walking short distances.
_____ You have musculoskeletal problems that limit your physical activity.
_____ You have concerns about the safety of exercise.
_____ You take prescription medication(s).
_____ You are pregnant.

Cardiovascular risk factors
_____ You are a man older than 45 years.
_____ You are a woman older than 55 years, have had a hysterectomy, or are postmenopausal.
_____ You smoke, or quit smoking within the previous 6 months.
_____ Your blood pressure is >140/90 mm Hg.
_____ You do not know your blood pressure.
_____ You take blood pressure medication.
_____ Your blood cholesterol level is >200 mg/dL.
_____ You do not know your cholesterol level.
_____ You have a close blood relative who had a heart attack or heart surgery before age 55 (father or brother) or age 65 (mother or sister).
_____ You are physically inactive (i.e., you get <30 minutes of physical activity on at least 3 days per week).
_____ You are >20 pounds overweight.

*If you marked two or more of the statements in this section you should consult your physician or other appropriate health care provider before engaging in exercise. You might benefit from using a facility with a **professionally qualified exercise staff†** to guide your exercise program.*

_____ None of the above

You should be able to exercise safely without consulting your physician or other appropriate health care provider in a self-guided program or almost any facility that meets your exercise program needs.

*Modified from American College of Sports Medicine and American Heart Association. ACSM/AHA Joint Position Statement: Recommendations for cardiovascular screening, staffing, and emergency policies at health/fitness facilities. Med Sci Sports Exerc 1998:1018.

†Professionally qualified exercise staff refers to appropriately trained individuals who possess academic training, practical and clinical knowledge, skills, and abilities commensurate with the credentials defined in Appendix F.

FIGURE 2-2. PAR-Q form.

Physical Activity Readiness
Questionnaire - PAR-Q
(revised 2002)

PAR-Q & YOU

(A Questionnaire for People Aged 15 to 69)

Regular physical activity is fun and healthy, and increasingly more people are starting to become more active every day. Being more active is very safe for most people. However, some people should check with their doctor before they start becoming much more physically active.

If you are planning to become much more physically active than you are now, start by answering the seven questions in the box below. If you are between the ages of 15 and 69, the PAR-Q will tell you if you should check with your doctor before you start. If you are over 69 years of age, and you are not used to being very active, check with your doctor.

Common sense is your best guide when you answer these questions. Please read the questions carefully and answer each one honestly: check YES or NO.

YES	NO		
☐	☐	1.	Has your doctor ever said that you have a heart condition <u>and</u> that you should only do physical activity recommended by a doctor?
☐	☐	2.	Do you feel pain in your chest when you do physical activity?
☐	☐	3.	In the past month, have you had chest pain when you were not doing physical activity?
☐	☐	4.	Do you lose your balance because of dizziness or do you ever lose consciousness?
☐	☐	5.	Do you have a bone or joint problem (for example, back, knee or hip) that could be made worse by a change in your physical activity?
☐	☐	6.	Is your doctor currently prescribing drugs (for example, water pills) for your blood pressure or heart condition?
☐	☐	7.	Do you know of <u>any other reason</u> why you should not do physical activity?

If

you

answered

YES to one or more questions

Talk with your doctor by phone or in person BEFORE you start becoming much more physically active or BEFORE you have a fitness appraisal. Tell your doctor about the PAR-Q and which questions you answered YES.

• You may be able to do any activity you want — as long as you start slowly and build up gradually. Or, you may need to restrict your activities to those which are safe for you. Talk with your doctor about the kinds of activities you wish to participate in and follow his/her advice.

• Find out which community programs are safe and helpful for you.

NO to all questions

If you answered NO honestly to <u>all</u> PAR-Q questions, you can be reasonably sure that you can:

• start becoming much more physically active – begin slowly and build up gradually. This is the safest and easiest way to go.

• take part in a fitness appraisal – this is an excellent way to determine your basic fitness so that you can plan the best way for you to live actively. It is also highly recommended that you have your blood pressure evaluated. If your reading is over 144/94, talk with your doctor before you start becoming much more physically active.

DELAY BECOMING MUCH MORE ACTIVE:

• if you are not feeling well because of a temporary illness such as a cold or a fever – wait until you feel better; or

• if you are or may be pregnant – talk to your doctor before you start becoming more active.

PLEASE NOTE: If your health changes so that you then answer YES to any of the above questions, tell your fitness or health professional. Ask whether you should change your physical activity plan.

<u>Informed Use of the PAR-Q</u>: The Canadian Society for Exercise Physiology, Health Canada, and their agents assume no liability for persons who undertake physical activity, and if in doubt after completing this questionnaire, consult your doctor prior to physical activity.

No changes permitted. You are encouraged to photocopy the PAR-Q but only if you use the entire form.

NOTE: If the PAR-Q is being given to a person before he or she participates in a physical activity program or a fitness appraisal, this section may be used for legal or administrative purposes.

"I have read, understood and completed this questionnaire. Any questions I had were answered to my full satisfaction."

NAME _____

SIGNATURE _____   DATE_____

SIGNATURE OF PARENT _____   WITNESS _____
or GUARDIAN (for participants under the age of majority)

Note: This physical activity clearance is valid for a maximum of 12 months from the date it is completed and becomes invalid if your condition changes so that you would answer YES to any of the seven questions.

CSEP
SCPE   © Canadian Society for Exercise Physiology   Supported by: [🍁]   Health   Santé   continued on other side...
                                                                        Canada   Canada

Source: Physical Activity Readiness Questionnaire (PAR-Q) © 2002. Reprinted with permission from the Canadian Society for Exercise Physiology. http://www.csep.ca/forms.asp.

Table 2-4. ACSM Risk Stratification Categories

1. Low risk	Men <45 years of age and women <55 years of age who are asymptomatic and meet no more than one risk factor threshold from Table 2-2
2. Moderate risk	Men ≥45 years and women ≥55 years *or* those who meet the threshold for two or more risk factors from Table 2-2
3. High risk	Individuals with one or more signs and symptoms listed in Table 2-3 *or* known cardiovascular,* pulmonary,† or metabolic‡ disease

*Cardiac, peripheral vascular, or cerebrovascular disease.

†Chronic obstructive pulmonary disease, asthma, interstitial lung disease, or cystic fibrosis (see Reference 24: American Association of Cardiovascular and Pulmonary Rehabilitation. Guidelines for pulmonary rehabilitation programs. 2nd ed. Champaign, IL: Human Kinetics, 1998:97–112.

‡Diabetes mellitus (IDDM, NIDDM), thyroid disorders, renal, or liver disease.

fitness and clinical exercise program facilities incorporate a more elaborate health/medical history questionnaire designed to provide additional detail regarding selected health habits and medical history.

Coronary Artery Disease Risk Factors

ACSM risk stratification is based, in part, on the presence or absence of the CAD risk factors listed in Table 2-2[6,12–15]. The risk factors in Table 2-2 should not be viewed as an all-inclusive list, but rather as a group with *clinically relevant thresholds* that should be considered collectively when making decisions about the level of medical clearance, the need for exercise testing prior to initiating participation, and the level of supervision for both exercise testing and exercise program participation. The *scope* of the list, and the *threshold* for each risk factor, should not be viewed as inconsistent with other risk factor lists that are intended for use in predicting coronary events prospectively during long-term follow-up[16], because the intended use for the list in Table 2-2 is to aid in the identification of occult coronary artery disease. Furthermore, other variables, such as major depression, also have been suggested as positive risk factors in the primary and secondary prevention of CAD[17–19].

Major Signs or Symptoms Suggestive of Cardiovascular, Pulmonary, and Metabolic Disease

Table 2-3 presents a listing of major signs or symptoms suggestive of cardiovascular, pulmonary and/or metabolic disease, along with additional information to aid the clinician in the clarification and significance of each sign or symptom[20]. The presence of most of these factors can be identified using the AHA/ACSM Questionnaire; however, a few (i.e., orthopnea, ankle edema, heart murmur) require a more thorough medical history and/or examination.

ACSM Risk Categories

Once symptom and risk factor information is known, candidates for exercise testing or training can be stratified based on the likelihood of untoward events during participation. This stratification becomes progressively more important as disease prevalence increases in the population under consideration. Using age, health status, symptom, and risk factor information, prospective participants can be classified into one of three risk strata (see Table 2-4) for triage to further screening prior to participation. Once risk strata are established, further screening recommendations are provided in Table 2-1.

Inherent within the concept of risk stratification is the impression that signs and symptoms (see Table 2-3) represent a higher-level concern for decision making as compared with risk factors (see Table 2-2). However, hypertension represents a unique risk factor in that it may be aggravated by acute exercise. Therefore, although it appears within Table 2-2, special consideration should be given to hypertensive patients when screening for exercise testing or training. The Seventh Report of the Joint National Committee on Prevention, Detection, Evaluation, and Treatment of High Blood Pressure (JNC7)[13] recommends a thorough medical history, physical examination, routine laboratory tests, and other diagnostic procedures in the evaluation of patients with documented hypertension. Because hypertension is commonly clustered with other risk factors associated with cardiovascular disease (i.e., dyslipidemia, obesity, diabetes), most hypertensive patients presenting for exercise testing or training fall into the *moderate-* or *high-*risk category as defined in Table 2-4. For such individuals, the requisite medical examination in Table 2-3 is consistent with the screening recommendations for hypertensive patients outlined in JNC7. However, in cases of isolated hypertension (i.e., hypertension is the only presenting risk factor from those in listed in Table 2-2), prudent recommendations for preparticipation screening should be based on the severity of the hypertension (see Table 3-1 for JNC7 classifications) and the desired intensity of exercise. For *low-*risk patients (see Table 2-4) with isolated stage 1 hypertension (<160/100 mm Hg), exercise testing generally is not necessary for clearance to engage in up to moderate intensity exercise (<60% of the $\dot{V}O_2R$). However, it is advisable for such patients to have physician clearance prior to participation. On the other hand, if the patient has documented stage 2 hypertension, or a patient with stage 1 hypertension desires to engage in more intense exercise training (>60% of the $\dot{V}O_2R$), an exercise assessment is recommended to quantify hemodynamic responses during exercise to aid in the establishment of prudent guidelines for exercise training[21].

ADDITIONAL PREPARTICIPATION ASSESSMENTS

Following risk stratification, additional fitness and/or clinical assessments and procedures may be incorporated into the preparticipation screening (Level 2 screening). The depth and breadth of these additional assessments vary as a function of:

- Type of program (i.e., *self-* or *professionally guided*)
- Intended training intensity (i.e., moderate versus vigorous) (see Table 1-1)
- Individual risk strata (see Table 2-4)

For self-guided physical activity regimens of light to moderate intensity, little additional assessment is needed beyond the ACSM-AHA Questionnaire provided that one adheres to all medical clearance recommendations contained within the form. Such regimens should incorporate the physical activity recommendations from the U.S. Surgeon General[6]. A specific self-guided regimen suitable for previously sedentary individuals can be found in the ACSM Fitness Book[10]. It should be noted that individuals in need of medical clearance as defined by the AHA/ACSM Questionnaire would likely benefit from participation in further fitness assessment and a professionally guided training regimen.

For individuals seeking a professionally guided exercise regimen, approved consent forms for exercise testing and training should be completed (see Chapter 3 for examples of forms), and any additional fitness and/or clinical assessments (including exercise testing) should follow procedures described in Chapters 3 through 5 for either *clinical* or *nonclinical* exercise settings.

EXERCISE TESTING AND TESTING SUPERVISION RECOMMENDATIONS

No set of guidelines for exercise testing and participation can cover all situations. Local circumstances and policies vary, and specific program procedures also are properly diverse. To provide some general guidance on the need for a medical examination and exercise testing prior to participation in a moderate to vigorous exercise program, ACSM suggests the recommendations presented in Level 3 of Table 2-1 for determining when a medical examination and diagnostic exercise test are appropriate and when physician supervision is recommended. Although the testing guidelines are less rigorous for those individuals considered to be low risk, the information gathered from an exercise test may be useful in establishing a safe and effective exercise prescription for these individuals. The exercise testing recommendations found in Table 2-1 reflect the notion that the risk of cardiovascular events increases as a function of physical activity intensity (i.e., moderate versus hard). Although Table 1-1 provides both absolute and relative thresholds for moderate and hard intensity physical activity, exercise professionals should choose the most applicable definition (i.e., relative or absolute) for their setting when making decisions about the level of screening prior to exercise training and physician supervision during exercise testing. It should be noted that the recommendations for medical examination and exercise testing for moderate risk individuals desiring vigorous exercise (Table 2-4) are consistent with those found within recent AHA Guidelines (See Box 2-2; categories A-2 and A-3).

The degree of medical supervision of exercise tests varies appropriately from physician-supervised tests to situations in which there may be no physician present[1]. The degree of physician supervision may differ with local policies and circumstances, the health status of the patient, and the experience of the laboratory staff. The appropriate protocol should be based on the age, health status, and physical activity level of the person to be tested. Physicians responsible for supervising exercise testing should meet or exceed the minimal competencies for supervision and interpretation of results as established by the AHA (see Box 5-3) [22]. In all situations where exercise testing is performed, site personnel should at least be certified at a level of basic life support; preferably, one or more staff should be certified in advanced cardiac life support (ACLS). Whenever possible, testing should be performed by ACSM-credentialed personnel, because these credentials document the individual's knowledge, skills, and abilities directly related to exercise testing.

Risk Stratification for Cardiac Patients

Cardiac patients may be further stratified regarding safety during exercise using published guidelines. Risk stratification criteria from the AACVPR are presented in Box 2-1[3]. Recommendations for the duration of monitored exercise training and/or education based on the risk factor profile have now been suggested[23]. The AHA has developed a more extensive risk classification system for medical clearance of cardiac patients (Box 2-2)[1]. The AHA guidelines provide recommendations for participant and/or patient monitoring and supervision and for activity restriction. Exercise program professionals should recognize that the AHA guidelines do not consider comorbidities (e.g., type 1 diabetes mellitus, morbid obesity, severe pulmonary disease, debilitating neurologic or orthopedic conditions) that could result in modification of the recommendations for monitoring and supervision during exercise training.

BOX 2-1	**American Association of Cardiovascular and Pulmonary Rehabilitation (AACVPR)**

Risk Stratification Criteria for Cardiac Patients*

LOWEST RISK

Characteristics of patients at lowest risk for exercise participation (all characteristics listed must be present for patients to remain at lowest risk)
- Absence of complex ventricular dysrhythmias during exercise testing and recovery
- Absence of angina or other significant symptoms (e.g., unusual shortness of breath, light-headedness, or dizziness, during exercise testing and recovery)
- Presence of normal hemodynamics during exercise testing and recovery (i.e., appropriate increases and decreases in heart rate and systolic blood pressure with increasing workloads and recovery)
- Functional capacity ≥7 METs

Nonexercise Testing Findings
- Resting ejection fraction ≥50%
- Uncomplicated myocardial infarction or revascularization procedure
- Absence of complicated ventricular dysrhythmias at rest
- Absence of congestive heart failure
- Absence of signs or symptoms of postevent/postprocedure ischemia
- Absence of clinical depression ▶

▶ **Box 2-1, continued**

MODERATE RISK

Characteristics of patients at moderate risk for exercise participation (any one or combination of these findings places a patient at moderate risk)

- Presence of angina or other significant symptoms (e.g., unusual shortness of breath, light-headedness, or dizziness occurring only at high levels of exertion [≥7 METs])
- Mild to moderate level of silent ischemia during exercise testing or recovery (ST-segment depression <2 mm from baseline)
- Functional capacity <5 METs

Nonexercise Testing Findings
- Rest ejection fraction = 40%–49%

HIGH RISK

Characteristics of patients at high risk for exercise participation (any one or combination of these findings places a patient at high risk)

- Presence of complex ventricular dysrhythmias during exercise testing or recovery
- Presence of angina or other significant symptoms (e.g., unusual shortness of breath, light-headedness, or dizziness at low levels of exertion [<5 METs] or during recovery)
- High level of silent ischemia (ST-segment depression ≥2 mm from baseline) during exercise testing or recovery
- Presence of abnormal hemodynamics with exercise testing (i.e., chronotropic incompetence or flat or decreasing systolic BP with increasing workloads) or recovery (i.e., severe postexercise hypotension)

Nonexercise Testing Findings
- Rest ejection fraction <40%
- History of cardiac arrest or sudden death
- Complex dysrhythmias at rest
- Complicated myocardial infarction or revascularization procedure
- Presence of congestive heart failure
- Presence of signs or symptoms of postevent/postprocedure ischemia
- Presence of clinical depression

*Reprinted from Williams MA. Exercise testing in cardiac rehabilitation: exercise prescription and beyond. Cardiol Clin 2001;19:415–431, with permission from Elsevier.

BOX 2-2	**American Heart Association (AHA)** **Risk Stratification Criteria***

Class A: Apparently Healthy Individuals

- Includes the following individuals
  1. Children, adolescents, men <age 45, and women <55 years who have no symptoms of or known presence of heart disease or major coronary risk factors
  2. Men ≥45 years and women ≥55 years who have no symptoms or known presence of heart disease and with <2 major cardiovascular risk factors.
  3. Men ≥45 years and women ≥55 years who have no symptoms or known presence of heart disease and with ≥2 major cardiovascular risk factors.
- *Activity guidelines*: No restrictions other than basic guidelines
- *ECG and blood pressure monitoring*: Not required
- *Supervision required*: None. *Although it is suggested that persons classified as Class A-2 and particularly Class A-3 undergo a medical examination and possibly a medically supervised exercise test before engaging in vigorous exercise.*

Class B: Presence of known, stable cardiovascular disease with low risk for complications with vigorous exercise, but slightly greater than for apparently healthy individuals

- Includes individuals with any of the following diagnoses:
  1. CAD (MI, CABGS, PTCA, angina pectoris, abnormal exercise test, and abnormal coronary angiograms) whose condition is stable and who have the clinical characteristics outlined below;
  2. Valvular heart disease, excluding severe valvular stenosis or regurgitation with the clinical characteristics outlined below;
  3. Congenital heart disease; risk stratification should be guided by the 27th Bethesda Conference recommendations.[25]
  4. Cardiomyopathy; ejection fraction ≤30%; includes stable patients with heart failure with any of the clinical characteristics as outlined below but not hypertrophic cardiomyopathy or recent myocarditis
  5. Exercise test abnormalities that do not meet the criteria outlined in Class C.
- *Clinical characteristics*:
  1. New York Heart Association class 1 or 2
  2. Exercise capacity ≤6 METs
  3. No evidence of congestive heart failure
  4. No evidence of myocardial ischemia or angina at rest or on the exercise test at or below 6 METs
  5. Appropriate rise in systolic blood pressure during exercise ▶

▶ **Box 2-2, continued**

6. Absence of sustained or nonsustained ventricular tachycardia at rest or with exercise
7. Ability to satisfactorily self-monitor intensity of activity
- *Activity guidelines*: Activity should be individualized, with exercise prescription by qualified individuals and approved by primary health care provider
- *Supervision required*: Medical supervision during initial prescription session is beneficial. Supervision by appropriate trained nonmedical personnel for other exercise sessions should occur until the individual understands how to monitor his or her activity. Medical personnel should be trained and certified in advanced cardiac life support. Nonmedical personnel should be trained and certified in basic life support (which includes CPR).
- *ECG and blood pressure monitoring*: Useful during the early prescription phase of training, usually 6 to 12 sessions.

Class C: Those at moderate to high risk for cardiac complications during exercise and/or unable to self-regulate activity or understand recommended activity level
- Includes individuals with any of the following diagnoses:
  1. CAD with the clinical characteristics outlined below
  2. Valvular heart disease, excluding severe valvular stenosis or regurgitation with the clinical characteristics outlined below
  3. Congenital heart disease; risk stratification should be guided by the 27th Bethesda Conference recommendations. (Fuster V, Gotto AM, Libby P. 27th Bethesda Conference: Matching the intensity of risk factor management with the hazard for coronary disease events. J Am Coll Cardiol 1996;27:964–976.)
  4. Cardiomyopathy; ejection fraction ≤30%; includes stable patients with heart failure with any of the clinical characteristics as outlined below but not hypertrophic cardiomyopathy or recent myocarditis
  5. Complex ventricular arrhythmias not well controlled
- *Clinical characteristics*:
  1. NYHA class 3 or 4
  2. Exercise test results:
     - Exercise capacity <6 METs
     - Angina or ischemia ST depression at workload <6 METs
     - Fall in systolic blood pressure below resting levels with exercise
     - Nonsustained ventricular tachycardia with exercise
  3. Previous episode of primary cardiac arrest (i.e., cardiac arrest that did not occur in the presence of an acute myocardial infarction or during a cardiac procedure)

▶ **Box 2-2, continued**

4. A medical problem that the physician believes may be life threatening
* *Activity guidelines*: Activity should be individualized, with exercise prescription provided by qualified individuals and approved by primary health care provider.
* *Supervision*: Medical supervision during all exercise sessions until safety is established.
* *ECG and blood pressure monitoring*: Continuous during exercise sessions until safety is established, usually ≥12 sessions.

Class D: Unstable disease with activity restriction†

* Includes individuals with
  1. Unstable ischemia
  2. Severe and symptomatic valvular stenosis or regurgitation;
  3. Congenital heart disease; criteria for risk that would prohibit exercise conditioning should be guided by the 27th Bethesda Conference recommendations.[25]
  4. Heart failure that is not compensated
  5. Uncontrolled arrhythmias
  6. Other medical conditions that could be aggravated by exercise
* *Activity guidelines*: No activity is recommended for conditioning purposes. Attention should be directed to treating the patient and restoring the patient to class C or better. Daily activities must be prescribed on the basis of individual assessment by the patient's personal physician.

*Modified from Fletcher GF, Balady GJ, Amsterdam EA, et al. Exercise standards for testing and training. A statement for health care professionals from the American Heart Association. Circulation 2001;104:1694–1740.

†Exercise for conditioning purposes is not recommended.

REFERENCES

1. Fletcher GF, Balady GJ, Amsterdam EA, et al. Exercise standards for testing and training. A statement for health care professionals from the American Heart Association. Circulation 2001;104:1694–1740.
2. American College of Sports Medicine and American Heart Association. ACSM/AHA Joint Position Statement: Recommendations for cardiovascular screening, staffing, and emergency policies at health/fitness facilities. Med Sci Sports Exerc 1998;1018.
3. American Association of Cardiovascular and Pulmonary Rehabilitation. Guidelines for Cardiac Rehabilitation and Secondary Prevention Programs. 4th ed. Champaign, IL: Human Kinetics, 2003.
4. Maron BJ, Araujo CG, Thompson PD, et al. Recommendations for preparticipation screening and the assessment of cardiovascular disease in masters athletes. Circulation 2001;103:327–334.
5. Maron BJ, Thompson PD, Puffer JC, et al. Cardiovascular preparticipation screening of competitive athletes. A statement for health professionals from the Sudden Death Committee (clinical cardiology) and Congenital Cardiac Defects Committee (cardiovascular disease in the young), American Heart Association. Circulation 1996;94:850–856.
6. United States Department of Health and Human Services. Physical activity and health: a report of the Surgeon General, 1996.

7. Pate RR, Pratt M, Blair SN, et al. Physical activity and public health. A recommendation from the Centers for Disease Control and Prevention and the American College of Sports Medicine. JAMA 1995;273:402–407.

8. Thompson PD, Buchner D, Pina IL, et al. Exercise and physical activity in the prevention and treatment of atherosclerotic cardiovascular disease. Circulation 2003;107:3109–3116.

9. American College of Sports Medicine. ACSM's health/fitness facility standards and guidelines. 2nd ed. Champaign, IL: Human Kinetics, 1997.

10. American College of Sports Medicine. ACSM fitness book. 3rd ed. Champaign, IL: Human Kinetics, 2003.

11. Canadian Society for Exercise Physiology. PAR-Q and you. Gloucester, Ontario: Canadian Society for Exercise Physiology, 1994.

12. National Cholesterol Education Program. Third Report of the National Cholesterol Education Program (NCEP) Expert Panel on Detection, Evaluation, and Treatment of High Blood Cholesterol in Adults (Adult Treatment Panel III). 2002. NIH Publication No. 02-5215, 2002.

13. National High Blood Pressure Education Program. The Seventh Report of the Joint National Committee on Prevention, Detection, Evaluation, and Treatment of High Blood Pressure (JNC7). 2003, 03-5233.

14. Expert Committee on the Diagnosis and Classification of Diabetes Mellitus. Follow-up report on the diagnosis of diabetes mellitus. Diabetes Care 2003;26:3160–3167.

15. Expert Panel on Detection Evaluation and Treatment of Overweight and Obesity in Adults. National Institutes of Health. Clinical guidelines on the identification, evaluation, and treatment of overweight and obesity in adults—the evidence report. Arch Int Med 1998;158:1855–1867.

16. Wilson PW, D'Agostino RB, Levy D, et al. Prediction of coronary heart disease using risk factor categories. Circulation 1998;97:1837–1847.

17. Barefoot JC, Helms MJ, Mark DB, et al. Depression and long-term mortality risk in patients with coronary artery disease. Am J Cardiol 1996;78:613–617.

18. Ford DE, Mead LA, Chang PP, et al. Depression is a risk factor for coronary artery disease in men: the precursors study. Arch Intern Med 1998;158:1422–1426.

19. Ferketich AK, Schwartzbaum JA, Frid, DJ, et al. Depression as an antecedent to heart disease among women and men in the NHANES I study. Arch Intern Med 2000;160:1261–1268.

20. Gordon S, Mitchell BS. Health appraisal in the non-medical setting. In: Durstine JL, King AC, Painter PL, eds. ACSM's resource manual for guidelines for exercise testing and prescription. Philadelphia: Lea & Febiger, 1993:219–228.

21. American College of Sports Medicine. Position stand: exercise and hypertension. Med Sci Sports Exerc 2004;36:533–553.

22. Rodgers GP, Ayanian JZ, Balady G, et al. American College of Cardiology/American Heart Association clinical competence statement on stress testing: a report of the American College of Cardiology/American Heart Association/American College of Physicians-American Society of Internal Medicine Task Force on Clinical Competence. Circulation 2000;102:1726–1738.

23. Roitman JL, LaFontaine T, Drimmer AM. A new model for risk stratification and delivery of cardiovascular rehabilitation services in the long-term clinical management of patients with coronary artery disease. J Cardio Rehab 1998;18:113–123.

24. American Association of Cardiovascular and Pulmonary Rehabilitation. Guidelines for pulmonary rehabilitation programs. 2nd ed. Champaign, IL: Human Kinetics, 1998:97–112.

25. Fuster V, Gotto AM, Libby P. 27th Bethesda Conference: Matching the intensity of risk factor management with the hazard for coronary disease events. J Am Coll Cardiol 1996;27:964–976.

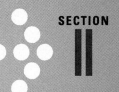

Exercise Testing

Pre-Exercise Evaluations

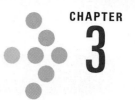

This chapter contains information related to pre-exercise testing procedures and serves as a bridge between the risk stratification concepts presented in Chapter 2, the fitness assessment (see Chapter 4), and/or clinical exercise testing concepts (see Chapters 5 and 6). Although each of the chapter elements (e.g., medical history, physical examination, identification of exercise contraindications, informed consent procedures) relate to both health and fitness and clinical exercise settings, the lower-risk population typically encountered in the health and fitness setting generally justifies a less sophisticated approach to the pre-exercise test procedures. Therefore, abbreviated versions of the medical history and physical examination procedures described within this chapter are reasonable within the health and fitness setting.

The extent of medical evaluation necessary before exercise testing depends on the assessment of risk as determined from the procedures outlined in Chapters 1 and 2. For many persons, especially those with coronary artery disease (CAD) and other cardiovascular disorders, the exercise test and accompanying physical examination are critical to the development of a safe and effective exercise program. In today's health care environment, not all persons warrant extensive testing; however, it is important to work with health care providers in understanding the importance of the baseline exercise evaluation. This evaluation provides greater assurance of exercise safety by identifying residual myocardial ischemia, significant dysrhythmias, and the effect of certain medical therapies.

A comprehensive pre-exercise test evaluation in the clinical setting generally includes a medical history, physical examination, and laboratory tests. The goal of this chapter is not to be totally inclusive or to supplant more specific references on each subject, but rather to provide a concise set of guidelines for the pre-exercise test participant assessment.

Medical History, Physical Examination, and Laboratory Tests

The pre-exercise test medical history should be thorough and include both past and current information. Appropriate components of the medical history are presented in Box 3-1. A preliminary physical examination should be performed by a physician or other qualified personnel before exercise testing moderate- and high-risk subjects (see Table 2-4). Appropriate components of the physical examination specific to subsequent exercise testing are presented in Box 3-2.

BOX 3-1	Components of the Medical History*

Appropriate components of the medical history may include the following:

- Medical diagnosis. Cardiovascular disease including myocardial infarction; percutaneous coronary artery procedures including angioplasty, coronary stent(s), and atherectomy; coronary artery bypass surgery; valvular surgery(s) and valvular dysfunction (e.g., aortic stenosis/mitral valve disease); other cardiac surgeries such as left ventricular aneurysmectomy and cardiac transplantation; pacemaker and/or implantable cardioverter defibrillator; presence of aortic aneurysm; ablation procedures for dysrhythmias; symptoms of ischemic coronary syndrome (angina pectoris); peripheral vascular disease; hypertension; diabetes; obesity; pulmonary disease including asthma, emphysema, and bronchitis; cerebrovascular disease, including stroke and transient ischemic attacks; anemia and other blood dyscrasias (e.g., lupus erythematosus); phlebitis, deep vein thrombosis or emboli; cancer; pregnancy; osteoporosis; musculoskeletal disorders; emotional disorders; eating disorders.
- Previous physical examination findings. Murmurs, clicks, gallop rhythms, other abnormal heart sounds, and other unusual cardiac and vascular findings; abnormal pulmonary findings (e.g., wheezes, rales, crackles); abnormal blood sugar, blood lipids and lipoproteins, or other significant laboratory abnormalities; high blood pressure; edema.
- History of symptoms. Discomfort (e.g., pressure, tingling, pain, heaviness, burning, tightness, squeezing, numbness) in the chest, jaw, neck, back, or arms; light-headedness, dizziness, or fainting; temporary loss of visual acuity or speech, transient unilateral numbness or weakness; shortness of breath; rapid heart beats or palpitations, especially if associated with physical activity, eating a large meal, emotional upset, or exposure to cold (or any combination of these activities).
- Recent illness, hospitalization, new medical diagnoses, or surgical procedures.
- Orthopedic problems, including arthritis, joint swelling, and any condition that would make ambulation or use of certain test modalities difficult.
- Medication use, drug allergies.
- Other habits, including caffeine, alcohol, tobacco, or recreational (illicit) drug use.
- Exercise history. Information on readiness for change and habitual level of activity: type of exercise, frequency, duration, and intensity.
- Work history with emphasis on current or expected physical demands, noting upper and lower extremity requirements.
- Family history of cardiac, pulmonary, or metabolic disease, stroke, or sudden death.

* For more detailed information see Bickley LS. Bate's pocket guide to physical examination and history taking. 4th ed. Philadelphia: Lippincott Williams & Wilkins, 2003.

BOX 3-2	Components of the Pre-exercise Test Physical Examination*

Appropriate components of the physical examination may include the following:

- Body weight; in many instances, determination of body mass index (BMI), waist girth, and/or body composition (percent body fat) is desirable
- Apical pulse rate and rhythm
- Resting blood pressure, seated, supine, and standing
- Auscultation of the lungs with specific attention to uniformity of breath sounds in all areas (absence of rales, wheezes, and other breathing sounds)
- Palpation of the cardiac apical impulse, point of maximal impulse (PMI)
- Auscultation of the heart with specific attention to murmurs, gallops, clicks, and rubs
- Palpation and auscultation of carotid, abdominal, and femoral arteries
- Evaluation of the abdomen for bowel sounds, masses, visceromegaly, and tenderness
- Palpation and inspection of lower extremities for edema and presence of arterial pulses
- Absence or presence of tendon xanthoma and skin xanthelasma
- Follow-up examination related to orthopedic or other medical conditions that would limit exercise testing
- Tests of neurologic function, including reflexes and cognition (as indicated)
- Inspection of the skin, especially of the lower extremities in known diabetics

*For more detailed information see Bickley LS. Bate's pocket guide to physical examination and history taking. 4th ed. Philadelphia: Lippincott Williams & Wilkins, 2003.

Identification and risk stratification of persons with CAD and those at high risk of developing CAD are facilitated by review of previous test results, such as coronary angiography or exercise nuclear or echocardiography studies[1]. Additional testing may include ambulatory ECG (Holter) monitoring and pharmacologic stress testing to further clarify the need for and extent of intervention, assess response to treatment such as medical therapies and revascularization procedures, or determine the need for additional assessment. As outlined in Box 3-3, other laboratory tests may be warranted based on the level of risk and clinical status of the patient. These laboratory tests may include, but are not limited to, serum chemistries, complete blood count, comprehensive lipoprotein profile, and pulmonary function.

BOX 3-3	Recommended Laboratory Tests by Level of Risk and Clinical Assessment

Apparently healthy (low risk) or individuals at increased risk, but without known disease (moderate risk)

- Fasting serum total cholesterol, LDL cholesterol, HDL cholesterol, and triglycerides.
- Fasting blood glucose, especially in individuals ≥45 years old and younger individuals who are overweight (BMI ≥25 kg·m^{-2}) and have one or more of the following risk factors for type 2 diabetes: a first-degree relative with diabetes, member of a high-risk ethnic population (e.g., Black, Hispanic American, Native American, Asian American, and Pacific Islander), delivered a baby weighing >9 lbs or history of gestational diabetes, hypertension (BP ≥140/90 mm Hg in adults), HDL cholesterol of ≤40 mg·dL^{-1} and/or triglyceride level ≥150 mg·dL^{-1}, previously identified impaired glucose tolerance or impaired fasting glucose (fasting glucose ≥100 mg·dL^{-1}), habitual physical inactivity, polycystic ovary disease, and history of vascular disease
- Thyroid function, as a screening evaluation especially if dyslipidemia is present

Patients with known or suspected cardiovascular disease (high risk)

- Preceding tests plus pertinent previous cardiovascular laboratory tests (e.g., resting 12-lead ECG, Holter monitoring, coronary angiography, radionuclide or echocardiography studies, previous exercise tests)
- Carotid ultrasound and other peripheral vascular studies
- Consider measures of homocysteine, Lp(a), high sensitivity C-reactive protein, fibrinogen, LDL particle size, HDL subspecies, and number (especially in young persons with a strong family history of CAD and in those persons without traditional coronary risk factors)
- Chest radiograph, if congestive heart failure is present or suspected
- Comprehensive blood chemistry panel and complete blood count as indicated by history and physical examination (see Table 3-3)

Patients with pulmonary disease

- Chest radiograph
- Pulmonary function tests (see Tables 3-4 and 3-5)
- Other specialized pulmonary studies (e.g., oximetry or blood gas analysis)

Although a detailed description of all the physical examination procedures listed in Box 3-2 and the recommended laboratory tests listed in Box 3-3 are beyond the scope of this text, additional information related to assessment of blood pressure, cholesterol and lipoproteins, other blood chemistries, and pulmonary function are provided in the following section. For more detailed descriptions of these assessments, the reader is referred to the work of Bickley[2].

BLOOD PRESSURE

Measurement of resting blood pressure (BP) is an integral component of the pre-exercise test evaluation. Subsequent decisions should be based on the average of two or more properly measured, seated BP readings recorded during each of two or more office visits[3]. Specific techniques for measuring BP are critical to accuracy and detection of high BP and are presented in Box 3-4. In addition to high BP readings, unusually low readings also should be evaluated for clinical significance. The Seventh Report of the Joint National Committee on Prevention, Detection, Evaluation, and Treatment of High Blood Pressure (JNC7) provides guidelines for hypertension detection and management[3]. Table 3-1 summarizes the JNC7 recommendations for the classification and management of BP for adults.

The relationship between BP and risk for cardiovascular events is continuous, consistent, and independent of other risk factors. For individuals 40 to 70 years of age, each increment of 20 mm Hg in systolic BP or 10 mm Hg in diastolic BP

BOX 3-4	Procedures for Assessment of Resting Blood Pressure*

1. Patients should be seated quietly for at least 5 minutes in a chair with back support (rather than on an examination table) with their feet on the floor and their arm supported at heart level. Patients should refrain from smoking cigarettes or ingesting caffeine during the 30 minutes preceding the measurement.
2. Measuring supine and standing values may be indicated under special circumstances.
3. Wrap cuff firmly around upper arm at heart level; align cuff with brachial artery.
4. The appropriate cuff size must be used to ensure accurate measurement. The bladder within the cuff should encircle at least 80% of the upper arm. Many adults require a large adult cuff.
5. Place stethoscope bell below the antecubital space over the brachial artery.
6. Quickly inflate cuff pressure to 20 mm Hg above first Korotkoff sound.
7. Slowly release pressure at rate equal to 2 to 5 mm Hg per second;
8. Systolic BP is the point at which the first of two or more Korotkoff sounds is heard (phase 1) and diastolic BP is the point before the disappearance of Korotkoff sounds (phase 5).
9. At least two measurements should be made (minimum of 1 minute apart).
10. Provide to patients, verbally and in writing, their specific BP numbers and BP goals.

*Modified from National High Blood Pressure Education Program. The Seventh Report of the Joint National Committee on Prevention, Detection, Evaluation, and Treatment of High Blood Pressure (JNC7). 2003. 03-5233.

TABLE 3-1. Classification and Management of Blood Pressure for Adults*†

BP Classification	SBP mm Hg	DPB mm Hg	Lifestyle Modification	Initial Drug Therapy Without Compelling Indication	Initial Drug Therapy With Compelling Indications
Normal	<120	And <80	Encourage		
Prehypertension	120–139	Or 80–89	Yes	No antihypertensive drug indicated	Drug(s) for compelling indications.‡
Stage 1 Hypertension	140–159	Or 90–99	Yes	Antihypertensive drug(s) indicated	Drug(s) for compelling indications.‡ Other antihypertensive drugs, as needed.
Stage 2 Hypertension	≥160	Or ≥100	Yes	Antihypertensive drug(s) indicated. Two-drug combination for most.§	

*From National High Blood Pressure Education Program. The Seventh Report of the Joint National Committee on Prevention, Detection, Evaluation, and Treatment of High Blood Pressure (JNC7). 2003. 03-5233.

†Treatment determined by highest BP category.

‡Compelling indications include heart failure, post myocardial infarction, high coronary heart disease risk, diabetes, chronic kidney disease, and recurrent stroke prevention. Treat patients with chronic kidney disease or diabetes to BP goal of <130/80 mm Hg.

§Initial combined therapy should be used cautiously in those at risk for orthostatic hypotension.

Abbreviations: DBP, diastolic blood pressure; SBP, systolic blood pressure.

doubles the risk of cardiovascular disease across the entire BP range from 115/75 to 185/115 mm Hg. According to JNC7, persons with a systolic BP of 120 to 139 mm Hg or a diastolic BP of 80 to 89 mm Hg should be considered as *prehypertensive* and require health-promoting lifestyle modifications to prevent cardiovascular disease.

Lifestyle modification, including physical activity, weight reduction (if needed), a DASH eating plan (i.e., a diet rich in fruits, vegetables, and low-fat dairy products with a reduced content of saturated and total fat) (see Box 9-3), dietary sodium reduction (no more than 100 mmol or 2.4 g sodium/day), and moderation of alcohol consumption, remains the cornerstone of antihypertensive therapy. However, JNC7 emphasizes the fact that most patients with hypertension who require drug therapy in addition to lifestyle modification require two or more antihypertensive medications to achieve the goal BP (i.e., <140/90 mm Hg, or <130/80 mm Hg for patients with diabetes or chronic kidney disease).

LIPIDS AND LIPOPROTEINS

The Third Report of the Expert Panel on Detection, Evaluation, and Treatment of High Blood Cholesterol in Adults (Adult Treatment Panel III, or ATP III) outlines the National Cholesterol Education Program's (NCEP's) recommendations for cholesterol testing and management (Table 3-2)[4]. ATP III identifies low-density lipoprotein (LDL) cholesterol as the primary target for cholesterol-lowering therapy. This designation is based on a wide variety of evidence indicating that elevated LDL cholesterol is a powerful risk factor for CAD and that lowering of LDL cholesterol results in a striking reduction in the incidence of CAD. Table 3-2 summarizes the ATP III classifications of LDL, total, and HDL-cholesterol and triglycerides.

According to ATP III, a low HDL cholesterol level is strongly and inversely associated with the risk for CAD. Clinical trials provide suggestive evidence that raising HDL cholesterol levels reduces the risk for CAD. However, it remains uncertain whether raising HDL cholesterol levels per se, independent of other changes in lipid and/or nonlipid risk factors, reduces the risk for CAD. In view of this, ATP III does not identify a specific HDL cholesterol goal level to reach with therapy. Rather, nondrug and drug therapies that raise HDL cholesterol that also are part of the management of other lipid and nonlipid risk factors are encouraged by ATP III.

There is growing evidence for a strong association between elevated triglyceride levels and CAD risk. Recent studies suggest that some species of triglyceride-

TABLE 3-2. ATP III Classification of LDL, Total, and HDL Cholesterol (mg·dL⁻¹)*

LDL Cholesterol	
<100	Optimal
100–129	Near optimal/above optimal
130–159	Borderline high
160–189	High
≥190	Very high
Total Cholesterol	
<200	Desirable
200–239	Borderline high
≥240	High
HDL Cholesterol	
<40	Low
≥60	High
Triglycerides	
<150	Normal
150–199	Borderline high
200–499	High
≥500	Very high

*From National Cholesterol Education Program. Third Report of the National Cholesterol Education Program (NCEP) Expert Panel on Detection, Evaluation, and Treatment of High Blood Cholesterol in Adults (Adult Treatment Panel III). 2002. NIH Publication No. 02-5215.

rich lipoproteins, notably, cholesterol-enriched remnant lipoproteins, promote atherosclerosis and predispose to CAD. Because these remnant lipoproteins appear to have atherogenic potential similar to that of LDL cholesterol, ATP III recommends that they be added to LDL cholesterol to become a secondary target of therapy for persons with elevated triglycerides. To accomplish this, non-HDL cholesterol is calculated by subtracting HDL cholesterol from the total cholesterol level.

The metabolic syndrome is characterized by a constellation of metabolic risk factors in one individual. Abdominal obesity, atherogenic dyslipidemia (i.e., elevated triglycerides, small LDL cholesterol particles, and reduced HDL cholesterol), elevated blood pressure, insulin resistance, prothrombotic state, and proinflammatory state generally are accepted as being characteristic of the metabolic syndrome. The root causes of the metabolic syndrome are overweight and obesity, physical inactivity, and genetic factors. Because the metabolic syndrome has emerged as an important contributor to CAD, ATP III places emphasis on the metabolic syndrome as a risk enhancer.

ATP III designates hypertension, cigarette smoking, diabetes, overweight and obesity, physical inactivity, and an atherogenic diet as modifiable nonlipid risk factors, whereas age, male gender, and family history of premature CAD are nonmodifiable nonlipid risk factors for CAD. Triglycerides, lipoprotein remnants, lipoprotein (a), small LDL particles, HDL subspecies, apolipoproteins B and A-1, and total cholesterol-to-HDL cholesterol ratio are designated by ATP III as emerging lipid risk factors. Homocysteine, thrombogenic and hemostatic factors, inflammatory markers (e.g., high sensitivity C-reactive protein), and impaired fasting glucose are designated by ATP III as emerging nonlipid risk factors.

The guiding principle of ATP III is that the intensity of LDL-lowering therapy should be adjusted to the individual's absolute risk for CAD. Since publication of ATP III, major clinical trials have been published that question the treatment thresholds for LDL. In particular, an LDL goal of <70 mg/dL appears to be appropriate for those in a category of "very high" risk.[5] The ATP III treatment guidelines are summarized in the ACSM Resource Manual. Additional guidelines for the primary and secondary prevention of cardiovascular diseases recently have been updated by the American Heart Association[6,7].

BLOOD PROFILE ANALYSES

Multiple analyses blood profiles are evaluated commonly in clinical exercise programs. Such profiles may provide useful information about an individual's overall health status and ability to exercise and may help to explain certain ECG abnormalities. Because of varied methods of assaying blood samples, some caution is advised when comparing blood chemistries from different laboratories. Table 3-3 gives normal ranges for selected blood chemistries, derived from a variety of sources. For many patients with CAD, medications for dyslipidemia and hypertension are common. Many of these medications act in the liver to lower blood cholesterol and in the kidneys to lower blood pressure. One should pay particular attention to liver function tests such as alanine transaminase (ALT), aspartate transaminase (AST), and bilirubin as well as to renal (kidney) function tests such as creatinine, blood urea nitrogen (BUN), and BUN/creatinine ratio in patients on such medications. Indication of volume depletion and potassium abnormalities can

TABLE 3-3. Typical Ranges of Normal Values for Selected Blood Variables in Adults*

Variable	Men	Neutral	Women
Hemoglobin (g·dL^{-1})	13.5–17.5		11.5–15.5
Hematocrit (%)	40–52		36–48
Red cell count (x10^{12}/L)	4.5–6.5		3.9–5.6
Mean cell hemoglobin concentration (MCHC)		30–35 (g·dL^{-1})	
White blood cell count		4–11 (x10^9/L)	
Platelet count		150–450 (x10^9/L)	
Fasting glucose†		60–99 mg·dL^{-1}	
Blood urea nitrogen (BUN)		4–24 mg·dL^{-1}	
Creatinine		0.3–1.4 mg·dL^{-1}	
BUN/creatinine ratio		7–27	
Uric acid (mg·dL^{-1})	4.0–8.9	2.3–7.8	
Sodium		135–150 mEq·dL^{-1}	
Potassium		3.5–5.5 mEq·dL^{-1}	
Chloride		98–110 mEq·dL^{-1}	
Osmolality		278–302 mOsm/kg	
Calcium		8.5–10.5 mg·dL^{-1}	
Calcium, ion		4.0–5.2 mg·dL^{-1}	
Phosphorus		2.5–4.5 mg·dL^{-1}	
Protein, total		6.0–8.5 g·dL^{-1}	
Albumin		3.0–5.5 g·dL^{-1}	
Globulin		2.0–4.0 g·dL^{-1}	
A/G ratio		1.0–2.2	
Iron, total (µg·dL^{-1})	40–190		35–180
Liver Function Tests			
Bilirubin		<1.5 mg·dL^{-1}	
(SGOT) (AST)	8–46 µ·L^{-1}		7–34 µ·L^{-1}
(SGPT) (ALT)	7–46 µ·L^{-1}		4–35 µ·L^{-1}

*Certain variables must be interpreted in relation to the normal range of the issuing laboratory.

†Fasting blood glucose ≥100 is considered impaired fasting glucose. Reference 13: Expert Committee on the Diagnosis and Classification of Diabetes Mellitus. Follow-up report on the diagnosis of diabetes mellitus. Diabetes Care 2003;26:3160–3167.

Abbreviations: SGOT, serum glutamic-oxaloacetic transaminase; AST, aspartate transaminase (formerly SGOT); SGPT, serum glutamic-pyruvic transaminase; ALT, alanine transaminase (formerly SGPT).

be seen in the sodium and potassium measurements. These tests should be applied judiciously and not used as finite ranges of normal.

PULMONARY FUNCTION

Pulmonary function testing with routine spirometry is recommended for all smokers over the age of 45 and in any person presenting with dyspnea (shortness of breath), chronic cough, wheezing, or excessive mucus production[8]. Spirometry is a relatively simple and noninvasive test that can be performed easily. When performing pulmonary function testing, standards for the performance of these tests should be followed[9]. Although many spirometric tests are available, the most commonly used include the forced vital capacity (FVC), the forced expiratory volume in 1 second (FEV_1), and the FEV_1/FVC ratio. Results from these tests can be used in the early identification of patients at risk for the development of both restrictive and obstructive pulmonary disease before symptoms developing. However, it should be emphasized that pulmonary function test results provide information that is closely related to symptoms and should not be interpreted in isolation. Additionally, Table 3-4 illustrates how these tests can be used to determine the severity of both obstructive and restrictive lung diseases. This spirometric classification of lung disease has proved useful in predicting health status, use of health care resources, development of exacerbations, and mortality. Additionally, abnormal pulmonary function test results can be indicative of an increased risk for

TABLE 3-4. Schema for Determining the Severity of Both Obstructive and Restrictive Lung Diseases from Pulmonary Function Tests*

Severity of Obstructive Disease: This interpretation is based on the assessment of both the FEV_1, expressed as a percent of predicted, and the FEV_1/FVC ratio.

Stage	Characteristics
0: At risk	FEV_1 ≥80% of predicted FEV_1/FVC ≥70% With chronic symptoms: cough, sputum production, dyspnea
I: Mild	FEV_1 ≥80% of predicted FEV_1/FVC <70% With or without chronic symptoms

II: Moderate	FEV_1 30% to 79% of predicted
	    IIA: FEV_1 50% to 79% of predicted
	    IIB: FEV_1 30% to 49% of predicted
	FEV_1/FVC <70%
	With or without chronic symptoms

III: Severe	FEV_1 <30% of predicted FEV_1/FVC <70%

Severity of Restrictive Disease: This interpretation is based on the assessment of the FVC, expressed as a percent of predicted. In patients where spirometry indicates a restrictive pattern, the measurement of total lung capacity is needed to confirm a restrictive defect.

Stage	Characteristics
Mild	FVC less than the lower limit of normal but ≥70% of predicted
Moderate	FVC 60% to 69% of predicted
Moderately severe	FVC 50% to 59% of predicted
Severe	FVC 34% to 49% of predicted
Very severe	FVC <34% of predicted

*References 14, 15, 16: From Pauwels RA, Buist AS, Calverley PM, et al. Global strategy for the diagnosis, management, and prevention of chronic obstructive pulmonary disease. NHLBI/WHO Global Initiative for Chronic Obstructive Lung Disease (GOLD) Workshop summary. Am J Respir Crit Care Med 2001;163:1256–1276; American Thoracic Society. Lung function testing: selection of reference values and interpretative strategies. Am Rev Respir Dis 1991;144:1202–1218; Aaron SD, Dales RE, Cardinal P. How accurate is spirometry at predicting restrictive pulmonary impairment? Chest 1999;115:869–873.

lung cancer, heart attack and stroke and can be used to identify patients in which interventions, such as smoking cessation, would be most beneficial. In addition to the preceding tests, the determination of the maximal voluntary ventilation (MVV) also should be obtained during routine spirometric testing. Results from this test often can be used to help evaluate ventilatory responses obtained during graded exercise testing[10].

Contraindications to Exercise Testing

For certain individuals the risks of exercise testing outweigh the potential benefits. For these patients it is important to carefully assess risk versus benefit when deciding whether the exercise test should be performed. Box 3-5 outlines both absolute and relative contraindications to exercise testing[11]. Performing the pre-exercise test evaluation and the careful review of prior medical history, as described earlier in this chapter, helps identify potential contraindications and increase the safety of the exercise test. Patients with absolute contraindications should not perform exercise tests until such conditions are stabilized or adequately treated. Patients with relative contraindications may be tested only after careful evaluation of the risk/benefit ratio. However, it should be emphasized that contraindications might not apply in certain specific clinical situations, such as soon after acute myocardial infarction, revascularization procedure, or bypass surgery or to determine the need for, or benefit of, drug therapy. Finally, conditions exist that preclude reliable diagnostic ECG information from exercise testing (e.g., left bundle-branch block, digitalis therapy). The exercise test may still provide useful information on exercise capacity, dysrhythmias, and hemodynamic responses to exercise. In these conditions, additional evaluative techniques such as echocardiography or nuclear imaging can be added to the exercise test to improve sensitivity, specificity, and diagnostic capabilities.

Emergency departments are increasingly performing an exercise test on low-risk patients who present with chest pain (i.e., within 4 to 8 hours) to rule out myocardial infarction[11,12]. Generally, these patients include those who are no longer symptomatic and who have unremarkable ECGs and no change in serial cardiac enzymes. However, exercise testing in this setting should be performed only as part of a carefully constructed patient management protocol and only after patients have been screened for high-risk features or other indicators for hospital admission. Table 3-5 is a quick reference source for serum concentrations of enzymes commonly used as indices of myocardial damage or necrosis.

Informed Consent

Obtaining adequate informed consent from participants before exercise testing and participation in an exercise program is an important ethical and legal consideration. Although the content and extent of consent forms may vary, enough information must be present in the informed consent process to ensure that the participant knows and understands the purposes and risks associated with the test or exercise program. The consent form should be verbally explained and include a statement indicating that the patient has been given an opportunity to ask questions about the

BOX 3-5 | Contraindications to Exercise Testing*

Absolute
- A recent significant change in the resting ECG suggesting significant ischemia, recent myocardial infarction (within 2 days), or other acute cardiac event
- Unstable angina
- Uncontrolled cardiac dysrhythmias causing symptoms or hemodynamic compromise
- Symptomatic severe aortic stenosis
- Uncontrolled symptomatic heart failure
- Acute pulmonary embolus or pulmonary infarction
- Acute myocarditis or pericarditis
- Suspected or known dissecting aneurysm
- Acute systemic infection, accompanied by fever, body aches, or swollen lymph glands

Relative†
- Left main coronary stenosis
- Moderate stenotic valvular heart disease
- Electrolyte abnormalities (e.g., hypokalemia, hypomagnesemia)
- Severe arterial hypertension (i.e., systolic BP of >200 mm Hg and/or a diastolic BP of >110 mm Hg) at rest
- Tachydysrhythmia or bradydysrhythmia
- Hypertrophic cardiomyopathy and other forms of outflow tract obstruction
- Neuromuscular, musculoskeletal, or rheumatoid disorders that are exacerbated by exercise
- High-degree atrioventricular block
- Ventricular aneurysm
- Uncontrolled metabolic disease (e.g., diabetes, thyrotoxicosis, or myxedema)
- Chronic infectious disease (e.g., mononucleosis, hepatitis, AIDS)
- Mental or physical impairment leading to inability to exercise adequately

*Modified from Gibbons RJ, Balady GJ, Bricker J, et al. ACC/AHA 2002 guideline update for exercise testing: a report of the American College of Cardiology/American Heart Association Task Force on Practice Guidelines (Committee on Exercise Testing). 2002. American College of Cardiology web site. www.acc.org/clinical/guidelines/exercise/dirIndex.htm

†Relative contraindications can be superseded if benefits outweigh risks of exercise. In some instances, these individuals can be exercised with caution and/or using low-level end points, especially if they are asymptomatic at rest.

TABLE 3-5. Serum Enzymes (Myocardial Tissue Damage or Necrosis)

Enzyme	Normal Value*	Time Course of Change (When Abnormally Elevated)
CK myocardial band (CK-MB)	<5% of total CK	Appears at 4–6 hours; peaks at 12–24 hours; returns to normal within 72 hours
Creatine phosphokinase (CPK or CK)	Females 10–70 U·L^{-1} Males 25–90 U·L^{-1}	Appears within hours and peaks at about 24 hours without reperfusion; returns to normal within 2–4 days
Troponin I	<0.5 ng·mL^{-1}	Appears about 4–6 hours; peaks at 24 hours, remains elevated 5–10 days

*Normal values vary depending on the laboratory and the method used. The SGOT and LDH enzymes are no longer used as "cardiac enzymes" and have been replaced by the others.

procedure and has sufficient information to give informed consent. Note specific questions from the participant on the form along with the responses provided. The consent form must indicate that the participant is free to withdraw from the procedure at any time. If the participant is a minor, a legal guardian or parent must sign the consent form. It is advisable to check with authoritative bodies (e.g., hospital risk management, institutional review boards, facility legal counsel) to determine what is appropriate for an acceptable informed consent process. Also, all reasonable efforts must be made to protect the privacy of the patient's health information (e.g., medical history, test results) as described in the Health Insurance Portability and Accountability Act (HIPPA) of 1996. A sample consent form for exercise testing is provided in Figure 3-1. No sample form should be adopted for a specific program unless approved by local legal counsel.

When the exercise test is for purposes other than diagnosis or prescription (i.e., for experimental purposes), this should be indicated during the consent process and reflected on the *Informed Consent Form*; and applicable policies for the testing of human subjects must be implemented. A copy of the Policy on Human Subjects for Research is periodically published in ACSM's journal, *Medicine and Science in Sports and Exercise*.

Because most consent forms include a statement that emergency procedures and equipment are available, the program must ensure that available personnel are appropriately trained and authorized to carry out emergency procedures that use such equipment. Written emergency policies and procedures should be in place, and emergency drills should be practiced at least once every 3 months or more often when there is a change in staff. See Appendix B for more information on emergency management.

PARTICIPANT INSTRUCTIONS

Explicit instructions for participants before exercise testing increase test validity and data accuracy. Whenever possible, written instructions along with a description of the evaluation should be provided well in advance of the appointment so

---

FIGURE 3-1. Sample of informed consent form for a symptom-limited exercise test.

Informed Consent for an Exercise Test

1. Purpose and Explanation of the Test

You will perform an exercise test on a cycle ergometer or a motor-driven treadmill. The exercise intensity will begin at a low level and will be advanced in stages depending on your fitness level. We may stop the test at any time because of signs of fatigue or changes in your heart rate, ECG, or blood pressure, or symptoms you may experience. It is important for you to realize that you may stop when you wish because of feelings of fatigue or any other discomfort.

2. Attendant Risks and Discomforts

There exists the possibility of certain changes occurring during the test. These include abnormal blood pressure, fainting, irregular, fast or slow heart rhythm, and in rare instances, heart attack, stroke, or death. Every effort will be made to minimize these risks by evaluation of preliminary information relating to your health and fitness and by careful observations during testing. Emergency equipment and trained personnel are available to deal with unusual situations that may arise.

3. Responsibilities of the Participant

Information you possess about your health status or previous experiences of heart-related symptoms (e.g., shortness of breath with low-level activity, pain, pressure, tightness, heaviness in the chest, neck, jaw, back, and/or arms) with physical effort may affect the safety of your exercise test. Your prompt reporting of these and any other unusual feelings with effort during the exercise test itself is very important. You are responsible for fully disclosing your medical history, as well as symptoms that may occur during the test. You are also expected to report all medications (including nonprescription) taken recently and, in particular, those taken today, to the testing staff.

4. Benefits to Be Expected

The results obtained from the exercise test may assist in the diagnosis of your illness, in evaluating the effect of your medications or in evaluating what type of physical activities you might do with low risk.

5. Inquiries

Any questions about the procedures used in the exercise test or the results of your test are encouraged. If you have any concerns or questions, please ask us for further explanations.

6. Use of Medical Records

The information that is obtained during exercise testing will be treated as privileged and confidential as described in the Health Insurance Portability and Accountability Act of 1996. It is not to be released or revealed to any person except your referring physician without your written consent. However, the information obtained may be used for statistical analysis or scientific purposes with your right to privacy retained.

FIGURE 3-1. continued

7. Freedom of Consent

I hereby consent to voluntarily engage in an exercise test to determine my exercise capacity and state of cardiovascular health. My permission to perform this exercise test is given voluntarily. I understand that I am free to stop the test at any point if I so desire.

I have read this form, and I understand the test procedures that I will perform and the attendant risks and discomforts. Knowing these risks and discomforts, and having had an opportunity to ask questions that have been answered to my satisfaction, I consent to participate in this test.

_____	_____
Date	Signature of Patient
_____	_____
Date	Signature of Witness
_____	_____
Date	Signature of Physician or Authorized Delegate

the client or patient can prepare adequately. The following points should be considered for inclusion in such preliminary instructions; however, specific instructions vary with test type and purpose.

- Participants should refrain from ingesting food, alcohol, or caffeine or using tobacco products within 3 hours of testing.
- Participants should be rested for the assessment, avoiding significant exertion or exercise on the day of the assessment.
- Clothing should permit freedom of movement and include walking or running shoes. Women should bring a loose-fitting, short-sleeved blouse that buttons down the front and should avoid restrictive undergarments.
- If the evaluation is on an outpatient basis, participants should be made aware that the evaluation may be fatiguing and that they may wish to have someone accompany them to the assessment to drive home afterward.
- If the test is for diagnostic purposes, it may be helpful for patients to discontinue prescribed cardiovascular medications, but only with physician approval. Currently prescribed antianginal agents alter the hemodynamic response to exercise and significantly reduce the sensitivity of ECG changes for ischemia. Patients taking intermediate- or high-dose β-blocking agents may be asked to taper their medication over a 2- to 4-day period to minimize hyperadrenergic withdrawal responses.
- If the test is for functional purposes, _patients should continue their medication regimen_ on their usual schedule so that the exercise responses will be consistent with responses expected during exercise training.

- Participants should bring a list of their medications, including dosage and frequency of administration, to the assessment and should report the last actual dose taken. As an alternative, participants may wish to bring their medications with them for the exercise testing staff to record.
- Drink ample fluids over the 24-hour period preceding the test to ensure normal hydration before testing.

REFERENCES

1. Fuster V, Pearson TA. 27th Bethesda Conference: Matching the intensity of risk factor management with the hazard for coronary disease events. September 14–15, 1995. J Am Coll Cardiol 1996;27: 957–1047.
2. Bickley LS. Bate's pocket guide to physical examination and history taking. 4th ed. Philadelphia: Lippincott Williams & Wilkins, 2003.
3. National High Blood Pressure Education Program. The Seventh Report of the Joint National Committee on Prevention, Detection, Evaluation, and Treatment of High Blood Pressure (JNC7). 2003. 03-5233.
4. National Cholesterol Education Program. Third Report of the National Cholesterol Education Program (NCEP) Expert Panel on Detection, Evaluation, and Treatment of High Blood Cholesterol in Adults (Adult Treatment Panel III). 2002. NIH Publication No. 02-5215.
5. Grundy SM, Cleeman JI, Noel Bairey Merz C et al. Implications of recent clinical trials for the National Cholesterol Education Program Adult Treatment Panel III Guidelines. J Am Coll Cardiol 2004;44:720–732.
6. Pearson TA, Blair SN, Daniels SR, et al. American Heart Association Science Advisory and Coordinating Committee. AHA Guidelines for Primary Prevention of Cardiovascular Disease and Stroke: 2002 Update: Consensus panel guide to comprehensive risk reduction for adult patients without coronary or other atherosclerotic vascular diseases. Circulation 2002;106:388–391.
7. Smith SC Jr, Blair SN, Bonow RO, et al. AHA/ACC Scientific Statement: AHA/ACC guidelines for preventing heart attack and death in patients with atherosclerotic cardiovascular disease: 2001 update. A statement for healthcare professionals from the American Heart Association and the American College of Cardiology. Circulation 2001;104:1577–1579.
8. Ferguson GT, Enright PL, Buist AS, et al. Office spirometry for lung health assessment in adults: a consensus statement from the National Lung Health Education Program. Chest 2000;117: 1146–1161.
9. American Thoracic Society. Standardization of spirometry, 1994 Update. Am J Respir Crit Care Med 1995;152:1107–1136.
10. American Thoracic Society and American College of Chest Physicians. ATS/ACCP Statement on cardiopulmonary exercise testing. Am J Respir Crit Care Med 2003;167(2):211–277.
11. Gibbons RJ, Balady GJ, Bricker J, et al. ACC/AHA 2002 guideline update for exercise testing: a report of the American College of Cardiology/American Heart Association Task Force on Practice Guidelines (Committee on Exercise Testing). 2002. American College of Cardiology web site. www.acc.org/clinical/guidelines/exercise/dirIndex.htm
12. Braunwald E, Antman EM, Beasley JW, et al. ACC/AHA 2002 guideline update for the management of patients with unstable angina and non-ST-segment elevation myocardial infarction: a report of the American College of Cardiology/American Heart Association task force on practice guidelines. 2002. http://www.acc.org/clinical/guidelines/unstable/unstable.pdf.
13. Expert Committee on the Diagnosis and Classification of Diabetes Mellitus. Follow-up report on the diagnosis of diabetes mellitus. Diabetes Care 2003;26:3160–3167.
14. Pauwels RA, Buist AS, Calverley PM, et al. Global strategy for the diagnosis, management, and prevention of chronic obstructive pulmonary disease. NHLBI/WHO Global Initiative for Chronic Obstructive Lung Disease (GOLD) Workshop summary. Am J Respir Crit Care Med 2001;163: 1256–1276.
15. American Thoracic Society. Lung function testing: selection of reference values and interpretative strategies. Am Rev Respir Dis 1991;144:1202–1218.
16. Aaron SD, Dales RE, Cardinal P. How accurate is spirometry at predicting restrictive pulmonary impairment? Chest 1999;115:869–873.

Health-Related Physical Fitness Testing and Interpretation

As evidence continues to evolve regarding the health benefits of physical activity and exercise, the focus on health-related physical fitness, and physiologic fitness appear to supersede that of skill-related physical fitness.[1,2] See Chapter 1 for a detailed description of the aforementioned terms. The health-related components of physical fitness have a strong relationship with good health, are characterized by an ability to perform daily activities with vigor, and demonstrate the traits and capacities associated with low risk of premature development of the hypokinetic diseases (e.g., those associated with physical inactivity).[1] Both health-related and physiologic fitness measures are closely allied with disease prevention and health promotion and can be modified through regular physical activity and exercise.

A fundamental goal of primary and secondary intervention programs is promotion of health; therefore, such programs should focus on enhancement of health-related and physiologic components of physical fitness. As part of the ACSM Pre-Participation Screening (Table 2-1), Level 2 recommends an additional Pre-Participation Assessment that precedes the development of an exercise prescription. This chapter provides guidelines for the Level 2 Pre-Participation Assessment through the measurement and evaluation of health-related physical fitness in presumably healthy adults.

Purposes of Health-Related Fitness Testing

Measurement of physical fitness is a common and appropriate practice in preventive and rehabilitative exercise programs. The purposes of health-related fitness testing in such programs include the following:

- Educating participants about their present health-related fitness status relative to health-related standards and age- and sex-matched norms
- Providing data that are helpful in development of exercise prescriptions to address all fitness components
- Collecting baseline and follow-up data that allow evaluation of progress by exercise program participants
- Motivating participants by establishing reasonable and attainable fitness goals
- Stratifying cardiovascular risk

Basic Principles and Guidelines

The information obtained from health-related physical fitness testing, in combination with the individual's health and medical information, is used by the health and fitness professional to help an individual achieve specific fitness goals. An ideal health-related physical fitness test is reliable, valid, relatively inexpensive, and easy to administer. The test should yield results that are indicative of the current state of fitness, reflect change from physical activity or exercise intervention, and be directly comparable to normative data.

PRETEST INSTRUCTIONS

All pretest instructions should be provided and adhered to prior to arrival at the testing facility. Certain steps should be taken to ensure client safety and comfort before administering a health-related fitness test. A minimal recommendation is that individuals complete a questionnaire such as the ACSM-AHA form (see Fig. 2-1). A listing of preliminary instructions for all clients can be found in Chapter 3 under Patient Instructions. These instructions may be modified to meet your needs.

TEST ORDER

The following should be accomplished before the participant arrives at the test site:

- Assure all forms, score sheets, tables, graphs, and other testing documents are organized and available for the test's administration.
- Calibrate all equipment a minimum of once each month to ensure accuracy (e.g., metronome, cycle ergometer, treadmill, sphygmomanometer, skinfold calipers)
- Organize equipment so that tests can follow in sequence without taxing the same muscle group repeatedly.
- Provide informed consent form (see Fig. 3-1).
- Maintain room temperature of 68°F to 72°F (20°C–22°C) and humidity of less than 60%.

When multiple tests are to be administered, the organization of the testing session can be very important, depending on what physical fitness components are to be evaluated. Resting measurements such as heart rate, blood pressure, height, weight, and body composition should be obtained first. When all fitness components are assessed in a single session, resting measurements should be followed (in order) by tests of cardiorespiratory (CR) endurance, muscular fitness, and flexibility. Testing CR endurance after assessing muscular fitness (which elevates heart rate) can produce inaccurate results about an individual's CR endurance status, particularly when tests using HR to predict aerobic fitness are used. Likewise, dehydration resulting from CR endurance tests might influence body composition values if measured by bioelectrical impedance analysis (BIA).

TEST ENVIRONMENT

The test environment is important for test validity and reliability. Test anxiety, emotional problems, food in the stomach, bladder distention, room temperature, and ventilation should be controlled as much as possible. To minimize anxiety, the test procedures should be explained adequately, and the test environment should be quiet and private. The room should be equipped with a comfortable seat and/or examination table to be used for resting blood pressure and heart rate and/or electrocardiographic (ECG) recordings. The demeanor of personnel should be one of relaxed confidence to put the subject at ease. Testing procedures should not be rushed, and all procedures must be explained clearly prior to initiating the process. These seemingly minor tasks are accomplished easily and are important in achieving valid and reliable test results.

Body Composition

It is well established that excess body fat is associated with hypertension, type 2 diabetes, stroke, coronary heart disease, and hyperlipidemia.[3] Approximately 65% of Americans are classified overweight (body mass index [BMI] >25) and almost 31% classified as obese (BMI >30).[4] In 1960 to 1962, 1971 to 1974, 1976 to 1980, 1988 to 1994, and 1999 to 2000 the incidence of obesity in the United States was 13.4%, 14.5%, 15%, 23.3%, and 30.9%, respectively. The twofold increase in adult obesity since 1980 coincides with an alarming trend in the incidence of overweight children in the United States, who displayed an increase from approximately 4% in 1970 to 15% in 2000.[5,6] This almost fourfold increase in 20 years shows no signs of abatement. Although there is almost no difference in obesity levels of males based on race and ethnicity, the incidence of obesity of Black women is 50%, Mexican-American women 40%, and White women approximately 30%.[4] Consequently, assessment of body composition should be emphasized throughout the life span.

Basic body composition can be expressed as the relative percentage of body mass that is fat and fat-free tissue using a two-compartment model. Body composition can be estimated with both laboratory and field techniques that vary in terms of complexity, cost, and accuracy. Different assessment techniques are briefly reviewed in this section; however, the detail associated with obtaining measurements and calculating estimates of body fat for all of these techniques is beyond the scope of this text. More detailed descriptions of each technique are available in Chapter 12 of the *ACSM Resource Manuals for Guidelines for Exercise Testing and Prescription*, 5th ed. and elsewhere.[7–9] Before collecting data for body composition assessment, the technician must be trained, routinely practiced in the techniques, and already have demonstrated reliability in his or her measurements, independent of the technique being used. Experience can be accrued under the direct supervision of a highly qualified mentor in a controlled testing environment.

ANTHROPOMETRIC METHODS

Measurements of height, weight, circumferences, and skinfolds are used to estimate body composition. Although skinfold measurements are more difficult than other anthropometric procedures, they provide a better estimate of body fatness than those based only on height, weight, and circumferences.[10]

Body Mass Index

The BMI, or Quetelet index, is used to assess weight relative to height and is calculated by dividing body weight in kilograms by height in meters squared ($kg \cdot m^{-2}$). For most people, obesity-related health problems increase beyond a BMI of 25, and the *Expert Panel on the Identification, Evaluation, and Treatment of Overweight and Obesity in Adults*[11] lists a BMI of 25.0 to 29.9 $kg \cdot m^{-2}$ for overweight and a BMI of greater than or equal to 30.0 $kg \cdot m^{-2}$ for obesity. Although, BMI fails to distinguish between body fat, muscle mass, or bone; an increased risk of hypertension, total cholesterol/HDL cholesterol ratio, coronary disease, and mortality rate are associated with a BMI greater than 30 $kg \cdot m^{-2}$ (Table 4-1).[12] A BMI of less than 18.5 $kg \cdot m^{-2}$ also increases the risk of cardiovascular disease and is responsible for the lower portion of the J-shaped curve of BMI versus cardiovascular risk. The use of specific BMI values to predict percentage body fat and health risk is in the initial stages of development (Table 4-2).[13] Because of the relatively large standard error of estimating percent fat from BMI ($\pm 5\%$ fat),[10] other methods of body composition assessment should be used to predict body fatness during a fitness assessment.

Circumferences

The pattern of body fat distribution is recognized as an important predictor of the health risks of obesity.[14] Android obesity which is characterized by more fat on the trunk (abdominal fat), provides an increased risk of hypertension, type 2 diabetes, dyslipidemia, coronary artery disease, and premature death compared with individuals who demonstrate gynoid obesity (fat distributed in the hip and thigh).[15]

Girth measurements may be used to predict body composition and equations are available for both genders and a range of age groups.[16,17] The accuracy may be within 2.5% to 4% of the actual body composition if the subject possesses similar characteristics of the original validation population and the girth measurements are

TABLE 4-1. Classification of Disease Risk Based on Body Mass Index (BMI) and Waist Circumference*

	BMI ($kg \cdot m^{-2}$)	Disease Risk† Relative to Normal Weight and Waist Circumference	
		Men, ≤102 cm Women, ≤88 cm	Men, >102 cm Women, >88 cm
Underweight	<18.5	—	—
Normal	18.5–24.9	—	—
Overweight	25.0–29.9	Increased	High
Obesity, class			
I	30.0–34.9	High	Very high
II	35.0–39.9	Very high	Very high
III	≥40	Extremely high	Extremely high

*See Reference 11: Modified from Expert Panel. Executive summary of the clinical guidelines on the identification, evaluation, and treatment of overweight and obesity in adults. Arch Intern Med 1998;158:1855–1867.

†Disease risk for Type 2 diabetes, hypertension, and cardiovascular disease. Dashes (—) indicate that no additional risk at these levels of BMI was assigned. Increased waist circumference can also be a marker for increased risk even in persons of normal weight.

TABLE 4-2. Predicted Body Fat Percentage based on Body Mass Index (BMI) for African-American and White Adults*†

BMI (kg·m⁻²)	Health Risk	20–39 yr	40–59 yr	60–79 yr
		Males		
<18.5	Elevated	<8%	<11%	<13%
18.6–24.9	Average	8%–19%	11%–21%	13%–24%
25.0–29.9	Elevated	20%–24%	22%–27%	25%–29%
>30	High	≥25%	≥28%	≥30%
		Females		
<18.5	Elevated	<21%	<23%	<24%
18.6–24.9	Average	21%–32%	23%–33%	24%–35%
25.0–29.9	Elevated	33%–38%	34%–39%	36%–41%
>30	High	≥39%	≥40%	≥42%

*See reference 13: From Gallagher D, Heymsfield SB, Heo M, et al. Healthy percentage body fat ranges: an approach for developing guidelines based on body mass index. Am J Clin Nutr 2000;72:694–701. Adapted with permission by the American Journal of Clinical Nutrition. © Am J Clin Nutr American Society for Clinical Nutrition.

†Note: Standard error of estimate is ±5% for predicting percent body fat from BMI (based on a four-compartment estimate of body fat percentage).

precise. A cloth tape measure with a spring-loaded handle (Gulick) reduces skin compression and improves consistency of measurement. Duplicate measurements are recommended at each site and should be obtained in a rotational instead of a consecutive order. The average of the two measures is used provided each measure is within 5 mm. Box 4-1 contains a description of the common sites.

The waist-to-hip ratio (WHR) is the circumference of the waist divided by the circumference of the hips (see Box 4-1, buttocks and hip measure) and has been used as a simple method for determining body fat distribution.[18] Health risk increases with WHR, and standards for risk vary with age and sex. For example, health risk is *very high* for young men when WHR is more than 0.95 and for young women when WHR is more than 0.86. For people 60 to 69 years old, the WHR values are greater than 1.03 for men and greater than 0.90 for women for the same risk classification.[8,15]

The waist circumference can be used alone as an indicator of health risk because abdominal obesity is the issue. The Expert Panel on the Identification, Evaluation and Treatment of Overweight and Obesity in Adults provided a classification of disease risk based on both BMI and waist circumference as shown in Table 4-1.[11] Furthermore, a new risk stratification scheme for adults based on waist circumference has been proposed (Table 4-3).[19] This can be used alone or in conjunction with BMI to evaluate chronic disease risk (see Table 4-1). All assessments should include a minimum of either waist circumference or BMI, but preferably both, for risk stratification.

Skinfold Measurements

Body composition determined from skinfold measurements correlates well ($r = .70$–$.90$) with body composition determined by hydrodensiometry.[9] The

BOX 4-1	Standardized Description of Circumference Sites and Procedures

Abdomen:	With the subject standing upright and relaxed, a horizontal measure taken at the greatest anterior extension of the abdomen, usually at the level of the umbilicus.
Arm:	With the subject standing erect and arms hanging freely at the sides with hands facing the thigh, a horizontal measure midway between the acromion and olecranon processes.
Buttocks/Hips:	With the subject standing erect and feet together, a horizontal measure is taken at the maximal circumference of buttocks. This measure is used for the hip measure in a waist/hip measure.
Calf:	With the subject standing erect (feet apart ~20 cm), a horizontal measure taken at the level of the maximum circumference between the knee and the ankle, perpendicular to the long axis.
Forearm:	With the subject standing, arms hanging downward but slightly away from the trunk and palms facing anteriorly, a measure perpendicular to the long axis at the maximal circumference.
Hips/Thigh:	With the subject standing, legs slightly apart (~10 cm), a horizontal measure is taken at the maximal circumference of the hip/proximal thigh, just below the gluteal fold.
Mid-Thigh	With the subject standing and one foot on a bench so the knee is flexed at 90 degrees, a measure is taken midway between the inguinal crease and the proximal border of the patella, perpendicular to the long axis.
Waist:	With the subject standing, arms at the sides, feet together, and abdomen relaxed, a horizontal measure is taken at the narrowest part of the torso (above the umbilicus and below the xiphoid process). The National Obesity Task Force (NOTF) suggests obtaining a horizontal measure directly above the iliac crest as a method to enhance standardization. Unfortunately, current formulae are not predicated on the NOTF suggested site. ▶

> ▶ **Box 4.1, continued**

Procedures
- All measurements should be made with a flexible yet inelastic tape measure.
- The tape should be placed on the skin surface without compressing the subcutaneous adipose tissue
- If a Gulick spring loaded handle is used, the handle should be extended to the same marking with each trial.
- Take duplicate measures at each site and retest if duplicate measurements are not within 5 mm.
- Rotate through measurement sites or allow time for skin to regain normal texture.

Modified from Callaway CW, et al. Circumferences: 39-80. In: Lohman TG, Roche AF, Martorell R. eds. Anthropometric Standardization Reference Manual. Champaign, IL: Human Kinetics, 1988.

principle behind this technique is that the amount of subcutaneous fat is proportional to the total amount of body fat. It is assumed that close to one-third of the total fat is located subcutaneously. The exact proportion of subcutaneous-to-total fat varies with sex, age, and ethnicity.[20] Therefore, regression equations used to convert sum of skinfolds to percent body fat must consider these variables for greatest accuracy. Box 4-2 presents a standardized description of skinfold sites and procedures. To improve the accuracy of the measurement, it is recommended that one train with a skilled technician, use video media that demonstrate proper technique, participate in workshops, and accrue experience in a supervised practical environment. The accuracy of predicting percent fat from skinfolds is approximately plus or minus 3.5% assuming that appropriate techniques and equations have been used.[8]

Factors that may contribute to measurement error within skinfold assessment include poor technique and/or an inexperienced evaluator, an extremely obese or

TABLE 4-3. New Criteria for Waist Circumference in Adults*

| | Waist Circumference cm (in) | |
Risk Category	Females	Males
Very low	<70 cm (<28.5 in)	<80 cm (31.5 in)
Low	70–89 (28.5–35.0)	80–99 (31.5–39.0)
High	90–109 (35.5–43.0)	100–120 (39.5–47.0)
Very High	>110 (>43.5)	>120 (47.0)

*See reference 19: From Bray GA. Don't throw the baby out with the bath water. Am J Clin Nutr 2004;70(3):347–349. Adapted with permission by the American Journal of Clinical Nutrition. © Am J Clin Nutr American Society for Clinical Nutrition.

BOX 4-2   Standardized Description of Skinfold Sites and Procedures

SKINFOLD SITE

Abdominal	Vertical fold; 2 cm to the right side of the umbilicus
Triceps	Vertical fold; on the posterior midline of the upper arm, halfway between the acromion and olecranon processes, with the arm held freely to the side of the body
Biceps	Vertical fold; on the anterior aspect of the arm over the belly of the biceps muscle, 1 cm above the level used to mark the triceps site
Chest/Pectoral	Diagonal fold; one-half the distance between the anterior axillary line and the nipple (men), or one-third of the distance between the anterior axillary line and the nipple (women)
Medial Calf	Vertical fold; at the maximum circumference of the calf on the midline of its medial border
Midaxillary	Vertical fold; on the midaxillary line at the level of the xiphoid process of the sternum. An alternate method is a horizontal fold taken at the level of the xiphoid/sternal border in the midaxillary line.
Subscapular	Diagonal fold (at a 45-degree angle); 1 to 2 cm below the inferior angle of the scapula
Suprailiac	Diagonal fold; in line with the natural angle of the iliac crest taken in the anterior axillary line immediately superior to the iliac crest
Thigh	Vertical fold; on the anterior midline of the thigh, midway between the proximal border of the patella and the inguinal crease (hip)

Procedures

- All measurements should be made on the right side of the body with the subject standing upright
- Caliper should be placed directly on the skin surface, 1 cm away from the thumb and finger, perpendicular to the skinfold, and halfway between the crest and the base of the fold
- Pinch should be maintained while reading the caliper
- Wait 1 to 2 seconds (not longer) before reading caliper
- Take duplicate measures at each site and retest if duplicate measurements are not within 1 to 2 mm
- Rotate through measurement sites or allow time for skin to regain normal texture and thickness

extremely lean subject, and an improperly calibrated caliper (tension should be set at ~ 12 g·mm^{-2}).[21] Various regression equations have been developed to predict body density or percent body fat from skinfold measurements. For example, Box 4-3 lists generalized equations that allow calculation of body density without a loss in prediction accuracy for a wide range of individuals.[21,22] However, if a population-specific equation is needed, Heyward and Stolarczyk provide a quick reference guide to match the client to the correct equation based on sex, age, ethnicity, fatness, and sport.[8]

BOX 4-3   Generalized Skinfold Equations*

MEN

- **Seven-Site Formula** (chest, midaxillary, triceps, subscapular, abdomen, suprailiac, thigh)
  Body density = 1.112 − 0.00043499 (sum of seven skinfolds)
  \qquad + 0.00000055 (sum of seven skinfolds)^2
  \qquad − 0.00028826 (age)   *[SEE 0.008 or ~3.5% fat]*
- **Three-Site Formula** (chest, abdomen, thigh)
  Body density = 1.10938 − 0.0008267 (sum of three skinfolds)
  \qquad + 0.0000016 (sum of three skinfolds)^2 − 0.0002574 (age)
  \qquad *[SEE 0.008 or ~3.4% fat]*
- **Three-Site Formula** (chest, triceps, subscapular)
  Body density = 1.1125025 − 0.0013125 (sum of three skinfolds)
  \qquad + 0.0000055 (sum of three skinfolds)^2 − 0.000244 (age)
  \qquad *[SEE 0.008 or ~3.6% fat]*

WOMEN

- **Seven-Site Formula** (chest, midaxillary, triceps, subscapular, abdomen, suprailiac, thigh)
  Body density = 1.097 − 0.00046971 (sum of seven skinfolds)
  \qquad + 0.00000056 (sum of seven skinfolds)^2
  \qquad − 0.00012828 (age)   *[SEE 0.008 or ~3.8% fat]*
- **Three-Site Formula** (triceps, suprailiac, thigh)
  Body density = 1.099421 − 0.0009929 (sum of three skinfolds)
  \qquad + 0.0000023 (sum of three skinfolds)^2 − 0.0001392 (age)
  \qquad *[SEE 0.009 or ~3.9% fat]*
- **Three-Site Formula** (triceps, suprailiac, abdominal)
  Body density = 1.089733 − 0.0009245 (sum of three skinfolds)
  \qquad + 0.0000025 (sum of three skinfolds)^2 − 0.0000979 (age)
  \qquad *[SEE 0.009 or ~3.9% fat]*

*See reference 22: Adapted from Jackson AS, Pollock ML. Practical assessment of body composition. Phys Sport Med 1985;13:76–90; Pollock ML, Schmidt DH, Jackson AS. Measurement of cardiorespiratory fitness and body composition in the clinical setting. Comp Ther 1980;6:12–17.

DENSITOMETRY

Body composition can be estimated from a measurement of whole-body density, using the ratio of body mass to body volume. In this technique, which has been used as a reference or criterion standard for assessing body composition, the body is divided into two components: the fat mass (FM) and the fat-free mass (FFM). The limiting factor in the measurement of body density is the accuracy of the body volume measurement because body mass is measured simply as body weight. Body volume can be measured by hydrodensiometry (underwater) weighing and by plethysmography.

Hydrodensiometry (Underwater) Weighing

This technique of measuring body composition is based on Archimedes' principle, which states that when a body is immersed in water, it is buoyed by a counterforce equal to the weight of the water displaced. This loss of weight in water allows calculation of body volume. Bone and muscle tissue are denser than water, whereas fat tissue is less dense. Therefore, a person with more FFM for the same total body mass weighs more in water and has a higher body density and lower percentage of body fat. Although hydrostatic weighing is a standard method for measuring body volume and hence, body composition, it requires special equipment, the accurate measurement of residual volume, and significant cooperation by the subject.[23] For a more detailed explanation of the technique (see Chapter 12 of *ACSM's Resource Manual for Guidelines for Exercise Testing and Prescription*, 5th ed.).

Plethysmography

Body volume also can be measured by air rather than water displacement. One commercial system uses a dual-chamber plethysmograph that measures body volume by changes in pressure in a closed chamber. This technology shows promise and generally reduces the anxiety associated with the technique of hydrodensiometry.[10,23,24] For a more detailed explanation of the technique, see Chapter 12 of *ACSM's Resource Manual for Guidelines for Exercise Testing and Prescription*, 5th ed.

Conversion of Body Density to Body Composition

Percent body fat can be estimated once body density has been determined. Two of the most common prediction equations used to estimate percent body fat from body density are derived from the two-component model of body composition:[25,26]

$$\% \text{ fat} = \frac{457}{\text{Body Density}} - 414.2$$

$$\% \text{ fat} = \frac{495}{\text{Body Density}} - 450$$

Each method assumes a slightly different density of both fat and fat free mass. Ongoing research, using the three- and four-component models of body compo-

TABLE 4-4. Population-Specific Formulas for Conversion of Body Density (Db) to Percent Body Fat*

Population	Age	Gender	% Body Fat†
Race			
American Indian	18–60	Female	(4.81/Db)–4.34
Black	18–32	Male	(4.37/Db)–3.93
	24–79	Female	(4.85/Db)–4.39
Hispanic	20–40	Female	(4.87/Db)–4.41
Japanese Native	18–48	Male	(4.97/Db)–4.52
		Female	(4.76/Db)–4.28
	61–78	Male	(4.87/Db)–4.41
		Female	(4.95/Db)–4.50
White	7–12	Male	(5.30/Db)–4.89
		Female	(5.35/Db)–4.95
	13–16	Male	(5.07/Db)–4.64
		Female	(5.10/Db)–4.66
	17–19	Male	(4.99/Db)–4.55
		Female	(5.05/Db)–4.62
	20–80	Male	(4.95/Db)–4.50
		Female	(5.01/Db)–4.57
Levels of Body Fatness			
Anorexia	15–30	Female	(5.26/Db)–4.83
Obese	17–62	Male	(5.00/Db)–4.56

*See reference 8: Adapted, with permission, from Heyward VH, Stolarczyk LM. Applied Body Composition Assessment. Champaign, IL: Human Kinetics, 1996;12.

†Percent body fat is obtained by multiplying the value calculated from the equation by 100.

sition provide a variety of new equations that should increase the accuracy of the estimate of percent fat when applied to different populations. These equations (Table 4-4) are likely to improve over time as additional studies are done on larger samples within each population group.[8]

OTHER TECHNIQUES

Additional assessment techniques of dual energy x-ray absorptiometry (DEXA) and total body electrical conductivity (TOBEC) are reliable and accurate measures of body composition, but these techniques are not popular for general health fitness testing because of cost and the need for highly trained personnel.[9] Techniques of bioelectrical impedance analysis (BIA) and near-infrared intercadence are used for general health fitness testing. Generally, the accuracy of BIA is similar to skinfolds, as long as a stringent protocol is followed and the equations programmed into the analyzer are valid and accurate for the populations being tested.[27] Near-infrared intercadence requires additional research to substantiate the validity and accuracy for body composition assessment.[28] Detailed explanations of these techniques are found in Chapter 12 of *ACSM's Resource Manual for Guidelines for Exercise Testing and Prescription*, 5th ed.

BODY COMPOSITION NORMS

There are no universally accepted norms for body composition; however, Tables 4-5 and 4-6, which are based on selected populations, provide percentile values for percent body fat in men and women, respectively. A consensus opinion for an exact percentage body fat value associated with optimal health risk has yet to be defined; however, a range 10% to 22% and 20% to 32% for men and women, respectively, is considered satisfactory for health.[29]

Cardiorespiratory Fitness

Cardiorespiratory fitness is related to the ability to perform large muscle, dynamic, moderate-to-high intensity exercise for prolonged periods. Performance of such exercise depends on the functional state of the respiratory, cardiovascular, and skeletal muscle systems. Cardiorespiratory fitness is considered health-related because: 1) low levels of CR fitness have been associated with a markedly increased risk of premature death from all causes and specifically from cardiovascular disease, 2) increases in CR fitness are associated with a reduction in death from all causes, and 3) high levels of CR fitness are associated with higher levels of habitual physical activity, which in turn are associated with many health benefits.[30–32] The assessment of CR fitness is an important part of a primary or secondary intervention program.

THE CONCEPT OF MAXIMAL OXYGEN UPTAKE

Maximal oxygen uptake ($\dot{V}O_{2max}$) is accepted as the criterion measure of CR fitness. Maximal oxygen uptake is the product of the maximal cardiac output (L blood·min^{-1}) and arterial-venous oxygen difference (mL O_2 per L blood). Significant variation in $\dot{V}O_{2max}$ (L·min^{-1}) across populations and fitness levels results primarily from differences in maximal cardiac output; therefore, $\dot{V}O_{2max}$ is closely related to the functional capacity of the heart.

TABLE 4-5. Body Composition (% Body Fat) for Men*

Percentile	Age				
	20–29	30–39	40–49	50–59	60+
90	7.1	11.3	13.6	15.3	15.3
80	9.4	13.9	16.3	17.9	18.4
70	11.8	15.9	18.1	19.8	20.3
60	14.1	17.5	19.6	21.3	22.0
50	15.9	19.0	21.1	22.7	23.5
40	17.4	20.5	22.5	24.1	25.0
30	19.5	22.3	24.1	25.7	26.7
20	22.4	24.2	26.1	27.5	28.5
10	25.9	27.3	28.9	30.3	31.2

*Data provided by the Institute of Aerobics Research, Dallas, TX (1994). Study population for the data set was predominantly White and college educated. The following may be used as descriptors for the percentile rankings: well above average (90), above average (70), average (50), below average (30), and well below average (10).

TABLE 4-6. Body Composition (% Body Fat) for Women*

Percentile	Age				
	20–29	30–39	40–49	50–59	60+
90	14.5	15.5	18.5	21.6	21.1
80	17.1	18.0	21.3	25.0	25.1
70	19.0	20.0	23.5	26.6	27.5
60	20.6	21.6	24.9	28.5	29.3
50	22.1	23.1	26.4	30.1	30.9
40	23.7	24.9	28.1	31.6	32.5
30	25.4	27.0	30.1	33.5	34.3
20	27.7	29.3	32.1	35.6	36.6
10	32.1	32.8	35.0	37.9	39.3

*Data provided by the Institute for Aerobics Research, Dallas, TX (1994). Study population for the data set was predominantly White and college educated. The following may be used as descriptors for the percentile rankings: well above average (90), above average (70), average (50), below average (30), and well below average (10).

Open-circuit spirometry is used to measure $\dot{V}O_{2max}$. In this procedure, the subject breathes through a low-resistance valve (with nose occluded) while pulmonary ventilation and expired fractions of O_2 and CO_2 are measured. Modern automated systems provide ease of use and a detailed printout of test results that save time and effort.[33] However, attention to detail relative to calibration is still essential to obtain accurate results. Administration of the test and interpretation of results should be reserved for professional personnel with a thorough understanding of exercise science. Because of the costs associated with the equipment, space, and personnel needed to carry out these tests, direct measurement of $\dot{V}O_{2max}$ generally is reserved for research or clinical settings.

When direct measurement of $\dot{V}O_{2max}$ is not feasible or desirable, a variety of submaximal and maximal exercise tests can be used to estimate $\dot{V}O_{2max}$. These tests have been validated by examining: 1) the correlation between directly measured $\dot{V}O_{2max}$ and the $\dot{V}O_{2max}$ estimated from physiologic responses to submaximal exercise (e.g., heart rate at a specified power output); or 2) the correlation between directly measured $\dot{V}O_{2max}$ and test performance (e.g., time to run 1 or 1.5 miles, or time to volitional fatigue using a standard graded exercise test protocol).

MAXIMAL VERSUS SUBMAXIMAL EXERCISE TESTING

The decision to use a maximal or submaximal exercise test depends largely on the reasons for the test and the availability of appropriate equipment and personnel. $\dot{V}O_{2max}$ can be estimated using conventional exercise test protocols, by considering test duration at a given workload on an ergometer and using the prediction equations found in Appendix D. The user would need to consider the population being tested and the standard error of the associated equation. Maximal tests have the disadvantage of requiring participants to exercise to the point of volitional fatigue and might require medical supervision (see Chapter 2) and emergency equipment. However, maximal exercise testing offers increased sensitivity in the diagnosis of coronary artery disease in asymptomatic individuals and provides a better estimate of $\dot{V}O_{2max}$ (see Chapter 5). Additionally, the use of open circuit spirometry during maximal exercise testing allows for the accurate assessment of anaerobic threshold and the measurement of $\dot{V}O_{2max}$.

Practitioners commonly rely on submaximal exercise tests to assess CR fitness because maximal exercise testing is not always feasible in the health and fitness setting. The basic aim of submaximal exercise testing is to determine the heart rate (HR) response to one or more submaximal work rates and use the results to predict $\dot{V}O_{2max}$. Although the primary purpose of the test has traditionally been to predict $\dot{V}O_{2max}$ from the HR-workload relationship, it is important to obtain additional indices of the client's response to exercise. The practitioner should use the various submaximal measures of heart rate, blood pressure, workload, RPE, and other subjective indices as valuable information regarding one's functional response to exercise. This information can be used to evaluate submaximal exercise responses over time in a controlled environment and to fine-tune an exercise prescription.

Estimates of $\dot{V}O_{2max}$ from the HR response to submaximal exercise tests are based on several assumptions:

- A steady-state heart rate is obtained for each exercise work rate and is consistent each day.
- A linear relationship exists between heart rate and work rate.
- The maximal work load is indicative of the maximal $\dot{V}O_2$.
- The maximal heart rate for a given age is uniform.
- Mechanical efficiency (i.e., $\dot{V}O_2$ at a given work rate) is the same for everyone.
- The subject is not on medications that alter heart rate.

Note: The most accurate estimate of $\dot{V}O_{2max}$ is achieved if all of the preceding assumptions are met.

MODES OF TESTING

Commonly used modes for exercise testing include field tests, treadmill tests, cycle ergometry tests, and step tests. Medical supervision may be required for moderate or high-risk individuals for each of these modes. Refer to Table 2-1 for exercise testing and supervision guidelines. There are advantages and disadvantages of each mode:

- *Field tests* consist of walking or running a certain distance in a given time (i.e., 12-minute and 1.5-mile run tests, and the 1- and 6-minute walk test). The advantages of field tests are that they are easy to administer to large numbers of individuals at one time and little equipment (e.g., a stopwatch) is needed. The disadvantages are that they all potentially could be maximal tests, and by their nature, are unmonitored for blood pressure and heart rate. An individual's level of motivation and pacing ability also can have a profound impact on test results. These all-out run tests may be inappropriate for sedentary individuals or individuals at increased risk for cardiovascular and musculoskeletal complications. However, $\dot{V}O_{2max}$ can be estimated from test results.
- *Motor driven treadmills* can be used for submaximal and maximal testing and often are used for diagnostic testing. They provide a common form of

exercise (i.e., walking) and can accommodate the least fit to the fittest individuals across the continuum of walking to running speeds. Nevertheless, a practice session might be necessary in some cases to permit habituation and reduce anxiety. On the other hand, treadmills usually are expensive, not easily transportable, and make some measurements (e.g., blood pressure) more difficult. Treadmills must be calibrated to ensure the accuracy of the test. In addition, holding on to the support rail should not be permitted to ensure accuracy of the metabolic work.

- **Mechanically braked cycle ergometers** are excellent test modalities for submaximal and maximal testing. They are relatively inexpensive, easily transportable, and allow blood pressure and the electrocardiogram (if appropriate) to be measured easily. The main disadvantage is that cycling is a less familiar mode of exercise for many Americans, often resulting in limiting localized muscle fatigue. Cycle ergometers provide a non–weight-bearing test modality in which work rates are easily adjusted in small work-rate increments, and subjects tend to be least anxious using this device. The cycle ergometer must be calibrated and the subject must maintain the proper pedal rate because most tests require that heart rate be measured at specific work rates. Electronic cycle ergometers can deliver the same work rate across a range of pedal rates, but calibration might require special equipment not available in most laboratories. Some electronic fitness cycles cannot be calibrated and should not be used for testing.

- **Step testing** is an inexpensive modality for predicting CR fitness by measuring the heart rate response to stepping at a fixed rate and/or a fixed step height or by measuring postexercise recovery heart rates. Step tests require little or no equipment; steps are easily transportable; stepping skill requires little practice; the test usually is of short duration; and stepping is advantageous for mass testing.[34] Postexercise (recovery) heart rates decrease with improved CR fitness and test results are easy to explain to participants.[35] Special precautions might be needed for those who have balance problems or are extremely deconditioned. Some single stage step tests require an energy cost of 7 to 9 metabolic equivalents (METs), which may exceed the maximal capacity of the participant.[36] The workload must be appropriate to the fitness level of the client. In addition, inadequate compliance to the step cadence and excessive fatigue in the lead limb may diminish the value of a step test. Most tests are unmonitored because of the difficulty of measuring heart rate and blood pressure during a step test.

Field Tests

Two of the most widely used running tests for assessing CR fitness are the Cooper 12-minute test and the 1.5-mile test for time. The objective in the 12-minute test is to cover the greatest distance in the allotted time period, and for the 1.5-mile test it is to run the distance in the shortest period of time. $\dot{V}O_{2max}$ can be estimated from the equations in Appendix D.

The Rockport One-Mile Fitness Walking Test has gained wide popularity as an effective means for estimating CR fitness. In this test, an individual walks 1 mile as fast as possible, preferably on a track or a level surface, and heart rate is obtained in the final minute. An alternative is to measure a 10-second heart rate immediately on completion of the 1-mile walk, but this may overestimate the $\dot{V}O_{2max}$ compared to when heart rate is measured during the walk. $\dot{V}O_{2max}$ is estimated from a regression equation (found in Appendix D) based on weight, age, sex, walk time, and heart rate.[37] In addition to independently predicting morbidity and mortality[38] the 6-minute walk test has been used to evaluate CR fitness within some clinical patient populations (e.g., persons with congestive heart failure or pulmonary disease). Even though the test is considered submaximal, it may result in near maximal performance for those with low fitness levels or disease. Several multivariate equations are available to predict peak oxygen consumption from the 6-minute walk; however, the following equation requires minimal clinical information:[39]

- Peak $\dot{V}O_2$ = VO_2 mL·kg^{-1}·min^{-1}= [0.02 × distance (m)] − [0.191 × age (yr)] − [0.07 × weight (kg)] + [0.09 × height (cm)] + [0.26 × RPP (× 10^{-3})] + 2.45
  - m = distance in meters; yr = year; kg = kilogram; cm = centimeter; RPP = rate pressure product (HR × systolic blood pressure in mm Hg)
- R^2 = 0.65 SEE = 2.68

Patients completing less than 300 meters during the 6-minute walk, demonstrate a limited short-term survival.[39]

Submaximal Exercise Tests

Both single-stage and multistage submaximal exercise tests are available to estimate $\dot{V}O_{2max}$ from simple heart rate measurements. Accurate measurement of heart rate is critical for valid testing. Although heart rate obtained by palpation is used commonly, the accuracy of this method depends on the experience and technique of the evaluator. It is recommended that an electrocardiograph, heart rate monitor, or a stethoscope be used to determine heart rate. The use of a relatively inexpensive heart rate monitor can reduce a significant source of error in the test. The submaximal heart rate response is easily altered by a number of environmental (e.g., heat and/or humidity, see Appendix E), dietary (e.g., caffeine, time since last meal), and behavioral (e.g., anxiety, smoking, previous activity) factors. These variables must be controlled to have a valid estimate that can be used as a reference point in a person's fitness program. In addition, the test mode (e.g., cycle, treadmill, or step) should be consistent with the primary activity used by the participant to address specificity of training issues. Standardized procedures for submaximal testing are presented in Box 4-4. Although there are no specific submaximal protocols for treadmill testing, several stages from any of the treadmill protocols found in Chapter 5 can be used to assess submaximal exercise responses. Preexercise test instructions were presented in Chapter 3.

Cycle Ergometer Tests

The Astrand-Rhyming cycle ergometer test is a single-stage test lasting 6 minutes.[40] For the population studied, these researchers observed that at 50% of $\dot{V}O_{2max}$, the average heart rate was 128 and 138 beats·min^{-1} for men and women, respectively. If a woman was working at a $\dot{V}O_2$ of 1.5 L·min^{-1} and her HR was

BOX 4-4	**General Procedures for Submaximal Testing of Cardiorespiratory Fitness**

1. Obtain resting HR and BP immediately prior to exercise in the exercise posture.
2. The client should be familiarized with the ergometer. If using a cycle ergometer properly position the client on the ergometer (i.e., upright posture, 5-degree bend in the knee at maximal leg extension, hands in proper position on handlebars).
3. The exercise test should begin with a 2- to 3-min warm-up to acquaint the client with the cycle ergometer and prepare him or her for the exercise intensity in the first stage of the test.
4. A specific protocol should consist of 2- or 3-minute stages with appropriate increments in work rate.
5. Heart rate should be monitored at least two times during each stage, near the end of the second and third minutes of each stage. If heart rate >110 beats·min^{-1}, steady-state heart rate (i.e., two heart rates within 5 beats·min^{-1}) should be reached before the workload is increased.
6. Blood pressure should be monitored in the last minute of each stage and repeated (verified) in the event of a hypotensive or hypertensive response.
7. Perceived exertion and additional rating scales should be monitored near the end of the last minute of each stage using either the 6–20 or 0–10 scale (see Table 4-8).
8. Client appearance and symptoms should be monitored and recorded regularly.
9. The test should be terminated when the subject reaches 70% heart rate reserve (85% of age-predicted maximal heart rate), fails to conform to the exercise test protocol, experiences adverse signs or symptoms, requests to stop, or experiences an emergency situation.
10. An appropriate cool-down/recovery period should be initiated consisting of either:
    a. continued exercise at a work rate equivalent to that of the first stage of the exercise test protocol or lower; or,
    b. a passive cool-down if the subject experiences signs of discomfort or an emergency situation occurs
11. All physiologic observations (e.g., heart rate, blood pressure, signs and symptoms) should be continued for at least 5 minutes of recovery unless abnormal responses occur, which would warrant a longer posttest surveillance period. Continue low-level exercise until HR and blood pressure stabilize, but not necessarily until they reach preexercise levels.

138 beats·min^{-1}, then her $\dot{V}O_{2max}$ was estimated to be 3.0 L·min^{-1}. The suggested work rate is based on sex and an individual's fitness status as follows:

men, unconditioned:	300 or 600 kg·m·min^{-1} (50 or 100 watts)
men, conditioned:	600 or 900 kg·m·min^{-1} (100 or 150 watts)
women, unconditioned:	300 or 450 kg·m·min^{-1} (50 or 75 watts)
women, conditioned:	450 or 600 kg·m·min^{-1} (75 or 100 watts)

The pedal rate is set at 50 rpm. The goal is to obtain HR values between 125 and 170 beats·min^{-1}, and HR is measured during the fifth and sixth minute of work. The average of the two heart rates is then used to estimate $\dot{V}O_{2max}$ from a nomogram (Fig. 4-1). This value must then be adjusted for age (because maximal HR decreases with age) by multiplying the $\dot{V}O_{2max}$ value by the following correction factors:[36]

Age	Correction Factor
15	1.10
25	1.00
35	0.87
40	0.83
45	0.78
50	0.75
55	0.71
60	0.68
65	0.65

In contrast to the single-stage test, Maritz et al.[41] measured HR at a series of submaximal work rates and extrapolated the response to the subject's age-predicted maximal heart rate. This has become one of the most popular assessment techniques to estimate $\dot{V}O_{2max}$, and the YMCA test is a good example.[42] The YMCA protocol uses two to four, 3-minute stages of continuous exercise (Fig. 4-2). The test is designed to raise the steady-state HR of the subject to between 110 beats·min^{-1} and 70% HRR (85% of the age-predicted maximal HR) for at least two consecutive stages. It is important to remember that two consecutive HR measurements must be obtained within this HR range to predict $\dot{V}O_{2max}$. In the YMCA protocol, each work rate is performed for at least 3 minutes, and heart rates are recorded during the final 15 to 30 seconds of the second and third minutes. If these two heart rates vary by more than 5 beats·min^{-1}, the work rate should be maintained for an additional minute. The test administrator should recognize the error associated with age-predicted maximal HR and monitor the subject throughout the test to ensure the test remains submaximal. The heart rate measured during the last minute of each steady-state stage is plotted against work rate. The line generated from the plotted points is then extrapolated to the age-predicted maximal heart rate (e.g., 220–age), and a perpendicular line is dropped to the x-axis to estimate the work rate that would have been achieved if the person had worked to maximum (Fig. 4-3). $\dot{V}O_{2max}$ can be estimated from the work rate using the formula in Appendix D. These equations are valid to estimate oxygen consumption at submaximal steady state workloads from 300 to 1,200 kg·m·min^{-1}, therefore caution must be used if extrapolating to workloads outside of this range. The two lines noted as ±1 SD in Figure 4-3 show what the estimated $\dot{V}O_{2max}$ would be if the

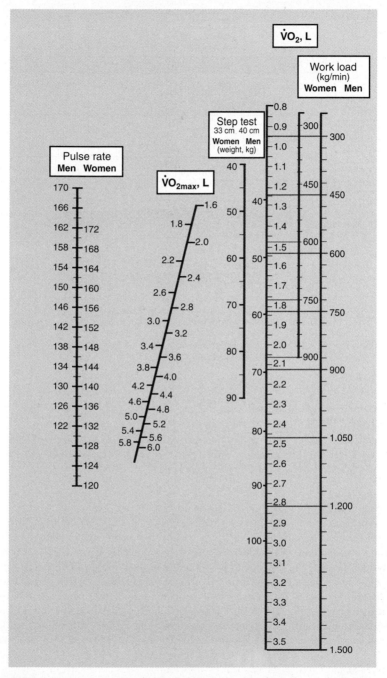

FIGURE 4-1. Modified Astrand-Ryhming nomogram. (Reprinted with permission from Astrand P-O, Ryhming I. A nomogram for calculation of aerobic capacity [physical fitness] from pulse rate during submaximal work. J Appl Physiol 1954;7:218–221.)

	1st stage	150 kgm/min (0.5 kg)		
	HR<80	HR: 80-90	HR: 90-100	HR>100
2nd stage	750 kgm/min (2.5 kg)*	600 kgm/min (2.0 kg)	450 kgm/min (1.5 kg)	300 kgm/min (1.0 kg)
3rd stage	900 kgm/min (3.0 kg)	750 kgm/min (2.5 kg)	600 kgm/min (2.0 kg)	450 kgm/min (1.5 kg)
4th stage	1050 kgm/min (3.5 kg)	900 kgm/min (3.0 kg)	750 kgm/min (2.5 kg)	600 kgm/min (2.0 kg)

Directions:
1 Set the 1st work rate at 150 kgm/min (0.5 kg at 50 rpm)
2 If the HR in the third minute of the stage is:
   <80, set the 2nd stage at 750 kgm/min (2.5 kg at 50 rpm)
   80-89, set the 2nd stage at 600 kgm/min (2.0 kg at 50 rpm)
   90-100, set the 2nd stage at 450 kgm/min (1.5 kg at 50 rpm)
   >100, set the 2nd stage at 300 kgm/min (1.0 kg at 50 rpm)
3 Set the 3rd and 4th (if required) according to the work rates in the columns below the 2nd loads

FIGURE 4-2. YMCA cycle ergometry protocol. Resistance settings shown here are appropriate for an ergometer with a flywheel of 6 m·rev^{-1}.

subject's true maximal HR were 168 or 192 beats·min^{-1}, rather than 180 beats·min^{-1}. Part of the error involved in estimating $\dot{V}O_{2max}$ from submaximal HR responses occurs because the formula (220 − age) can provide only an estimate of maximal HR. In addition, errors can be attributed to inaccurate pedaling cadence (workload) and imprecise steady-state heart rates.

Treadmill Tests

The primary exercise modality for submaximal exercise testing traditionally has been the cycle ergometer, although treadmills have been used in many settings. The same endpoint (70% HRR or 85% of age-predicted maximal HR) is used, and the stages of the test should be 3 minutes or longer to ensure a steady-state HR response at each stage. The HR values are extrapolated to age-predicted maximal HR, and $\dot{V}O_{2max}$ is estimated using the formula in Appendix D from the highest speed and/or grade that would have been achieved if the person had worked to maximum. Most common treadmill protocols (see Chapter 5) can be used, but the duration of each stage should be at least 3 minutes.

Step Tests

Step tests have also been used to estimate $\dot{V}O_{2max}$. Astrand and Ryhming[36] used a single-step height of 33 cm for women and 40 cm for men at a rate of

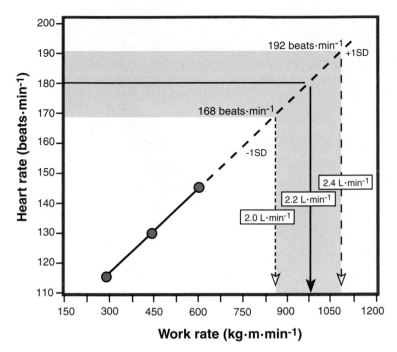

FIGURE 4-3. Heart rate responses to three submaximal work rates for a 40-year old, sedentary woman weighing 64 kg. $\dot{V}O_{2max}$ was estimated by extrapolating the heart rate (HR) response to the age-predicted maximal HR of 180 beats·min^{-1} (based on 220–age). The work rate that would have been achieved at that HR was determined by dropping a line from that HR value to the x-axis. $\dot{V}O_{2max}$, estimated using the formula in Appendix D and expressed in L·min^{-1}, was 2.2 L·min^{-1}. The other two lines estimate what the $\dot{V}O_{2max}$ would have been if the subject's true maximal HR was ±1 SD from the 180 beats·min^{-1} value.

22.5 steps·min^{-1}. These tests require oxygen uptakes of about 25.8 and 29.5 mL·kg^{-1}·min^{-1}, respectively. Heart rate is measured as described for the cycle test, and $\dot{V}O_{2max}$ is estimated from the nomogram (see Fig. 4-1). In contrast, Maritz et al.[41] used a single-step height (30.5 cm) and four-step rates to systematically increase the work rate. A steady-state HR was measured for each step rate and a line formed from these HR values was extrapolated to age-predicted maximal HR; the maximal work rate was determined as described for the YMCA cycle test. $\dot{V}O_{2max}$ can be estimated from the formula for stepping in Appendix D. Such step tests should be modified to suit the population being tested. The Canadian Home Fitness Test has demonstrated that such testing can be performed on a large scale and at low cost.[35–37,40–43]

Instead of estimating VO$_{2max}$ from HR responses to several submaximal work rates, a wide variety of step tests have been developed to categorize cardiovascular fitness on the basis of a person's recovery HR following a standardized step test. The 3-Minute YMCA Step Test is a good example of such a test. This test uses a 12-inch (30.5-cm) bench, with a stepping rate of 24 steps·min^{-1} (estimated oxygen cost of 25.8 mL·kg^{-1}·min^{-1}). After exercise is completed, the subject immediately sits down and heart rate is counted for 1 minute. Counting must start within 5 seconds of the end of exercise. Heart rate values are used to obtain a qualitative rating of fitness from published normative tables.[42]

CARDIORESPIRATORY TEST SEQUENCE AND MEASURES

A minimum of heart rate, blood pressure, and rating of perceived exertion (RPE) should be measured during exercise tests. After the initial screening process, selected baseline measurements should be obtained prior to the start of the exercise test. Taking a resting ECG prior to exercise testing assumes that trained personnel are available to interpret the ECG and provide medical guidance. An ECG is not necessary when diagnostic testing is not being done, and when apparently healthy individuals are being tested with submaximal tests. The sequence of measures is listed in Box 4-4.

Heart rate can be determined using several techniques, including radial or carotid pulse palpation, auscultation with a stethoscope, or the use of heart rate monitors. The pulse palpation technique involves "feeling" the pulse by placing the first and second fingers over an artery (usually the radial artery located near the thumb side of the wrist or the carotid artery located in the neck near the larynx). The pulse is typically counted for 15 seconds, and then multiplied by 4, to determine the per-minute HR. Although the carotid pulse might be easier to obtain, one should not press too hard with the palpating fingers because this could produce a marked bradycardia in the presence of a hypersensitive carotid sinus reflex. For the auscultation method, the bell of the stethoscope should be placed to the left of the sternum just above the level of the nipple. This method is most accurate when the heart sounds are clearly audible and the subject's torso is relatively stable. Heart rate telemetry monitors ("heart rate watches") with chest electrodes have proved to be accurate and reliable, provided there is no outside electrical interference (e.g., emissions from the display consoles of computerized exercise equipment).[44] Many electronic cycles and treadmills have embedded this HR technology into the equipment.

Blood pressure should be measured at heart level with the subject's arm relaxed and not grasping a handrail (treadmill) or handlebar (cycle ergometer). To help ensure accurate readings, the use of an appropriate-sized blood pressure cuff is important. The rubber bladder of the blood pressure cuff should encircle at least 80% of the subject's upper arm. If the subject's arm is large, a normal-size adult cuff will be too small, thus resulting in an erroneous elevated reading (the converse is also true). Blood pressure measurements should be taken with a mercury sphygmomanometer adjusted to eye level or a recently calibrated aneroid manometer. Systolic and diastolic blood pressure measurements can be used as indicators for stopping an exercise test (see next section). To obtain accurate blood pressure measures during exercise, follow the guidelines in Chapter 3 (Box 3-4) for resting blood pressure; however, obtain blood pressure in the exercise position. In addition, if the fourth Korotkoff sound can not be discerned, the fifth

Korotkoff sound should be obtained. During exercise, it is advisable to obtain the first, fourth, and fifth Korotkoff sounds.

RPE can be a valuable indicator for monitoring an individual's exercise tolerance. Although, perceived exertion ratings correlate with exercise heart rates and work rates, large interindividual variability in RPE with both healthy as well as cardiac patients mandates caution in the universal application of the scales.[45] Borg's RPE scale was developed to allow the exerciser to subjectively rate his or her feelings during exercise, taking into account personal fitness level, environmental conditions, and general fatigue levels.[46] Ratings can be influenced by psychological factors, mood states, environmental conditions, exercise modes, and age, which reduce its utility.[47] Currently, two RPE scales are widely used: the original or category scale, which rates exercise intensity on a scale of 6 to 20, and the revised or category-ratio scale of 0 to 10. Both RPE scales are shown in Table 4-7. Either scale is appropriate as a subjective tool.

During exercise testing, the RPE can be used as an indication of impending fatigue. Most apparently healthy subjects reach their subjective limit of fatigue at an RPE of 18 to 19 (very, very hard) on the category Borg scale or 9 to 10 (very, very strong) on the category-ratio scale; therefore, RPE can be used to monitor progress toward maximal exertion during exercise testing. It is important to

TABLE 4-7. Category and Category-Ratio Scales for Ratings of Perceived Exertion*

Category Scale	Category-Ratio Scale†		
6	0	Nothing at all	"No I"
7 Very, very light	0.3		
8	0.5	Extremely weak	Just noticeable
9 Very light	0.7		
10	1	Very weak	
11 Fairly light	1.5		
12	2	Weak	Light
13 Somewhat hard	2.5		
14	3	Moderate	
15 Hard	4		
16	5	Strong	Heavy
17 Very Hard	6		
18	7	Very strong	
19 Very, very hard	8		
20	9		
	10	Extremely strong	"Strongest I"
	11		
	•	Absolute maximum	Highest possible

*Copyright Gunnar Borg. Reproduced with permission. For correct usage of the Borg scales, it is necessary to follow the administration and instructions given in Borg G. Borg's Perceived Exertion and Pain Scales. Champaign, IL: Human Kinetics, 1998.

†Note: ON the Category-Ratio Scale, "I" represents intensity.

use standardized instructions to reduce problems of misinterpretation of RPE. The following are recommended instructions for using the RPE scale during exercise testing:[48]

> *During the exercise test we want you to pay close attention to how hard you feel the exercise work rate is. This feeling should reflect your total amount of exertion and fatigue, combining all sensations and feelings of physical stress, effort, and fatigue. Don't concern yourself with any one factor such as leg pain, shortness of breath or exercise intensity, but try to concentrate on your total, inner feeling of exertion. Try not to underestimate or overestimate your feelings of exertion; be as accurate as you can.*

TEST TERMINATION CRITERIA

Graded exercise testing, whether maximal or submaximal, is a safe procedure when subject screening and testing guidelines (see Chapter 2) are adhered to. Occasionally, for safety reasons, the test may have to be terminated prior to the subject reaching a measured $\dot{V}O_{2max}$, volitional fatigue, or a predetermined endpoint (i.e., 50% to 70% HRR or 70% to 85% age-predicted maximal HR). Because of the individual variation in maximal heart rate, the upper limit of 85% of an estimated maximal heart rate may result in a maximal effort for some individuals. General indications—those that do not rely on physician involvement or ECG monitoring—for stopping an exercise test are outlined in Box 4-5. More specific termination criteria for clinical or diagnostic testing are provided in Chapter 5.

BOX 4-5	**General Indications for Stopping an Exercise Test in Low-Risk Adults***

- Onset of angina or angina-like symptoms
- Drop in systolic blood pressure of >10 mm Hg from baseline blood pressure despite an increase in workload
- Excessive rise in blood pressure: systolic pressure >250 mm Hg or diastolic pressure >115 mm Hg
- Shortness of breath, wheezing, leg cramps, or claudication
- Signs of poor perfusion: light-headedness, confusion, ataxia, pallor, cyanosis, nausea, or cold and clammy skin
- Failure of heart rate to increase with increased exercise intensity
- Noticeable change in heart rhythm
- Subject requests to stop
- Physical or verbal manifestations of severe fatigue
- Failure of the testing equipment

*Assumes that testing is nondiagnostic and is being performed without direct physician involvement or ECG monitoring. For clinical testing, Box 5-2 provides more definitive and specific termination criteria.

INTERPRETATION OF RESULTS

Table 4-8 provides normative values for $\dot{V}O_{2max}$ ($mL \cdot kg^{-1} \cdot min^{-1}$), with specific reference to age and sex. Research suggests that a $\dot{V}O_{2max}$ below the 20th percentile for age and sex, which is often indicative of a sedentary lifestyle, is associated with an increased risk of death from all causes.[30] In a comparison of the fitness status of

TABLE 4-8. Percentile Values for Maximal Aerobic Power ($mL \cdot kg^{-1} \cdot min^{-1}$)*

Percentile values for maximal oxygen uptake ($mL \cdot kg^{-1} \cdot min^{-1}$) in men.

Percentile	Age (yr)				
	20–29 (N = 2,234)	30–39 (N = 11,158)	40–49 (N = 13,109)	50–59 (N = 5,641)	60+ (N = 1,244)
90	55.1	52.1	50.6	49.0	44.2
80	52.1	50.6	49.0	44.2	41.0
70	49.0	47.4	45.8	41.0	37.8
60	47.4	44.2	44.2	39.4	36.2
50	44.2	42.6	41.0	37.8	34.6
40	42.6	41.0	39.4	36.2	33.0
30	41.0	39.4	36.2	34.6	31.4
20	37.8	36.2	34.6	31.4	28.3
10	34.6	33.0	31.4	29.9	26.7

*Data were obtained from the initial examination of apparently healthy men enrolled in the Aerobics Center Longitudinal Study (ACLS), 1970 to 2002. The study population for the data set was predominantly White and college educated. Maximal treadmill exercise tests were administered using a modified Balke protocol. Maximal oxygen uptake was estimated from the final treadmill speed and grade using the current ACSM equations found in this edition of the *Guidelines*. The data are provided courtesy of the ACLS investigators, The Cooper Institute, Dallas, TX. The ACLS is supported in part by a grant from the National Institute on Aging (AG06945), SN Blair, Principal Investigator. The following may be used as descriptors for the percentile rankings: well above average (90), above average (70), average (50), below average (30), and well below average (10).

Percentile values for maximal oxygen uptake ($mL \cdot kg^{-1} \cdot min^{-1}$) in women.

Percentile	Age (yr)				
	20–29 (N = 1,223)	30–39 (N = 3,895)	40–49 (N = 4,001)	50–59 (N = 2,032)	60+ (N = 465)
90	49.0	45.8	42.6	37.8	34.6
80	44.2	41.0	39.4	34.6	33.0
70	41.0	39.4	36.2	33.0	31.4
60	39.4	36.2	34.6	31.4	28.3
50	37.8	34.6	33.0	29.9	26.7
40	36.2	33.0	31.4	28.3	25.1
30	33.0	31.4	29.9	26.7	23.5
20	31.4	29.9	28.3	25.1	21.9
10	28.3	26.7	25.1	21.9	20.3

*Data were obtained from the initial examination of apparently healthy women enrolled in the Aerobics Center Longitudinal Study (ACLS), 1970 to 2002. The study population for the data set was predominantly White and college educated. Maximal treadmill exercise tests were administered using a modified Balke protocol. Maximal oxygen uptake was estimated from the final treadmill speed and grade using the current ACSM equations found in this edition of the *Guidelines*. The data are provided courtesy of the ACLS investigators, The Cooper Institute, Dallas, TX. The ACLS is supported in part by a grant from the National Institute on Aging (AG06945), SN Blair, Principal Investigator. The following may be used as descriptors for the percentile rankings: well above average (90), above average (70), average (50), below average (30), and well below average (10).

any one individual to published norms, the accuracy of the classification is dependent on the similarities between the populations and methodology (estimated vs measured $\dot{V}O_{2max}$, maximal versus submaximal, etc.). Although submaximal exercise testing is not as precise as maximal exercise testing, it provides a reasonably accurate reflection of an individual's fitness at a lower cost and reduced risk, and requires less time and effort on the part of the subject.

Some of the assumptions inherent in a submaximal test are more easily met (e.g., steady-state heart rate can be verified), whereas others (e.g., estimated maximal heart rate) introduce unknown errors into the prediction of $\dot{V}O_{2max}$. When an individual is given repeated submaximal exercise tests over a period of weeks or months and the heart rate response to a fixed work rate decreases over time, it is likely that the individual's CR fitness has improved, independent of the accuracy of the $\dot{V}O_{2max}$ prediction. Despite differences in test accuracy and methodology, virtually all evaluations can establish a baseline and be used to track relative progress.

Muscular Strength and Muscular Endurance

Muscular strength and endurance are health-related fitness components that may improve or maintain the following:

- Bone mass, which is related to osteoporosis
- Glucose tolerance, which is related to type 2 diabetes
- Musculotendinous integrity, which is related to a lower risk of injury, including low-back pain
- The ability to carry out the activities of daily living, which is related to self-esteem
- The fat-free mass and resting metabolic rate, which are related to weight management

The ACSM has melded the terms muscular strength and muscular endurance into a category termed "muscular fitness" and included it as an integral portion of total health-related fitness in a position stand on the quantity and quality of exercise to achieve and maintain fitness.[49] Muscular strength refers to *the ability of the muscle to exert force*.[1] Muscular endurance is *the muscle's ability to continue to perform for successive exertions or many repetitions*.[1] Traditionally, tests allowing few (<3) repetitions of a task prior to reaching momentary muscular fatigue have been considered strength measures, whereas those in which numerous repetitions (>12) are performed prior to momentary muscular fatigue were considered measures of muscular endurance. However, the performance of a maximal repetition range (i.e., 4, 6, 8) also can be used to assess strength.

Muscle function tests are very specific to the muscle group tested, the type of contraction, the velocity of muscle movement, the type of equipment, and the joint range of motion. Results of any one test are specific to the procedures used, and no single test exists for evaluating total body muscular endurance or muscular strength. Unfortunately, few muscle endurance or strength tests control for repetition duration (speed of movement) or range of motion, thus results are difficult to interpret. Individuals should participate in familiarization/practice sessions with the equipment, and adhere to a specific protocol (including a predetermined repetition duration and range of motion) in order to obtain a reliable score that can be used to track true physiologic adaptations over time. The standardized conditions or protocol should include:

- Strict posture
- Consistent repetition duration (movement speed)
- Full range of motion
- Use of spotters (when necessary)
- Equipment familiarization
- Proper warm-up

A change in one's muscular fitness over time can be based on the absolute value of the external load or resistance (e.g., newtons, kilograms [kg], or pounds [lb]), but when comparisons are made between individuals, the values should be expressed as relative values (per kilogram of body weight [kg/kg]). In both cases, caution must be used in the interpretation of the scores because the norms may not include a representative sample of the individual being measured, a standardized protocol may be absent, or the exact test being used (free weight versus machine weight) may differ.

MUSCULAR STRENGTH

Although muscular strength refers to the external force (properly expressed in newtons, although kilograms and pounds are commonly used as well) that can be generated by a specific muscle or muscle group, it is commonly expressed in terms of resistance lifted. Strength can be assessed either statically (no overt muscular movement or limb movement) or dynamically (movement of an external load or body part, in which the muscle changes length). Static or isometric strength can be measured conveniently using a variety of devices, including cable tensiometers and handgrip dynamometers. Unfortunately, measures of static strength are specific to both the muscle group and joint angle involved in testing; therefore, their utility in describing overall muscular strength is limited. Peak force development in such tests is commonly referred to as the maximum voluntary contraction (MVC).

Traditionally, the 1-repetition maximum (1-RM), the greatest resistance that can be moved through the full range of motion in a controlled manner with good posture, has been the standard for dynamic strength assessment. However, a multiple RM can be used, such as 4- or 8-RM, as a measure of muscular strength, which may allow the participant to integrate evaluation into their training program. For example, if one were training with 6 to 8 RM, the performance of a 6 RM to momentary muscular fatigue would provide an index of strength changes over time, independent of the true 1-RM. Estimating a 1-RM from such tests is problematic, and generally not necessary. The number of lifts one can perform at a fixed percent of a 1-RM for different muscle groups (e.g., leg press versus bench press) varies tremendously, thus rendering an estimate of 1-RM impractical.[50,51] However, the true 1-RM is still a popular measure.[52] Valid measures of general upper body strength include the 1-RM values for bench press or military press. Corresponding indices of lower body strength include 1-RM values for leg press or leg extension. Norms, based on resistance lifted divided by body mass for the bench press and leg press are provided in Tables 4-9 and 4-10, respectively. The following represents the basic steps in 1-RM (or any multiple RM) testing following familiarization/practice sessions:[52]

1. The subject should warm-up by completing a number of submaximal repetitions.
2. Determine the 1 RM (or any multiple RM) within four trials with rest periods of 3 to 5 minutes between trials.
3. Select an initial weight that is within the subject's perceived capacity (~50%–70% of capacity).
4. Resistance is progressively increased by 2.5 to 20 kg until the subject cannot complete the selected repetition(s). All repetitions should be performed at the same speed of movement and range of motion to instill consistency between trials.
5. The final weight lifted successfully is recorded as the absolute 1-R or multiple RM.

Isokinetic testing involves the assessment of maximal muscle tension throughout a range of joint motion set at a constant angular velocity (e.g., 60 angles per

TABLE 4-9. Upper Body Strength*†

	Age				
Percentile	20–29	30–39	40–49	50–59	60+
Men					
90	1.48	1.24	1.10	0.97	0.89
80	1.32	1.12	1.00	0.90	0.82
70	1.22	1.04	0.93	0.84	0.77
60	1.14	0.98	0.88	0.79	0.72
50	1.06	0.93	0.84	0.75	0.68
40	0.99	0.88	0.80	0.71	0.66
30	0.93	0.83	0.76	0.68	0.63
20	0.88	0.78	0.72	0.63	0.57
10	0.80	0.71	0.65	0.57	0.53
Women					
90	0.90	0.76	0.71	0.61	0.64
80	0.80	0.70	0.62	0.55	0.54
70	0.74	0.63	0.57	0.52	0.51
60	0.70	0.60	0.54	0.48	0.47
50	0.65	0.57	0.52	0.46	0.45
40	0.59	0.53	0.50	0.44	0.43
30	0.56	0.51	0.47	0.42	0.40
20	0.51	0.47	0.43	0.39	0.38
10	0.48	0.42	0.38	0.37	0.33

*One repetition maximum bench press, with bench press weight ratio = weight pushed/body weight.

†Adapted from Institute for Aerobics Research, Dallas, 1994. Study population for the data set was predominantly White and college educated. A Universal DVR machine was used to measure the 1-RM. The following may be used as descriptors for the percentile rankings: well above average (90), above average (70), average (50), below average (30), and well below average (10).

TABLE 4-10. Leg Strength* †

Percentile	Age 20–29	30–39	40–49	50–59	60+
Men					
90	2.27	2.07	1.92	1.80	1.73
80	2.13	1.93	1.82	1.71	1.62
70	2.05	1.85	1.74	1.64	1.56
60	1.97	1.77	1.68	1.58	1.49
50	1.91	1.71	1.62	1.52	1.43
40	1.83	1.65	1.57	1.46	1.38
30	1.74	1.59	1.51	1.39	1.30
20	1.63	1.52	1.44	1.32	1.25
10	1.51	1.43	1.35	1.22	1.16
Women					
90	1.82	1.61	1.48	1.37	1.32
80	1.68	1.47	1.37	1.25	1.18
70	1.58	1.39	1.29	1.17	1.13
60	1.50	1.33	1.23	1.10	1.04
50	1.44	1.27	1.18	1.05	0.99
40	1.37	1.21	1.13	0.99	0.93
30	1.27	1.15	1.08	0.95	0.88
20	1.22	1.09	1.02	0.88	0.85
10	1.14	1.00	0.94	0.78	0.72

*One repetition maximum leg press with leg press weight ratio = weight pushed/body weight.

†Adapted from Institute for Aerobics Research, Dallas, 1994. Study population for the data set was predominantly White and college educated. A Universal DVR machine was used to measure the 1-RM. The following may be used as descriptors for the percentile rankings: well above average (90), above average (70), average (50), below average (30), and well below average (10).

second). Equipment that allows control of the speed of joint rotation (degrees/sec) as well as the ability to test movement around various joints (e.g., knee, hip, shoulder, elbow) is available from commercial sources. Such devices measure peak rotational force or torque, but an important drawback is that this equipment is extremely expensive compared to other strength-testing modalities.[53]

MUSCULAR ENDURANCE

Muscular endurance is the ability of a muscle group to execute repeated contractions over a period of time sufficient to cause muscular fatigue, or to maintain a specific percentage of the maximum voluntary contraction for a prolonged period of time. If the total number of repetitions at a given amount of resistance is measured, the result is termed absolute muscular endurance. If the number of repetitions performed at a percentage of the 1-RM (e.g., 70%) is used both pre- and posttesting, the result is termed relative muscular endurance. Simple field tests such as a curl-up (crunch) test[53,54] or the maximum number of push-ups that can be performed without rest[54] may be used to evaluate the endurance of the abdominal muscle groups and upper body muscles, respectively. Although

BOX 4-6	Push-up and Curl-up (Crunch) Test Procedures for Measurement of Muscular Endurance

PUSH-UP

1. The push-up test is administered with male subjects starting in the standard "down" position (hands pointing forward and under the shoulder, back straight, head up, using the toes as the pivotal point) and female subjects in the modified "knee push-up" position (legs together, lower leg in contact with mat with ankles plantar-flexed, back straight, hands shoulder width apart, head up, using the knees as the pivotal point).
2. The subject must raise the body by straightening the elbows and return to the "down" position, until the chin touches the mat. The stomach should not touch the mat.
3. For both men and women, the subject's back must be straight at all times and the subject must push up to a straight arm position.
4. The maximal number of push-ups performed consecutively without rest is counted as the score.
5. The test is stopped when the client strains forcibly or unable to maintain the appropriate technique within two repetitions.

CURL-UP (CRUNCH)

1. Individual assumes a supine position on a mat with the knees at 90 degrees. The arms are at the side, palms facing down with the middle fingers touching a piece of masking tape. A second piece of masking tape is placed 10 cm apart.† Shoes remain on during the test.
2. A metronome is set to 50 beats·min^{-1} and the individual does slow, controlled curl-ups to lift the shoulder blades off the mat (trunk makes a 30-degree angle with the mat) in time with the metronome at a rate of 25 per minute. The test is done for 1 minute. The low back should be flattened before curling up.
3. Individual performs as many curl-ups as possible without pausing, to a maximum of 25.‡

*See reference 54: Canadian Society for Exercise Physiology. The Canadian Physical Activity, Fitness & Lifestyle Approach: CSEP-Health & Fitness Program's Health-Related Appraisal & Counseling Strategy. 3rd ed. Canadian Society for Exercise Physiology, 2003.

†Alternatives include: 1) having the hands held across the chest, with the head activating a counter when the trunk reaches a 30-degree position [55] and placing the hands on the thighs and curling up until the hands reach the knee caps.[56] Elevation of the trunk to 30 degrees is the important aspect of the movement.

‡An alternative includes doing as many curl-ups as possible in 1 minute.

scientific data to support a cause-effect relationship between abdominal strength and low back pain are lacking, poor abdominal strength or endurance is commonly thought to contribute to muscular low back pain.[55,56] Procedures for conducting the push-up and curl-up (crunch) muscular endurance tests are given in Box 4-6, and fitness categories are provided in Tables 4-11 and 4-12, respectively.

Resistance training equipment also can be adapted to measure muscular endurance by selecting an appropriate submaximal level of resistance and measuring the number of repetitions or the duration of static contraction before fatigue. For example, the YMCA bench press test involves performing standardized repetitions at a rate of 30 lifts or reps·min^{-1}. Men are tested using an 80-pound barbell and women using a 35-pound barbell. Subjects are scored by the number of successful repetitions completed.[42] The YMCA test is an excellent example of a test that attempts to control for repetition duration and posture alignment, thus possessing high reliability. Normative data for the YMCA bench press test are presented in Table 4-13.

Flexibility

Flexibility is the ability to move a joint through its complete range of motion. It is important in athletic performance (e.g., ballet, gymnastics) and in the ability to carry out the activities of daily living. Consequently, maintaining flexibility of all joints facilitates movement; in contrast, when an activity moves the structures of a joint beyond a joint's shortened range of motion, tissue damage can occur.

Flexibility depends on a number of specific variables, including distensibility of the joint capsule, adequate warm-up, and muscle viscosity. Additionally, compliance ("tightness") of various other tissues such as ligaments and tendons affects the range of motion. Just as muscular strength is specific to the muscles involved, flexibility is joint specific; therefore, no single flexibility test can be used to evaluate total body flexibility. Laboratory tests usually quantify flexibility in terms of range

TABLE 4-11. Fitness Categories by Age Groups and Gender for Push-ups*

Category	Age									
	20–29		30–39		40–49		50–59		60–69	
Gender	M	F	M	F	M	F	M	F	M	F
Excellent	36	30	30	27	25	24	21	21	18	17
Very good	35	29	29	26	24	23	20	20	17	16
	29	21	22	20	17	15	13	11	11	12
Good	28	20	21	19	16	14	12	10	10	11
	22	15	17	13	13	11	10	7	8	5
Fair	21	14	16	12	12	10	9	6	7	4
	17	10	12	8	10	5	7	2	5	2
Needs Improvement	16	9	11	7	9	4	6	1	4	1

*See reference 54: The Canadian Physical Activity, Fitness & Lifestyle Approach: CSEP-Health & Fitness Program's Health-Related Appraisal and Counseling Strategy. 3rd ed. Reprinted with permission from the Canadian Society for Exercise Physiology, 2003.

TABLE 4-12. Fitness Categories by Age Groups and Gender for Partial Curl-up*

Category	Age									
	20–29		30–39		40–49		50–59		60–69	
Gender	M	F	M	F	M	F	M	F	M	F
Excellent	25	25	25	25	25	25	25	25	25	25
Very good	24	24	24	24	24	24	24	24	24	24
	21	18	18	19	18	19	17	19	16	17
Good	20	17	17	18	17	18	16	18	15	16
	16	14	15	10	13	11	11	10	11	8
Fair	15	13	14	9	12	10	10	9	10	7
	11	5	11	6	6	4	8	6	6	3
Needs Improvement	10	4	10	5	5	3	7	5	5	2

*See reference 54: The Canadian Physical Activity, Fitness & Lifestyle Approach: CSEP-Health & Fitness Program's Health-Related Appraisal and Counseling Strategy. 3rd ed. Reprinted with permission from the Canadian Society for Exercise Physiology, 2003.

of motion, expressed in degrees. Common devices for this purpose include various goniometers, electrogoniometers, the Leighton flexometer, inclinometers, and tape measures. Comprehensive instructions are available for the evaluation of flexibility of most anatomic joints.[57,58] Visual estimates of range of motion can be useful in fitness screening, but are inaccurate relative to directly measured range of motion. These estimates can include neck and trunk flexibility, hip flexibility, lower extremity flexibility, shoulder flexibility, and postural assessment. A more precise measurement of joint range of motion can be assessed at most anatomic joints following strict procedures[57,58] and the proper use of a goniometer. Accurate measurements require in-depth knowledge of bone, muscle, and joint anatomy, as well as experience in administering the evaluation. Table 4-14 provides normative range of motion values for select anatomic joints. Additional information can be found in the ACSM Resource Manual.

The sit-and-reach test has been used commonly to assess low back and hip-joint flexibility; however, its relationship to predict the incidence of low back pain is limited.[59] The sit-and-reach test is suggested to be a better measure of hamstring flexibility than low-back flexibility.[60] However, the relative importance of hamstring flexibility to activities of daily living and sports performance requires the inclusion of the sit-and-reach test for health-related fitness testing until a criterion measure evaluation of low back flexibility is available. Although limb and torso length disparity may impact on the sit-and-reach scoring, modified testing that establishes an individual zero point for each participant has not enhanced the predictive index for low back flexibility or low back pain.[61,62]

The back saver unilateral sit and reach test measures each limb independently as opposed to the standard simultaneous measurement of both limbs. One limb is held straight while the knee of the other limb is flexed and the plantar surface of the foot on the flexed limb is placed on the floor adjacent to the medial surface of the knee of the straight limb. The back saver test is purported to reduce excessive disk compression, posterior ligament tension, and erector spinae muscle strain,

TABLE 4-13. YMCA Bench Press Test: Total Lifts*

Category	Age											
	18–25		26–35		36–45		46–55		56–65		>65	
Gender	M	F	M	F	M	F	M	F	M	F	M	F
Excellent	64	66	61	62	55	57	47	50	41	42	36	30
	44	42	41	40	36	33	28	29	24	24	20	18
Good	41	38	37	34	32	30	25	24	21	21	16	16
	34	30	30	29	26	26	21	20	17	17	12	12
Above average	33	28	29	28	25	24	20	18	14	14	10	10
	29	25	26	24	22	21	16	14	12	12	9	8
Average	28	22	24	22	21	20	14	13	11	10	8	7
	24	20	21	18	18	16	12	10	9	8	7	5
Below average	22	18	20	17	17	14	11	9	8	6	6	4
	20	16	17	14	14	12	9	7	5	5	4	3
Poor	17	13	16	13	12	10	8	6	4	4	3	2
	13	9	12	9	9	6	5	2	2	2	2	0
Very poor	<10	6	9	6	6	4	2	1	1	1	1	0

*Reprinted from YMCA Fitness Testing and Assessment Manual with permission of the YMCA of the USA, 101 N. Wacker Drive, Chicago, IL 60606.

TABLE 4-14. Range of Motion of Select Single Joint Movements (degrees)*

Shoulder Girdle
Flexion	90–120	Extension	20–60
Abduction	80–100		
Horizontal Abduction	30–45	Horizontal Adduction	90–135
Medial Rotation	70–90	Lateral Rotation	70–90

Elbow
Flexion	135–160		
Supination	75–90	Pronation	75–90

Trunk
Flexion	120–150	Extension	20–45
Lateral Flexion	10–35	Rotation	20–40

Hip
Flexion	90–135	Extension	10–30
Abduction	30–50	Adduction	10–30
Medial Rotation	30–45	Lateral Rotation	45–60

Knee
Flexion	130–140	Extension	5–10

Ankle
Dorsiflexion	15–20	Plantarflexion	30–50
Inversion	10–30	Eversion	10–20

*Reprinted with Permission from Norkin C, Levangie P. Joint Structure and Function: A Comprehensive Approach, 2nd Ed. Philadelphia: F.A. Davis, 1992.

while permitting the assessment of limb asymmetry.[63] A comparison of the two versions of the sit and reach test found no difference in movement in the sit and reach and in Cailliet's protective-hamstring stretch.[64] Although asymmetric stretching is appropriate for flexibility training, a lack of normative data for adults precludes the inclusion of the back saver unilateral sit and reach test at this time.

BOX 4-7   Trunk Flexion (Sit-and-Reach) Test Procedures*

Pretest: Participant should perform a short warm-up prior to this test and include some stretches (e.g., modified hurdler's stretch). It is also recommended that the participant refrain from fast, jerky movements, which may increase the possibility of an injury. The participant's shoes should be removed.

1. For the Canadian Trunk Forward Flexion test, the client sits without shoes and the soles of the feet flat against the flexometer (sit-and-reach box) at the 26-cm mark. Inner edges of the soles are placed within 2 cm of the measuring scale. For the YMCA sit-and-reach test, a yardstick is placed on the floor and tape is placed across it at a right angle to the 15-inch mark. The participant sits with the yardstick between the legs, with legs extended at right angles to the taped line on the floor. Heels of the feet should touch the edge of the taped line and be about 10 to 12 inches apart. (Note the zero point at the foot/box interface and use the appropriate norms.)

2. The participant should slowly reach forward with both hands as far as possible, holding this position approximately 2 seconds. Be sure that the participant keeps the hands parallel and does not lead with one hand. Fingertips can be overlapped and should be in contact with the measuring portion or yardstick of the sit-and-reach box.

3. The score is the most distant point (in centimeters or inches) reached with the fingertips. The best of two trials should be recorded. To assist with the best attempt, the participant should exhale and drop the head between the arms when reaching. Testers should ensure that the knees of the participant stay extended; however, the participant's knees should not be pressed down. The participant should breathe normally during the test and should not hold his or her breath at any time. Norms for the Canadian test are presented in Table 4-15. Note that these norms use a sit-and-reach box in which the "zero" point is set at the 26-cm mark. If you are using a box in which the zero point is set at 23 cm (e.g., Fitnessgram), subtract 3 cm from each value in this table. The norms for the YMCA test are presented in Table 4-16.

*Diagrams of these procedures are available from Golding LA, Myers CR, Sinning WE. YMCA Fitness Testing and Assessment Manual, 4th ed. YMCA of the USA, 101 N. Wacker Drive, Chicago, IL 60606. Canadian Society for Exercise Physiology. The Canadian Physical Activity, Fitness & Lifestyle Approach: CSEP-Health & Fitness Program's Health-Related Appraisal & Counseling Strategy. 3rd ed. Canadian Society for Exercise Physiology, 2003.

TABLE 4-15. Fitness Categories by Age Groups for Trunk Forward Flexion Using a Sit-and-Reach Box (cm)*†

	Age									
Category	20–29		30–39		40–49		50–59		60–69	
Gender	M	F	M	F	M	F	M	F	M	F
Excellent	40	41	38	41	35	38	35	39	33	35
Very Good	39	40	37	40	34	37	34	38	32	34
	34	37	33	36	29	34	28	33	25	31
Good	33	36	32	35	28	33	27	32	24	30
	30	33	28	32	24	30	24	30	20	27
Fair	29	32	27	31	23	29	23	29	19	26
	25	28	23	27	18	25	16	25	15	23
Needs Improvement	24	27	22	26	17	24	15	24	14	22

*The Canadian Physical Activity, Fitness & Lifestyle Approach: CSEP-Health & Fitness Program's Health-Related Appraisal & Counseling Strategy. 3rd ed. Reprinted with permission from the Canadian Society for Exercise Physiology, 2003.

†Note: These norms are based on a sit-and-reach box in which the "zero" point is set at 26 cm. When using a box in which the zero point is set at 23 cm, subtract 3 cm from each value in this table.

Poor lower back and hip flexibility may, in conjunction with poor abdominal strength/endurance or other causative factors, contribute to development of muscular low back pain; however, this hypothesis remains to be substantiated.[65] Methods for administering the sit-and-reach test are presented in Box 4-7. Normative data for two sit-and-reach tests are presented in Tables 4-15 and 4-16.

A Comprehensive Health Fitness Evaluation

A typical fitness assessment includes the following:

- Prescreening/risk stratification
- Resting HR, BP, height, body mass, ECG (if appropriate)
- Body composition
  - Waist circumference
  - Skinfold assessment
- Cardiorespiratory Fitness
  - Submaximal YMCA cycle ergometer test
- Muscular Strength
  - 1-, 4-, 6-, or 8-RM upper body (bench press) and lower body (leg press)
- Muscular Endurance
  - Curl-up test
  - Push-up test
- Flexibility
  - Sit-and-reach test or goniometric measures of isolated anatomic joints

Additional evaluations may be administered; however, the aforementioned components of a fitness evaluation represent a comprehensive assessment that can be performed within 1 hour. The data accrued from the evaluation should be

TABLE 4-16. Percentiles by Age Groups and Gender for YMCA Sit-and-Reach Test (Inches)*

Percentile	Age											
	18–25		26–35		36–45		46–55		56–65		>65	
Gender	M	F	M	F	M	F	M	F	M	F	M	F
90	22	24	21	23	21	22	19	21	17	20	17	20
80	20	22	19	21	19	21	17	20	15	19	15	18
70	19	21	17	20	17	19	15	18	13	17	13	17
60	18	20	17	20	16	18	14	17	13	16	12	17
50	17	19	15	19	15	17	13	16	11	15	10	15
40	15	18	14	17	13	16	11	14	9	14	9	14
30	14	17	13	16	13	15	10	14	9	13	8	13
20	13	16	11	15	11	14	9	12	7	11	7	11
10	11	14	9	13	7	12	6	10	5	9	4	9

*Reprinted from YMCA Fitness Testing and Assessment Manual with permission of the YMCA of the USA, 101 N. Wacker Drive, Chicago, IL 60606. The following may be used as descriptors for the percentile rankings: well above average (90), above average (70), average (50), below average (30), and well below average (10).

interpreted by a competent professional and conveyed to the client. This information is central to the development of a client's short- and long-term goals, as well as forming the basis for the initial exercise prescription and subsequent evaluations to monitor progress.

REFERENCES

1. President's Council on Physical Fitness. Definitions: health, fitness, and physical activity. Research Digest, 2000.
2. Caspersen CJ, Powell KE, Christenson GM. Physical activity, exercise, and physical fitness: definitions and distinctions for health-related research. Public Health Rep 1985;100:126–131.
3. National Institutes of Health. Health implications of obesity. Annals of Internal Medicine 1985;163:1073–1077.
4. Flegal KM, Carroll MD, Ogden CL, et al. Prevalence and trends in obesity among US adults, 1999–2000. JAMA 2002;288:1723–1727.
5. Ogden CL, Flegal KM, Carroll MD, et al. Prevalence and trends in overweight among US children and adolescents, 1999–2000. JAMA 2002;288:1728–1732.
6. Troiano RP, Flegal KM. Overweight children and adolescents: description, epidemiology, and demographics. Pediatrics 1998;101:497–504.
7. Kaminsky LA, ed. ACSM's Resource Manual for Guidelines for Exercise Testing and Prescription. Baltimore: Lippincott Williams & Wilkins, 2005.
8. Heyward VH, Stolarczyk LM, eds. Applied Body Composition Assessment. Champaign, IL: Human Kinetics, 1996;12.
9. Roche AF, Heymsfield SB, Lohman TG, eds. Human Body Composition. Champaign, IL: Human Kinetics, 1996.
10. Lohman TG, Houtkooper L, Going SB. Body fat measurement goes high-tech. ACSM's Health Fitness J 1997;1(1):30–35.
11. Panel E. Executive summary of the clinical guidelines on the identification, evaluation, and treatment of overweight and obesity in adults. Arch Intern Med 1998;158:1855–1867.
12. Rimm EB, Stampfer MJ, Giovannucci E, et al. Body size and fat distribution as predictors of coronary heart disease among middle-aged and older US men. Am J Epidemiol 1995;141:1117–1127.
13. Gallagher D, Heymsfield SB, Heo M, et al. Healthy percentage body fat ranges: an approach for developing guidelines based on body mass index. Am J Clin Nutr 2000;72:694-701.
14. Van Itallie TB, ed. Topography of body fat: relationship to risk of cardiovascular and other diseases. In: Lohman TG, Roche AF, Martorell R, eds. Anthropometric Standardization Reference Manual. Champaign, IL: Human Kinetics, 1988.

15. Folsom AR, Kaye SA, Sellers TA, et al. Body fat distribution and 5-year risk of death in older women. JAMA 1993;269:483–487.
16. Tran ZV, Weltman A. Generalized equation for predicting body density of women from girth measurements. Med Sci Sports Exerc 1989;21:101–104.
17. Tran ZV, Weltman A. Predicting body composition of men from girth measurements. Hum Biol 1988;60:167–175.
18. Bray GA, Gray DS. Obesity. Part I. Pathogenesis. West J Med 1988;149:429–441.
19. Bray GA. Don't throw the baby out with the bath water. Am J Clin Nutr 2004;79:347–349.
20. Roche AF. Anthropometry and ultrasound. In: Roche AF, Heymsfield SB, Lohman TG, eds. Human Body Composition. Champaign, IL: Human Kinetics, 1996:167–189.
21. Heyward VH. Practical body composition assessment for children, adults, and older adults. Int J Sport Nutr 1998;8:285–307.
22. Jackson AS, Pollock ML. Practical assessment of body composition. Phys Sport Med 1985;13(3):76–90.
23. Going BS. Densitometry. In: Roche AF, Heymsfield SB, Lohman TG, eds. Human Body Composition. Champaign, IL: Human Kinetics, 1996:3–23.
24. Dempster P, Aitkens S. A new air displacement method for the determination of human body composition. Med Sci Sports Exerc 1995;27:1692–1697.
25. Brozek J, Grade F, Anderson J. Densitometric analysis of body composition: revision of some quantitative assumptions. Ann NY Acad Sci 1963;110:113–140.
26. Siri WE. Body composition from fluid spaces and density. Univ Calif Donner Lab Med Phys Rep, 1956.
27. Hendel HW, Gotfredsen A, Hojgaard L, et al. Change in fat-free mass sed by bioelectrical impedance, total body potassium and dual energy X-ray absorptiometry during prolonged weight loss. Scand J Clin Lab Invest 1996;56:671–679.
28. Mclean KP, Skinner JS. Validity of Futrex-5000 for body composition determination. Med Sci Sports Exerc 1992;24:253–258.
29. Lohman TG. Body composition methodology in sports medicine. Phys Sportsmed 1982;10:47–58.
30. Blair SN, Kohl HW 3rd, Barlow CE, et al. Changes in physical fitness and all-cause mortality. A prospective study of healthy and unhealthy men. JAMA 1995;273:1093–1098.
31. Blair SN, Kohl HW 3rd, Paffenbarger RS Jr, et al. Physical fitness and all-cause mortality. A prospective study of healthy men and women. JAMA 1989;262:2395–2401.
32. Sesso HD, Paffenbarger RS Jr, Lee IM. Physical activity and coronary heart disease in men: The Harvard Alumni Health Study. Circulation 2000;102:975–980.
33. Davis JA, ed. Direct determination of aerobic power. In: Maud PJ, Foster C, eds. Physiological Assessment of Human Fitness. Champaign, IL: Human Kinetics, 1995:9–17.
34. McConnell TR. Cardiorespiratory assessment of apparently healthy populations. In: Roitman JL, ed. ACSM Resource Manual for Guidelines for Exercise Testing and Prescription. 4th ed. Baltimore: Williams & Wilkins: Baltimore, 2001:361–375.
35. Jette M, Campbell J, Mongeon J, et al. The Canadian Home Fitness Test as a predictor for aerobic capacity. Can Med Assoc J 1976;114:680–682.
36. Astrand P-O. Aerobic work capacity in men and women with special reference to age. Acta Physiol Scand 1960;49(suppl):45–60.
37. Kline GM, Porcari JP, Hintermeister R, et al. Estimation of $\dot{V}O_{2max}$ from a one-mile track walk, gender, age, and body weight. Med Sci Sports Exerc 1987;19:253–259.
38. Bittner V, Weiner DH, Yusuf S, et al. Prediction of mortality and morbidity with a 6-minute walk test in patients with left ventricular dysfunction. JAMA 1993;270:1702–1707.
39. Cahalin LP, Mathier MA, Semigran MJ, et al. The six minute walk test predicts peak oxygen uptake and survival in patients with advanced heart failure. Chest 1996;110:325–332.
40. Astrand P-O, Ryhming I. A nomogram for calculation of aerobic capacity (physical fitness) from pulse rate during submaximal work. J Appl Physiol 1954;7:218–221.
41. Maritz JS, Morrison JF, Peter J. A practical method of estimating an individual's maximal oxygen uptake. Ergonomics 1961;4:97–122.
42. Golding LA. YMCA Fitness Testing and Assessment Manual. Champaign, IL: Human Kinetics, 1989.
43. Shephard RJ, Thomas S, Weller I. The Canadian Home Fitness Test. 1991 update. Sports Med 1991;11:358–366.
44. Leger L, Thivierge M. Heart rate monitors: validity, stability and functionality. Phys Sport Med 1988;16:143–151.

45. Whaley MH, Brubaker PH, Kaminsky LA, et al. Validity of rating of perceived exertion during graded exercise testing in apparently healthy adults and cardiac patients. J Cardiopul Rehabil 1997;17:261–267.

46. Noble BJ, Borg GA, Jacobs I, et al. A category-ratio perceived exertion scale: relationship to blood and muscle lactates and heart rate. Med Sci Sports Exerc 1983;15:523–528.

47. Robertson RJ, Noble BJ. Perception of physical exertion: methods, mediators, and applications. Exerc Sport Sci Rev 1997;25:407–452.

48. Morgan W, Borg GA, eds. Perception of effort in the prescription of physical activity. Nelson T, ed. Mental Health and Emotional Aspects of Sports. Chicago: American Medical Association, 1976:126–129.

49. American College of Sports Medicine. Position Stand: The recommended quantity and quality of exercise for developing and maintaining cardiorespiratory and muscular fitness, and flexibility in healthy adults. Med Sci Sports Exerc 1998;30:975–991.

50. Hoeger WW, Barette SL, Hale DR. Relationship between repetition and selected percentages of one repetition maximum. J Appl Sport Sci Res 1987;1(1):11–13.

51. Hoeger WW, Hopkins DR, Bareete SL. Relationship between repetitions and selected percentages of one repetition maximum: a comparison between untrained and trained males and females. J Appl Sport Sci Res 1990;4(2):47–54.

52. Logan P, Fornasiero D, Abernathy P, et al, eds. Protocols for the assessment of isoinertial strength. In: Fore CJ, ed. Physiological tests for elite athletes. Champaign, IL: Human Kinetics, 2000: 200–221.

53. Graves JE, Pollock ML, Bryant CX, eds. Assessment of muscular strength and endurance, 4th ed. In: Roitman JL, ed. ACSM's Resource Manual for Guidelines for Exercise Testing and Prescription. Baltimore: Lippincott Williams & Wilkins, 2001:376–380.

54. Canadian Society for Exercise Physiology. The Canadian Physical Activity, Fitness & Lifestyle Approach: CSEP-Health & Fitness Program's Health-Related Appraisal & Counseling Strategy. 3rd ed. Canadian Society for Exercise Physiology, 2003.

55. Diener MH, Golding LA, Diener D. Validity and reliability of a one-minute half sit-up test of abdominal muscle strength and endurance. Sports Med Training Rehab 1995;6:5–119.

56. Faulkner RA, Sprigings EJ, McQuarrie A, et al. A partial curl-up protocol for adults based on an analysis of two procedures. Can J Sport Sci 1989;14:135–141.

57. Clarkson H. Musculoskeletal Assessment, Joint Range of Motion and Manual Muscle Strength. Baltimore: Lippincott Williams & Wilkins, 1999.

58. Palmer ML, Epler ME, eds. Fundamentals of Musculoskeletal Assessment Techniques. 2nd ed. Philadelphia: Lippincott-Raven, 1998.

59. Jackson AW, Morrow JR Jr, Brill PA, et al. Relations of sit-up and sit-and-reach tests to low back pain in adults. J Orthop Sports Phys Ther 1998;27:22–26.

60. Jackson AW, Baker AA. The relationship of the sit and reach test to criterion measures of hamstring and back flexibility in young females. Res Q Exerc Sport 1986;57(3):183–186.

61. Hoeger WW, Hopkins DR. A comparison of the sit and reach and the modified sit and reach in the measurement of flexibility in women. Res Q Exerc Sport 1992;63:191–195.

62. Minkler S, Patterson P. The validity of the modified sit-and-reach test in college-age students. Res Q Exerc Sport 1994;65:189–192.

63. Cailliet R. Low Back Pain Syndrome. Philadelphia: FA Davis, 1988:175–179.

64. Liemohn WP, Sharpe GL, Wasserman JF. Lumbosacral movement in the sit-and-reach and in Cailliet's protective-hamstring stretch. Spine 1994;19:2127–2130.

65. Protas EJ, ed. Flexibility and range of motion. In: Roitman JL, ed. ACSM's Resource Manual for Guidelines for Exercise Testing and Prescription. Baltimore: Lippincott Williams & Wilkins, 2001: 381–390.

Clinical Exercise Testing

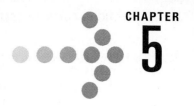

Standard graded exercise tests are used in clinical applications to assess a patient's ability to tolerate increasing intensities of exercise while electrocardiographic (ECG), hemodynamic, and symptomatic responses are monitored for manifestations of myocardial ischemia, electrical instability, or other exertion-related abnormalities. Gas exchange and ventilatory responses also are commonly assessed during the exercise test, particularly in patients with chronic heart failure, in those whom preoperative risk is indeterminate, among postmyocardial infarction (post-MI) patients who wish to return to moderate heavy occupations, or in patients with known or suspected pulmonary limitations.

Indications and Applications

The exercise test may be used for diagnostic, prognostic, and therapeutic applications, especially in regard to exercise prescription (see Chapters 7 and 8).

DIAGNOSTIC EXERCISE TESTING

Diagnostic exercise testing is best used in patients with an intermediate probability of angiographically significant coronary artery disease (CAD) as determined by age, gender, and symptoms (Table 5-1). Asymptomatic individuals generally represent those with a low likelihood (i.e., <10%) of significant CAD. Diagnostic exercise testing in asymptomatic individuals generally is not indicated. However, exercise testing may be useful in asymptomatic persons when multiple risk factors are present,[1] indicating at least a moderate risk of experiencing a serious cardiovascular event within 5 years.[2] It also may be indicated in those who are about to start a vigorous exercise program (see Chapter 2), or those involved in occupations in which cardiovascular events may affect public safety. In general, patients with a high probability of disease (e.g., typical angina, prior coronary revascularization or myocardial infarction [MI]) are tested to assess residual myocardial ischemia and prognosis rather than for diagnostic purposes. Exercise electrocardiography for diagnostic purposes is less accurate in women largely because of a greater number of false-positive responses. Although differences in test accuracy between men and women may be in the order of 10% on average, the standard exercise test is considered the initial diagnostic evaluation of choice regardless of gender.[1]

TABLE 5-1. Pretest Likelihood of Coronary Artery Disease*†

Age	Gender	Typical Definite Angina Pectoris	Atypical/Probable Angina Pectoris	Nonanginal Chest Pain	Asymptomatic
30–39	Men	Intermediate	Intermediate	Low	Very low
	Women	Intermediate	Very low	Very low	Very low
40–49	Men	High	Intermediate	Intermediate	Low
	Women	Intermediate	Low	Very low	Very low
50–59	Men	High	Intermediate	Intermediate	Low
	Women	Intermediate	Intermediate	Low	Very low
60–69	Men	High	Intermediate	Intermediate	Low
	Women	High	Intermediate	Intermediate	Low

*See reference 1: Reprinted with permission from Gibbons RJ, Balady GJ, Bricker JT, et al. ACC/AHA 2002 Guideline Update for Exercise Testing; a report of the American College of Cardiology/ American Heart Association Task Force on Practice Guidelines; Committee on Exercise Testing, 2002. American College of Cardiology web site: www.acc.org/clinical/guidelines/exercise/dirIndex.htm

†No data exist for patients who are <30 or >69 years, but it can be assumed that prevalence of CAD increases with age. In a few cases, patients with ages at the extremes of the decades listed may have probabilities slightly outside the high or low range. High indicates >90%; intermediate, 10%–90%; low, <10%; and very low, <5%.

The use of maximal or sign/symptom-limited exercise testing has expanded greatly to help guide decisions regarding medical management and surgical therapy in a broad spectrum of patients. For example, immediate exercise testing of selected low-risk patients presenting to the emergency department with chest pain is now increasingly employed to "rule out myocardial infarction,"[3] and help make decisions regarding which patients require hospital admission.[4] Generally, patients who may be safely discharged include those who are no longer symptomatic, and those with unremarkable ECGs and normal serial cardiac enzyme assays (e.g., no appreciable rise in the level of troponin).

EXERCISE TESTING FOR DISEASE SEVERITY AND PROGNOSIS

Exercise testing is useful for the evaluation of disease severity among persons with known or suspected CAD. Data derived from the exercise test are most useful when considered in context with other clinical data. Information related to risk factors, symptoms, functional capacity, and myocardial ischemia during the exercise test must be considered together. The magnitude of ischemia caused by a coronary lesion generally is proportional to the degree of ST-segment depression, the number of electrocardiographic (ECG) leads involved, and the duration of ST-segment depression in recovery. It is inversely proportional to the ST slope, the double product at which the ST-segment depression occurs, and the maximal heart rate, systolic blood pressure, and metabolic equivalent (MET) level achieved. Several numeric indices of prognosis have been published and are discussed in Chapter 6.[5,6]

EXERCISE TESTING AFTER MYOCARDIAL INFARCTION

Exercise testing after MI can be performed before or soon after hospital discharge (as early as 4 days after MI) for prognostic assessment, activity prescription, and evaluation of medical therapy. Submaximal tests may be used before hospital discharge at 4 to 6 days after acute MI. Low-level exercise testing provides sufficient data to make recommendations about the patient's ability to safely perform activities of daily living and serves as a guide for early ambulatory exercise therapy. Symptom-limited tests are usually performed at more than 14 days after MI.[1] As contemporary therapies have led to dramatic reductions in mortality after MI, the use of exercise testing in the evaluation of prognosis has changed. Patients who have not undergone coronary revascularization and are unable to undergo exercise testing appear to have the worst prognosis. Other indicators of adverse prognosis in the post-MI patient include ischemic ST-segment depression at a low level of exercise (particularly if accompanied by reduced left ventricular systolic function); functional capacity of less than 5 METs; and a hypotensive blood pressure response to exercise.

FUNCTIONAL EXERCISE TESTING

Exercise testing is useful to determine functional capacity. This information can be valuable for activity counseling, exercise prescription, return to work evaluations, disability assessment, and to help estimate prognosis. Functional capacity can be evaluated based on percentile ranking (based on apparently healthy men and women) as presented in Table 4-8. Exercise capacity also may be reported as the percentage of expected METs for age using a nomogram (Fig. 5-1), with 100% being normal (separate nomograms are provided for referred men with suspected CAD and in healthy men).[7] Normal standards for exercise capacity based on directly measured $\dot{V}O_{2max}$ are also available for women and by age.[8] When using a particular regression equation for estimating percentage of normal exercise capacity achieved, factors such as population specificity, exercise mode, and whether exercise capacity was measured directly or estimated should be considered.

Previous studies in persons without known coronary artery disease have identified a low level of aerobic fitness as an independent risk factor for all-cause and cardiovascular mortality.[9,10] Recently, investigators extended these analyses to 527 men with cardiovascular disease who were referred to an outpatient cardiac rehabilitation program.[11] Oxygen uptake at peak exercise on a cycle ergometer was directly measured 13 weeks after acute myocardial infarction ($N = 312$) or coronary artery bypass surgery ($N = 215$). All tests were terminated at a comparable endpoint, that is, volitional fatigue. During an average follow-up of 6.1 years, 33 and 20 patients died of cardiovascular and noncardiovascular cases, respectively. Figure 5-2 shows the inverse relationship between peak oxygen uptake and subsequent mortality. Those with the highest cardiovascular and all-cause mortality averaged ≤4.4 METs. In contrast, there were no deaths among patients who averaged ≥9.2 METs.

Another study[12] reported on 3,679 men with coronary disease who were referred for treadmill exercise testing for clinical reasons. Those with an exercise capacity of ≤4.9 METs had a relative risk of death of 4.1 compared to those with a fitness level ≥10.7 METs over the average follow-up of 6.2 years. For every 1-MET increase in exercise capacity there was a 12% improvement in survival. Similarly, findings from the National Exercise and Heart Disease Project among post-MI patients demonstrated that every 1-MET increase after the training

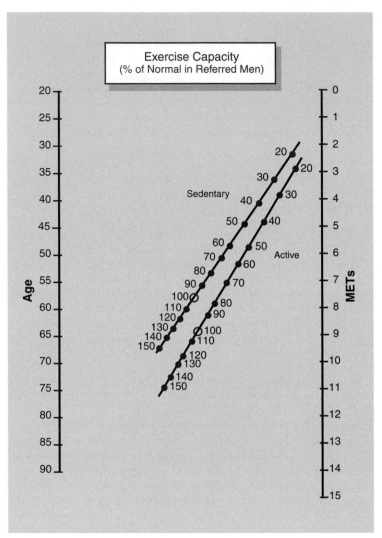

(**FIGURE 5-1.** Nomograms of percent normal exercise capacity in men with suspected coronary artery disease who were referred for clinical exercise testing (this page) and in healthy men (page 97).

period conferred an approximate 10% reduction in mortality from any cause, regardless of the study group assignment, over a 19-year follow-up.[13]

Exercise Test Modalities

The treadmill and cycle ergometer are the most commonly used devices for clinical exercise testing. Treadmill testing provides a more common form of physiologic stress (e.g., walking) in which subjects are more likely to attain a slightly

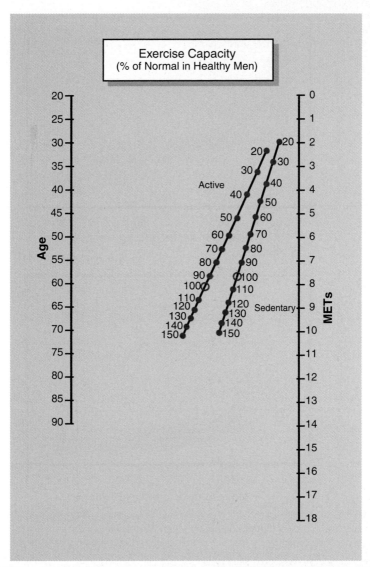

FIGURE 5-1. (continued) See reference 7: Reprinted from Morris CK, Myers J, Froelicher VF, et al. Nomogram based on metabolic equivalents and age for assessing aerobic exercise capacity in men. J Am Coll Cardiol 1993;22:175–182, with permission from the American College of Cardiology Foundation.

higher oxygen consumption ($\dot{V}O_2$) and peak heart rate than during cycle ergometer testing.[14,15] The treadmill should have handrails for patients to steady themselves, but holding the handrails can reduce the accuracy of estimated exercise capacity and the quality of the ECG recording, and should be discouraged. However, it may be necessary for some individuals to hold the handrails

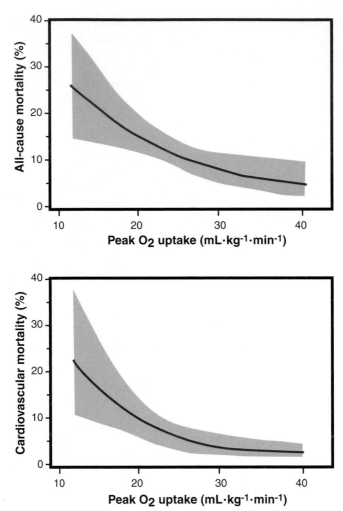

FIGURE 5-2. Relation between peak oxygen uptake with all cause mortality (top) and cardiovascular mortality (bottom) in patients with coronary artery disease. Shaded area represents 95% confidence limits. See reference 11: Modified from Journal of the American College of Cardiology, 23(2): 358–363, Vanhees L, Fagard R, Thijs L, et al. Prognostic significance of peak exercise capacity in patients with coronary artery disease. © 1994 American College of Cardiology Foundation.

lightly for balance. An emergency stop button should be readily available to supervising staff.

Cycle ergometers are less expensive, require less space, and make less noise than treadmills. Incremental work rates on an electronically braked cycle ergometer are more sensitive than mechanically braked ergometers because the work rate can be maintained over a wide range of pedal rates. Because there is less movement of the patient's arms and thorax during cycling, it is easier to obtain better quality ECG recordings and blood pressure measurements. However, stationary cycling is an unfamiliar method of exercise for many and is highly dependent on patient motivation. Thus, the test may end prematurely (i.e., because of localized leg fatigue) before a cardiopulmonary endpoint has been achieved. Lower values for $\dot{V}O_{2max}$ during cycle ergometer testing (versus treadmill testing) can range from 5% to 25%, depending on the participant's conditioning and leg strength.[14–16]

Arm ergometry is an alternative method of exercise testing for patients who cannot perform leg exercise. Because a smaller muscle mass is used during arm ergometry, $\dot{V}O_{2max}$ during arm exercise is generally 20% to 30% lower than that obtained during treadmill testing.[17] Although this test has diagnostic utility,[18] it has been largely replaced by the nonexercise pharmacologic stress techniques that are described later in this chapter. Arm ergometer tests can be used for activity counseling and exercise prescription for certain disabled populations (e.g., spinal cord injury), and individuals who perform primarily dynamic upper body work during occupational or leisure-time activities.

Exercise Protocols

The protocol employed for an exercise test should consider the purpose of the test, the specific outcomes desired, and the characteristics of the individual being tested. Some of the most common exercise protocols and the predicted $\dot{V}O_2$ for each stage are illustrated in Figure 5-3. The Bruce treadmill test remains the most commonly used protocol; however, it employs relatively large increments (i.e., METs per stage) every 3 minutes. Consequently, changes in physiologic responses tend to be less uniform and exercise capacity may be markedly overestimated when it is predicted from exercise time or workload. Protocols with larger increments (e.g., Bruce, Ellestad) are better suited for screening younger and/or physically active individuals, whereas protocols with smaller increments, such as Naughton or Balke-Ware (i.e., 1 MET per stage or lower), are preferable for older or deconditioned individuals and patients with chronic diseases.

The ramp protocol is an alternative approach to incremental exercise testing that has gained popularity in recent years, in which the work rate increases in a constant and continuous manner.[15,19,20] Although ramp testing using a cycle ergometer has been available for many years, many of the major treadmill manufacturers recently developed controllers that ramp speed and grade. Both individualized[19] and standardized ramp tests, such as the BSU/Bruce ramp,[20] have been used. The former test individualizes the rate of increase in intensity based on the subject, and the latter matches work rates to equivalent time periods on the commonly used Bruce protocol, but increases in ramp fashion. Advantages of the ramp approach include the following:[15]

- Avoidance of large and unequal increments in workload
- Uniform increase in hemodynamic and physiologic responses
- More accurate estimates of exercise capacity and ventilatory threshold
- Individualizing the test protocol (individualized ramp rate)
- Targeted test duration (applies only to individualized ramp protocols)

FUNCTIONAL CLASS	CLINICAL STATUS	O₂ COST ml/kg/min	METS	BICYCLE ERGOMETER	BRUCE 3 MIN STAGES MPH / %AGR		RAMP

FUNCTIONAL CLASS	CLINICAL STATUS	O₂ COST ml/kg/min	METS	BICYCLE ERGOMETER	BRUCE MPH	BRUCE %AGR	RAMP MPH / %GR
NORMAL AND I	HEALTHY, DEPENDENT ON AGE, ACTIVITY	73.5	21				
		70	20	FOR 70 KG BODY WEIGHT Kpm/min (WATTS)	5.5	20	
		66.5	19				
		63	18				
		59.5	17		5.0	18	
		56.0	16				
		52.5	15				
		49.0	14	1500 (246)			PER 30 SEC MPH / %GR
		45.5	13		4.2	16	3.0 25.0
							3.0 24.0
		42.0	12	1350 (221)			3.0 23.0
							3.0 22.0
		38.5	11	1200 (197)			3.0 21.0
							3.0 20.0
							3.0 19.0
	SEDENTARY HEALTHY	35.0	10	1050 (172)	3.4	14	3.0 18.0
							3.0 17.0
		31.5	9				3.0 16.0
				900 (148)			3.0 15.0
		28.0	8				3.0 14.0
				750 (123)			3.0 13.0
		24.5	7		2.5	12	3.0 12.0
							3.0 11.0
				600 (98)			3.0 10.0
		21.0	6				3.0 9.0
II	LIMITED SYMPTOMATIC			450 (74)			3.0 8.0
		17.5	5				3.0 7.0
					1.7	10	3.0 6.0
III		14.0	4	300 (49)			3.0 5.0
							3.0 4.0
		10.5	3	150 (24)			3.0 3.0
							3.0 2.0
		7.0	2				3.0 1.0
							3.0 0
							2.5 0
IV		3.5	1				2.0 0
							1.5 0
							1.0 0
							0.5 0

FIGURE 5-3. Common exercise protocols and associated metabolic costs of each stage.

BRUCE RAMP (MIN / %GR)	BALKE-WARE	USAFSAM (MPH / %GR)	"SLOW" USAFSAM (MPH / %GR)	MODIFIED BALKE (MPH / %GR)	ACIP (MPH / %GR)	MOD. NAUGHTON (CHF) (MPH / %GR)	METS
20							21
19	%GRADE						20
	AT 3.3						19
18	MPH						18
	1 MIN						17
18	STAGES						16
17	26	3.3 25			3.4 24.0		15
	25						
	24						
16	23			3.0 25	3.1 24.0	3.0 25	14
16	22						
	21			3.0 22.5		3.0 22.5	13
15	20	3.3 20					
	19			3.0 20	3.0 21.0	3.0 20	12
14	18						
	17			3.0 17.5	3.0 17.5	3.0 17.5	11
	16	3.3 15					
14	15		2 25	3.0 15		3.0 15	10
	14				3.0 14.0		
	13			3.0 12.5		3.0 12.5	9
13	12						
	11	3.3 10	2 20	3.0 10	3.0 10.5	3.0 10	8
12	10						
	9						7
	8		2 15	3.0 7.5		3.0 7.5	
12	7				3.0 7.0		6
11	6	3.3 5	2 10	3.0 5		2.0 10.5	
10	5						5
	4			3.0 2.5	3.0 3.0	2.0 7.0	
10	3		2 5		2.5 2.0	2.0 3.5	4
	2	3.3 0		3.0 0			3
5	1	2.0 0	2 0	2.0 0	2.0 0.0	1.5 0	2
0						1.0 0	1

Whichever exercise protocol is chosen, it should be individualized so that the treadmill speed and increments in grade are based on the subject's capability. Ideally, increments in work rate should be chosen so that the total test time ranges between 8 and 12 minutes.[1,8,21] For example, increments of 10 to 15 watts (1 W = 6.12 kg·m·min^{-1}) per minute can be used on the cycle ergometer for elderly persons, deconditioned individuals, and patients with cardiovascular or pulmonary disease. Increases in grade of 1% to 3% per minute, with constant belt speeds of 1.5 to 2.5 mph, can be used for treadmill tests for these same populations.

Although no longer widely used, submaximal testing can be an appropriate choice for predischarge, post-MI evaluations, and for patients who may be at high risk for serious rhythm disturbances, abnormal blood pressure responses, or other adverse signs or symptoms. Submaximal tests can be useful for making activity recommendations, adjusting the medical regimen, and identifying the need for further interventions. These tests are stopped frequently at a predetermined level, such as a heart rate of 120 beats·min^{-1} or a MET level of 5, but this may vary based on the patient and clinical judgment. When performed in this manner, submaximal tests have been useful in risk stratifying post-MI patients.

UPPER BODY EXERCISE TESTING

An arm cycle ergometer can be purchased as such, or modified from an existing stationary cycle ergometer by replacing the pedals with handles and mounting the unit on a table at shoulder height. Similar to leg cycle ergometers, these can be braked either mechanically or electrically. Work rates are adjusted by altering the cranking rates and/or resistance against the flywheel. Work rate increments of 10 W every 2 to 3 minutes, at a cranking rate of 50 to 60 rpm, have been applied to a broad spectrum of patients.[22] Arm ergometry is best performed in the seated position with the fulcrum of the handle adjusted to shoulder height. Electrocardiographic leads should be placed to minimize muscle artifact from upper body movement. Blood pressure can be measured with the individual dropping one arm and continuing to arm crank with the other, or during brief rest periods between stages. However, systolic blood pressures taken by the standard cuff method immediately after arm crank ergometry are likely to underestimate "true" physiologic responses.[23] Blood pressures can also be measured at the thigh during arm ergometry testing.

Testing for Return to Work

The decision to return to work after a cardiac event is a complex one, with about 15% to 20% of patients failing to resume work.[24] Both medical and nonmedical factors contribute to this loss of employment.

Work assessment and counseling are useful in optimizing return-to-work decisions. Early discussion of work-related issues with patients, preferably before hospital discharge, may help establish reasonable return-to-work expectations. Discussion with the patient could include a job history analysis to: 1) ascertain job demands and concerns, 2) establish tentative time lines for work evaluation and return, 3) individualize rehabilitation according to job demands, and 4) determine special work-related needs or job contacts.[24] The appropriate time to return to work varies with type of cardiac event or interventional procedure, associated complications, and prognosis.

The value of a symptom-limited treadmill or cycle ergometer graded exercise test (GXT) in evaluating and counseling patients on return-to-work status is well established.[24] First, the patient's responses can help assess prognosis. Second, measured or estimated peak MET capacity can be compared to the estimated aerobic requirements of the patient's job to assess expected relative energy demands.[25] For most patients, physical demands are considered appropriate if the 8-hour energy expenditure requirement averages less than or equal to 50% peak METs and peak job demands (e.g., 5–45 minutes) are within guidelines prescribed for a home exercise program (e.g., 80% peak METs or lower). Most job tasks require less than 5 METs.[24]

The GXT is the only type of exercise test needed to provide realistic advice on return-to-work status for the majority of cardiac patients. However, some patients may benefit from further functional testing if job demands differ substantially from that evaluated with the GXT, especially patients with borderline physical work capacity in relationship to the anticipated job demands, those with concomitant left ventricular dysfunction, and/or those concerned about resuming a physically demanding job. Job tasks that produce disproportionate myocardial demands compared to a GXT include those requiring static muscular contraction, work combined with temperature stress, and intermittent heavy work.[24] Typical physiologic responses include a greater pressor response to work involving a static muscular contraction, a progressive rise in heart rate and decrease in stroke volume over time for work in a hot environment, and a sudden increase in myocardial oxygen demands with intermittent heavy work.

Tests simulating the task(s) in question can be administered when insufficient information is available to determine a patient's ability to resume work within a reasonable degree of safety. For patients at risk for serious arrhythmias or ischemia on the job, ambulatory ECG monitoring may be considered. Specialized work simulators (e.g., Baltimore Therapeutic and Valpar work simulators) also are available,[26] although simple, inexpensive tests can be set up to evaluate types of work not evaluated with a GXT.[24] A weight-carrying test can be used to evaluate tolerance for light to heavy static work combined with light dynamic work and is typically performed to assess appropriateness for returning to occupational activities.

Measurements During Exercise Testing

Common variables assessed during clinical exercise testing include heart rate and blood pressure, ECG changes, subjective ratings, as well as signs and symptoms. Expired gases and ventilatory responses also are commonly evaluated during the exercise test, particularly in certain groups, such as heart failure and pulmonary disease patients.

HEART RATE AND BLOOD PRESSURE

Heart rate and blood pressure should be measured before, during, and after the graded exercise test. Table 5-2 indicates the recommended frequency and

TABLE 5-2. Recommended Monitoring Intervals Associated with Exercise Testing*

Variable	Before Exercise Test	During the Test	After Exercise Test
ECG	Monitored continuously; recorded supine position and posture of exercise	Monitored continuously; recorded during the last 15 sec of each stage (interval protocol) or the last 15 sec of each 2 min time period (ramp protocols)	Monitored continuously; recorded immediately post-exercise, during the last 15 sec of first minute of recovery, and then every 2 min thereafter
HR‡	Monitored continuously; recorded supine position and posture of exercise	Monitored continuously; recorded during the last 5 sec of each minute	Monitored continuously; recorded during the last 5 sec of each minute
BP†‡	Measured and recorded in supine position and posture of exercise	Measured and recorded during the last 45 sec of each stage (interval protocol) or the last 45 sec of each 2 min time period (ramp protocols)	Measured and recorded immediately postexercise and then every 2 min thereafter
Signs and symptoms	Monitored - continuously; recorded as observed	Monitored continuously; recorded as observed	Monitored continuously; recorded as observed
RPE	Explain scale	Recorded during the last 5 sec of each minute	Obtain peak exercise value then not measured in recovery
Gas exchange	Baseline reading to assure proper operational status	Measured continuously	Generally not needed in recovery

*See Reference 44: Adapted, by permission, from Brubaker PH, Kaminsky LA, Whaley MH. Coronary Artery Disease: Champaign, IL: Human Kinetics 2002:182.

†Notes: An unchanged or decreasing systolic blood pressure with increasing workloads should be retaken (i.e., verified immediately).

‡In addition BP and HR should be assessed and recorded whenever adverse symptoms or abnormal ECG changes occur.

Abbreviations: HR, heart rate; BP, blood pressure; RPE, ratings of perceived exertion; sec, seconds.

sequence of these measures. A standardized procedure should be adopted for each laboratory so that baseline measures can be assessed more accurately when repeat testing is performed.

Although numerous devices have been developed to automate blood pressure measurements during exercise, they are generally prone to artifact, thus manual measurements remain the preferred method. Boxes 3-4 and 5-1 suggest methods

---

BOX 5-1 | Potential Sources of Error in Blood Pressure Assessment

- Inaccurate sphygmomanometer
- Improper cuff size
- Auditory acuity of technician
- Rate of inflation or deflation of cuff pressure
- Experience of technician
- Reaction time of technician
- Faulty equipment
- Improper stethoscope placement or pressure
- Background noise
- Allowing patient to hold treadmill handrails or flex elbow
- Certain physiologic abnormalities (e.g., damaged brachial artery, subclavian steal syndrome, arteriovenous fistula)

---

for blood pressure assessment at rest and potential sources of error during exercise, respectively. If systolic blood pressure appears to be decreasing with increasing exercise intensity, it should be retaken immediately.[27] If a drop in systolic blood pressure of 10 mm Hg or more occurs with an increase in work rate, or if it drops below the value obtained in the same position before testing, the test should be stopped, particularly if accompanied by adverse signs or symptoms. (See Box 5-2 for test termination criteria.) Anxious patients who demonstrate a drop in systolic blood pressure during the onset of exercise, without corresponding signs and symptoms, do not warrant test termination.

ELECTROCARDIOGRAPHIC MONITORING

A high-quality ECG is of paramount importance in an exercise test. Proper skin preparation is essential for recording the electrocardiogram. It is important to lower the resistance at the skin–electrode interface and thereby improve the signal-to-noise ratio. The general areas for electrode placement should be shaved, if hair is present, and cleansed with an alcohol-saturated gauze pad. The superficial layer of skin then should be removed using light abrasion with fine-grain emery paper or gauze. The electrodes then are placed according to standardized anatomic landmarks (see Appendix C). Twelve leads are available; however, three leads, representing the inferior, anterior, and lateral distribution are routinely monitored throughout the test. Because electrodes placed on wrists and ankles obstruct exercise and cause artifact, the limb electrodes commonly are affixed to the torso at the base of the limbs for exercise testing.[28] Because torso leads may give a slightly different ECG configuration when compared with the standard 12-lead resting ECG, use of torso leads should be noted on the ECG.[23] Substantial breast tissue or abdominal adiposity may warrant modification of standard electrode placement to minimize movement artifact.

Signal processing techniques have made it possible to average ECG waveforms and remove noise, but caution is urged because signal averaging can actually distort

| BOX 5-2 | Indications for Terminating Exercise Testing* |

ABSOLUTE INDICATIONS
- Drop in systolic blood pressure of >10 mm Hg from baseline[†] blood pressure despite an increase in workload, when accompanied by other evidence of ischemia
- Moderately severe angina (defined as 3 on standard scale)
- Increasing nervous system symptoms (e.g., ataxia, dizziness, or near syncope)
- Signs of poor perfusion (cyanosis or pallor)
- Technical difficulties monitoring the ECG or systolic blood pressure
- Subject's desire to stop
- Sustained ventricular tachycardia
- ST elevation (+1.0 mm) in leads without diagnostic Q-waves (other than V_1 or aVR)

RELATIVE INDICATIONS
- Drop in systolic blood pressure of >10 mm Hg from baseline[†] blood pressure despite an increase in workload, in the absence of other evidence of ischemia
- ST or QRS changes such as excessive ST depression (>2 mm horizontal or downsloping ST-segment depression) or marked axis shift
- Arrhythmias other than sustained ventricular tachycardia, including multifocal PVCs, triplets of PVCs, supraventricular tachycardia, heart block, or bradyarrhythmias
- Fatigue, shortness of breath, wheezing, leg cramps, or claudication
- Development of bundle-branch block or intraventricular conduction delay that cannot be distinguished from ventricular tachycardia
- Increasing chest pain
- Hypertensive response (systolic blood pressure of >250 mm Hg and/or a diastolic blood pressure of >115 mm Hg).

*See reference 1: Modified from Gibbons RJ, Balady GJ, Bricker JT, et al. ACC/AHA 2002 Guideline Update for Exercise Testing; a report of the American College of Cardiology/American Heart Association Task Force on Practice Guidelines Committee on Exercise Testing, 2002. American College of Cardiology web site: www.acc.org/clinical/guidelines/exercise/dirIndex.htm

†Baseline refers to a measurement obtained immediately before the test and in the same posture as the test is being performed.

the signal.[29] Moreover, most manufacturers do not specify how such procedures modify the ECG. Therefore, it is important to consider the "real time" ECG data first, using filtered data to aid in the interpretation if no distortion is obvious.

SUBJECTIVE RATINGS AND SYMPTOMS

The measurement of perceptual responses during exercise testing can provide useful clinical information. Somatic ratings of perceived exertion (RPE) and/or specific symptomatic complaints (e.g., degree of chest pain, burning, discomfort, dyspnea, leg discomfort/pain) should be assessed routinely during clinical exercise tests. Patients are asked to provide subjective estimates during the last 5 seconds of each exercise stage (or every 2 minutes during Ramp protocols) either verbally or manually. For example, the individual can provide a number verbally or point to a number if a mouthpiece or face mask is being used. The exercise technician should state the number out loud to confirm the correct rating. Either the 6–20 category scale or the 0–10 category-ratio scale (see Chapter 4) may be used to assess RPE during exercise testing.[25] Before the start of the exercise test, the patient should be given clear and concise instructions for use of the selected scale. Generic instructions for explaining either scale are provided in Chapter 4.

Use of alternative rating scales that are specific to subjective symptoms are recommended when subjects become symptomatic during exercise testing. Frequently used scales for assessing the patients' level of angina, claudication, and/or dyspnea are as follows:

Angina

1. Mild, barely noticeable
2. Moderate, bothersome
3. Moderately severe, very uncomfortable
4. Most severe or intense pain ever experienced

Claudication

1. Definite discomfort or pain, but only of initial or modest levels (established, but minimal)
2. Moderate discomfort or pain from which the patients attention can be diverted (e.g., by conversation)
3. Intense pain (short of grade 4) from which the patients attention cannot be diverted
4. Excruciating and unbearable pain

Dyspnea

1. Light, barely noticeable
2. Moderate, bothersome
3. Moderately severe, very uncomfortable
4. Most severe or intense dyspnea ever experienced

In general, reaching a rating of 3 on the angina scale or a degree of chest discomfort that would cause the patient to stop normal daily activities, are reasons to terminate the exercise test. However, higher levels of dyspnea or claudication may be acceptable during the exercise test.[30]

GAS EXCHANGE AND VENTILATORY RESPONSES

Because of the inaccuracies associated with estimating oxygen consumption and METs from work rate (i.e., treadmill speed and grade), many laboratories directly measure expired gases. The direct measurement of $\dot{V}O_2$ has been shown to be more reliable and reproducible than estimated values from treadmill or cycle ergometer work rate. Peak $\dot{V}O_2$ is the most accurate measurement of functional capacity and is a useful index of overall cardiopulmonary health.[8] In addition, the measurement of $\dot{V}O_2$, carbon dioxide ($\dot{V}CO_2$) and the subsequent calculation of the respiratory exchange ratio (RER) can be used to determine total energy expenditure and specific substrate contribution during physical activity. The measurement of minute ventilation also should be collected whenever gas exchange responses are measured. Measurement of gas exchange and ventilation is not necessary for all clinical exercise testing, but the additional information can provide useful physiologic data. Because heart and lung diseases frequently manifest as ventilatory or gas exchange abnormalities during exercise, an integrated analysis of these measures can be useful for differential diagnosis.[8] Furthermore, collection of gas exchange and ventilatory responses are increasingly being used in clinical trials to objectively assess the response to specific interventions. Situations in which gas exchange and ventilation measurements are appropriate include the following:[1]

- When a precise cardiopulmonary response to a specific therapeutic intervention is required
- When the etiology of exercise limitation or dyspnea is uncertain
- When evaluation of exercise capacity in patients with heart failure is used to assist in the estimation of prognosis and assess the need for transplantation
- When a precise cardiopulmonary response is needed within a research context
- When assisting in the development of an appropriate exercise prescription for cardiac and/or pulmonary rehabilitation

BLOOD GASES

Pulmonary disease should be considered in patients who exhibit with dyspnea on exertion. As such, it is also important to measure gas partial pressures in these patients because oxygen desaturation may occur during exertion. Although measurement of P_aO_2 and P_aCO_2 from arterial blood has been the standard in the past, the availability of oximetry has replaced the need to routinely draw arterial blood in most patients. In patients with pulmonary disease, measurements of oxygen saturation (S_aO_2) from oximetry at rest correlate reasonably well with S_aO_2 measured from arterial blood (95% confidence limits are $\pm$ 3% to 5% saturation).[31] Carboxyhemoglobin (COHb) levels greater than 4% and black skin may adversely affect the accuracy of pulse oximeters,[32,33] and most oximeters are inaccurate at an S_aO_2 of 85% or less. Arterial blood gases may be obtained if clinically warranted.

INDICATIONS FOR EXERCISE TEST TERMINATION

The absolute and relative indications for termination of an exercise test are listed in Box 5-2. Absolute indications are unambiguous, whereas relative indications sometimes may be superseded by clinical judgment.

Postexercise Period

If maximal sensitivity is to be achieved with an exercise test, patients should be placed supine during the postexercise period,[34] although it is advantageous to

BOX 5-3	Cognitive Skills Required to Competently Supervise Exercise Tests*

- Knowledge of appropriate indications for exercise testing
- Knowledge of alternative physiologic cardiovascular tests
- Knowledge of appropriate contraindications, risks, and risk assessment of testing
- Knowledge to promptly recognize and treat complications of exercise testing
- Competence in cardiopulmonary resuscitation and successful completion of an American Heart Association–sponsored course in advance cardiovascular life support and renewal on a regular basis
- Knowledge of various exercise protocols and indications for each
- Knowledge of basic cardiovascular and exercise physiology, including hemodynamic response to exercise
- Knowledge of cardiac arrhythmia and the ability to recognize and treat serious arrhythmias
- Knowledge of cardiovascular drugs and how they can affect exercise performance, hemodynamics, and the electrocardiogram
- Knowledge of the effects of age and disease on hemodynamic and the electrocardiographic response to exercise
- Knowledge of principles and details of exercise testing, including proper lead placement and skin preparation
- Knowledge of endpoints of exercise testing and indications to terminate exercise testing

*See reference 35: Adapted from Rodgers GP, Ayanian JZ, Balady GJ, et al. American College of Cardiology/American Heart Association clinical competance statement on stress testing. Circulation 2000;102:1726–1738.

record about 10 seconds of ECG data while the patient is in the upright position immediately after exercise for ECG clarity at peak exercise heart rate. Having the patient perform a cool-down walk after the test may decrease the risk of hypotension but can attenuate the magnitude of ST-segment depression. When the test is being performed for nondiagnostic purposes, an active cool-down usually is preferable; for example, slow walking (1.0–1.5 mi·h^{-1}) or continued cycling against minimal resistance. Monitoring should continue for at least 5 minutes after exercise or until ECG changes return to baseline and significant signs and symptoms resolve. Hemodynamic variables (heart rate and blood pressure) also should return to near-baseline levels before discontinuation of monitoring. ST-segment changes that occur only during the postexercise period are currently recognized to be an important diagnostic part of the test.[35] In addition, the rate in which heart rate recovers from exercise recently has been demonstrated to be an important prognostic marker and is discussed in Chapter 6.[36,37] In patients who are severely dyspneic, the supine posture may exacerbate the condition, and sitting may be a more appropriate posture.

Exercise Testing With Imaging Modalities

Cardiac imaging modalities are indicated when ECG changes from standard exercise testing are nondiagnostic, it is important to quantify the extent and distribution of myocardial ischemia, or a positive or negative exercise ECG needs to be confirmed.

EXERCISE ECHOCARDIOGRAPHY

Imaging modalities such as echocardiography can be combined with exercise ECG in an attempt to increase the sensitivity and specificity of stress testing, as well as to determine the extent of myocardium at risk as a result of ischemia. Echocardiographic images at rest are compared with those obtained during cycle ergometry or immediately after treadmill exercise. Images must be obtained within 1 to 2 minutes after exercise because abnormal wall motion begins to normalize after this point.

Rest and stress images are compared side-by-side in a cine-loop display that is gated during systole from the QRS complex. Myocardial contractility normally increases with exercise, whereas ischemia causes hypokinetic, dyskinetic, or akinetic wall motion to develop or worsen in the affected segments.[38] Advantages of exercise echocardiography over nuclear testing include a lower cost, the absence of exposure to low-level ionizing radiation, and a shorter amount of time for testing. Limitations include dependence on the operator for obtaining adequate, timely images. In addition, approximately 5% of patients have inadequate echocardiographic windows secondary to body habitus or lung interference,[38] although sonicated contrast agents can be helpful to enhance endocardial definition in these conditions.

EXERCISE NUCLEAR IMAGING

Exercise tests with nuclear imaging are performed with ECG monitoring. There are several different imaging protocols using only technetium (Tc)-99m or thallous (thallium) chloride-201. A common protocol with technetium is to perform rest images 30 to 60 minutes after intravenous administration of technetium followed by exercise (or pharmacologic stress) 1 to 3 hours later. Stress images are obtained 30 to 60 minutes after injecting technetium approximately 1 minute before completion of peak exercise. Comparison of the rest and stress images permit differentiation of fixed versus transient perfusion abnormalities.

Technetium-99m permits higher dosing with less radiation exposure than thallium and results in improved images that are sharper and have less artifact and attenuation. Consequently, technetium is the preferred imaging agent when performing tomographic images of the heart using single photon emission computed tomography (SPECT). SPECT images are obtained with a gamma camera, which rotates 180 degrees around the patient, stopping at preset angles to record the image. Cardiac images then are displayed in slices from three different axes to allow visualization of the heart in three dimensions. Thus, multiple myocardial segments can be viewed individually, without the overlap of segments that occurs with planar imaging.[39] Perfusion defects that are present during exercise but not seen at rest suggest myocardial ischemia. Perfusion defects that are present during exercise and persist at rest suggest previous MI or scar. The extent and distribution of ischemic myocardium can be identified in this manner.

The limitations of nuclear imaging include the exposure to low-level ionizing radiation. Furthermore, additional equipment and personnel are required for image acquisition and interpretation, including a nuclear technician to administer the radioactive isotope and acquire the images, and a physician trained in nuclear medicine to reconstruct and interpret the images.

PHARMACOLOGIC STRESS TESTING

Patients unable to undergo exercise stress testing for reasons such as deconditioning, peripheral vascular disease, orthopedic disabilities, neurologic disease, and concomitant illness often benefit from pharmacologic stress testing. The two most commonly used pharmacologic tests are dobutamine stress echocardiography and dipyridamole or adenosine stress nuclear scintigraphy. Indications for these tests include establishing a diagnosis of CAD, determining myocardial viability before revascularization, assessing prognosis after MI or in chronic angina, and evaluating cardiac risk preoperatively. Some protocols include light exercise in combination with pharmacologic infusion.

Dobutamine elicits wall motion abnormalities by increasing heart rate and therefore myocardial oxygen demand. It is infused intravenously and the dose is increased gradually until the maximal dose or an endpoint is achieved. Endpoints may include new or worsening wall-motion abnormalities, an adequate heart rate response, serious arrhythmias, angina, significant ST depression, intolerable side effects, and a significant increase or decrease in blood pressure. Atropine may be given if an adequate heart rate is not achieved or other endpoints have not been reached at peak dobutamine dose. Heart rate, blood pressure, ECG, and echocardiographic images are obtained throughout the infusion. Echocardiographic images are obtained similar to exercise echocardiography. A new or worsening wall motion abnormality constitutes a positive test for ischemia.[40]

Vasodilators such as dipyridamole and adenosine commonly are used to assess coronary perfusion in conjunction with a nuclear imaging agent. Dipyridamole and adenosine cause maximal coronary vasodilation in normal epicardial arteries, but not in stenotic segments. As a result, a coronary steal phenomenon occurs, with a relatively increased flow to normal arteries and a relatively decreased flow to stenotic arteries. Nuclear perfusion imaging under resting conditions is then compared with imaging obtained after coronary vasodilation.[40] Interpretation is similar to that for exercise nuclear testing.

ELECTRON BEAM COMPUTED TOMOGRAPHY

Although not an exercise test per se, electron beam computed tomography (EBCT) is being used increasingly to screen asymptomatic and high-risk individuals to detect CAD. EBCT is highly sensitive for detecting coronary artery calcium; and the presence and extent of calcium is closely related to atherosclerosis. However, calcium also may stabilize plaque, particularly in elderly people, among whom it is most often noted. Although EBCT has been highly promoted in the media, it has not been shown to produce test results that are superior to existing modalities. In studies reviewed by a recent AHA consensus writing panel,[41] EBCT had an overall predictive accuracy (percentage of subjects correctly classified) of approximately 70% for detecting CAD, which is no better than standard exercise testing. Because of this, the panel did not recommend the routine use of EBCT for screening individuals who are asymptomatic or suspected to be at risk for CAD.

Supervision of Exercise Testing

Although exercise testing generally is considered a safe procedure, both acute MI and cardiac arrest have been reported and can be expected to occur at a combined rate of up to 1 per 2,500 tests.[1] Accordingly, individuals who supervise exercise tests must have the cognitive and technical skills necessary to be competent to do so. The American College of Cardiology, American Heart Association, and American College of Physicians with broad involvement from other professional organizations involved with exercise testing (including the American College of Sports Medicine) have outlined those cognitive skills needed to competently supervise exercise tests.[35] These are presented in Box 5-3. In most cases, exercise tests can be supervised by properly trained exercise physiologists, physical therapists, nurses, physician assistants, or medical technicians who are working under the direct supervision of a physician; that is, the physician must be in the immediate vicinity and available for emergencies.[35] Several studies have demonstrated that the incidence of cardiovascular complications during exercise testing is no higher with experienced paramedical personnel than with direct physician supervision.[42,43] In situations where the patient is deemed to be at increased risk for an adverse event during exercise testing, the physician should be physically present in the exercise testing room to personally supervise the test. Such cases include, but are not limited to, patients undergoing symptom limited testing following recent acute events (i.e., acute coronary syndrome or myocardial infarction within 7–10 days), severe left ventricular dysfunction, severe valvular stenosis (e.g., aortic stenosis), or known complex arrhythmias.[35]

REFERENCES

1. Gibbons RJ, Balady GJ, Bricker J, et al. ACC/AHA 2002 guideline update for exercise testing: a report of the American College of Cardiology/American Heart Association Task Force on Practice Guidelines (Committee on Exercise Testing). 2002. American College of Cardiology web site. available at: www.acc.org/clinical/guidelines/exercise/dirIndex.htm
2. Wilson PW, D'Agostino RB, Levy D, et al. Prediction of coronary heart disease using risk factor categories. Circulation 1998;97:1837–1847.
3. Lewis WR, Amsterdam EA. Evaluation of the patient with 'rule out myocardial infarction.' Arch Intern Med 1996;156:41–45.
4. Amsterdam EA, Kirk JD, Diercks DB, et al. Immediate exercise testing to evaluate low-risk patients presenting to the emergency department with chest pain. J Am Coll Cardiol 2002;40:251–256.
5. Mark DB, Shaw L, Harrell FE Jr, et al. Prognostic value of a treadmill exercise score in outpatients with suspected coronary artery disease. N Engl J Med 1991;325:849–853.
6. Ashley E, Myers J, Froelicher V. Exercise testing scores as an example of better decisions through science. Med Sci Sports Exerc 2002;34:1391–1398.

7. Morris CK, Myers J, Froelicher VF, et al. Nomogram based on metabolic equivalents and age for assessing aerobic exercise capacity in men. J Am Coll Cardiol 1993;22:175–182.

8. American Thoracic Society and American College of Chest Physicians. American Thoracic Society/American College of Chest Physicians Statement on Cardiopulmonary Exercise Testing. Am J Respir Crit Care Med 2003;167:211–277.

9. Blair SN, Kohl HW 3rd, Paffenbarger RS Jr, et al. Physical fitness and all-cause mortality. A prospective study of healthy men and women. JAMA 1989;262:2395–2401.

10. Blair SN, Kohl HW 3rd, Barlow CE, et al. Changes in physical fitness and all-cause mortality. A prospective study of healthy and unhealthy men. JAMA 1995;273:1093–1098.

11. Vanhees L, Fagard R, Thijs L, et al. Prognostic significance of peak exercise capacity in patients with coronary artery disease. J Am Coll Cardiol 1994;23:358–363.

12. Myers J, Prakash M, Froelicher V, et al. Exercise capacity and mortality among men referred for exercise testing. N Engl J Med 2002;346:793–801.

13. Dorn J, Naughton J, Imamura D, et al. Results of a multicenter randomized clinical trial of exercise and long-term survival in myocardial infarction patients: the National Exercise and Heart Disease Project (NEHDP). Circulation 1999;100:1764–1769.

14. Hambrecht RP, Schuler GC, Muth T, et al. Greater diagnostic sensitivity of treadmill versus cycle exercise testing of asymptomatic men with coronary artery disease. Am J Cardiol 1992;70:141–146.

15. Myers J, Buchanan N, Walsh D, et al. Comparison of the ramp versus standard exercise protocols. J Am Coll Cardiol 1991;17:1334–1342.

16. Pollock ML, Wilmore JH, Fox SM. Exercise in Health and Disease: Evaluation and Prescription for Prevention and Rehabilitation. Philadelphia: WB Saunders, 1990.

17. Franklin BA. Exercise testing, training and arm ergometry. Sports Med 1985;2:100–119.

18. Balady GJ, Weiner DA, McCabe CH, et al. Value of arm exercise testing in detecting coronary artery disease. Am J Cardiol 1985;55:37–39.

19. Myers J, Buchanan N, Smith D, et al. Individualized ramp treadmill. Observations on a new protocol. Chest 1992;101:236S–241S.

20. Kaminsky LA, Whaley MH. Evaluation of a new standardized ramp protocol: the BSU/Bruce Ramp protocol. J Cardiopulm Rehabil 1998;18:438–444.

21. Buchfuhrer MJ, Hansen JE, Robinson TE, et al. Optimizing the exercise protocol for cardiopulmonary assessment. J Appl Physiol 1983;55:1558–1564.

22. Balady GJ, Weiner DA, Rose L, et al. Physiologic responses to arm ergometry exercise relative to age and gender. J Am Coll Cardiol 1990;16:130–135.

23. Hollingsworth V, Bendick P, Franklin B, et al. Validity of arm ergometer blood pressures immediately after exercise. Am J Cardiol 1990;65:1358–1360.

24. Sheldahl LM, Wilke NA, Tristani FE. Evaluation and training for resumption of occupational and leisure-time physical activities in patients after a major cardiac event. Med Exerc Nutr Health 1995;4: 273–289.

25. Ainsworth BE, Haskell WL, Whitt MC, et al. Compendium of physical activities: an update of activity codes and MET intensities. Med Sci Sports Exerc 2000;32:S498–S516.

26. Wilke NA, Sheldahl LM, Dougherty SM, et al. Baltimore Therapeutic Equipment work simulator: energy expenditure of work activities in cardiac patients. Arch Phys Med Rehabil 1993;74:419–424.

27. Dubach P, Froelicher VF, Klein J, et al. Exercise-induced hypotension in a male population. Criteria, causes, and prognosis. Circulation 1988;78:1380–1387.

28. Mason RE, Likar I. A new system of multiple-lead exercise electrocardiography. Am Heart J 1966; 71:196–205.

29. Milliken JA, Abdollah H, Burggraf GW. False-positive treadmill exercise tests due to computer signal averaging. Am J Cardiol 1990;65:946–948.

30. Myers JN. Perception of chest pain during exercise testing in patients with coronary artery disease. Med Sci Sports Exerc 1994;26:1082–1086.

31. Ries AL, Farrow JT, Clausen JL. Accuracy of two ear oximeters at rest and during exercise in pulmonary patients. Am Rev Respir Dis 1985;132:685–689.

32. Zeballos RJ, Weisman IM. Reliability of noninvasive oximetry in black subjects during exercise and hypoxia. Am Rev Respir Dis 1991;144:1240–1244.

33. Orenstein DM, Curtis SE, Nixon PA, et al. Accuracy of three pulse oximeters during exercise and hypoxemia in patients with cystic fibrosis. Chest 1993;104:1187–1190.

34. Lachterman B, Lehmann KG, Abrahamson D, et al. "Recovery only" ST-segment depression and the predictive accuracy of the exercise test. Ann Intern Med 1990;112:11–16.

35. Rodgers GP, Ayanian JZ, Balady G, et al. American College of Cardiology/American Heart Association Clinical Competence Statement on Stress Testing: A Report of the American College of Cardiology/American Heart Association/American College of Physicians-American Society of Internal Medicine Task Force on Clinical Competence. Circulation 2000;102:1726–1738.
36. Cole CR, Blackstone EH, Pashkow FJ, et al. Heart-rate recovery immediately after exercise as a predictor of mortality. N Engl J Med 1999;341:1351–1357.
37. Shetler K, Marcus R, Froelicher VF, et al. Heart rate recovery: validation and methodologic issues. J Am Coll Cardiol 2001;38:1980–1987.
38. Armstrong W, Marcovitz PA. Stress echocardiography. In: Braunwald E, ed. Heart Disease Updates. Philadelphia: WB Saunders, 1993:1–10.
39. Ritchie JL, Bateman TM, Bonow RO. Guidelines for clinical use of cardiac radionuclide imaging. Report of the American College of Cardiology/American Heart Association Task Force on Assessment of Diagnostic and Therapeutic Cardiovascular Procedures (Committee on Radionuclide Imaging, developed in conjunction with the American Society of Nuclear Cardiology). J Am Coll Cardiol 1995:521–547.
40. Poldermans D, Fioretti PM, Forster T, et al. Dobutamine stress echocardiography for assessment of perioperative cardiac risk in patients undergoing major vascular surgery. Circulation 1993;87:1506–1512.
41. O'Rourke RA, Brundage BH, Froelicher VF, et al. American College of Cardiology/American Heart Association Expert Consensus document on electron-beam computed tomography for the diagnosis and prognosis of coronary artery disease. Circulation 2000;102:126–140.
42. Franklin BA, Gordon S, Timmis GC, et al. Is direct physician supervision of exercise stress testing routinely necessary? Chest 1997;111:262–265.
43. Knight JA, Laubach CA Jr, Butcher RJ, et al. Supervision of clinical exercise testing by exercise physiologists. Am J Cardiol 1995;75:390–391.
44. Brubaker PH, Kaminsky LA, Whaley MH. Coronary Artery Disease. Champaign, IL: Human Kinetics, 2002:182.

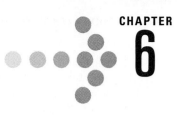

Interpretation of Clinical Exercise Test Data

This chapter addresses the interpretation and clinical significance of exercise test results, with specific reference to screening for coronary artery disease (CAD), hemodynamic electrocardiographic (ECG) gas exchange and ventilatory responses, as well as the diagnostic and prognostic value of the exercise test.

Exercise Testing As a Screening Tool for Coronary Artery Disease

The probability of a patient having CAD cannot be estimated accurately from the exercise test result and the diagnostic characteristics of the test alone. It also depends on the likelihood of the patient having disease before the test is administered. Bayes theorem states that the posttest probability of a patient having disease is determined by the disease probability *before* the test and the probability that the test will provide a true result. The probability of a patient having disease before the test is related, most importantly, to the patient's chest pain characteristics, but also to the patient's age, gender, and the presence of major risk factors for cardiovascular disease.

Exercise testing in individuals with known CAD (prior myocardial infarction, angiographically documented coronary stenoses, and/or prior coronary revascularization) is not regularly used for diagnostic purposes. However, the description of symptoms can be most helpful among individuals in whom the diagnosis is in question. Typical or definite angina (substernal chest discomfort that may radiate to the back, jaw, or arms; symptoms provoked by exertion or emotional stress and relieved by rest and/or nitroglycerin) makes the pretest probability so high that the test result does not dramatically change the probability of underlying CAD. Atypical angina (chest discomfort that lacks one of the mentioned characteristics of typical angina) generally indicates an intermediate pretest likelihood of CAD in men more than 30 years old and women more than 50 years old (see Table 5-1).

The use of exercise testing in screening asymptomatic individuals, particularly among individuals without diabetes or other risk factors for coronary artery disease, is problematic in view of the low to very low pretest likelihood of CAD, even among symptom-free men and women more than 60 years old (see Table 5-1). Exercise testing as a part of routine health screening in apparently healthy individuals is not recommended.[1] Such testing can have potential adverse consequences (e.g., psychological, work and insurance status, costs for subsequent testing) by misclassifying a large percentage of those without CAD as having disease. Testing in asymptomatic persons with multiple risk factors may provide some useful information, although this practice cannot be strongly recommended based on available data.[1] It is likewise difficult to choose a chronological age beyond which exercise testing becomes valuable as a screening tool prior to beginning an exercise program because physiologic age often differs from chronological age. In general, the guidelines presented in Table 2-1 are recommended if the exercise is more strenuous than brisk walking. The potential ramifications resulting from mass screening must be considered and the results of such testing must be applied using the predictive model and Bayesian analyses. Test results should be considered as probability statements and not as absolutes.

Interpretation of Responses to Graded Exercise Testing

Before interpreting clinical test data, it is important to consider the purpose of the test (e.g., diagnostic or prognostic) and patient conditions that may influence the exercise test or its interpretation. Medical conditions influencing test interpretation include orthopedic limitations, pulmonary disease, obesity, neurologic disorders, and significant deconditioning. Medication effects (see Appendix A) and resting ECG abnormalities also must be considered, especially resting ST-segment changes secondary to conduction defects, left ventricular hypertrophy, and other factors that may contribute to spurious ST-segment depression.

Although total body and myocardial oxygen consumption are directly related, the relationship between these variables can be altered by exercise training, drugs, and disease. For example, exercise-induced myocardial ischemia may cause left ventricular dysfunction, exercise intolerance, and a hypotensive blood pressure response. Although the severity of symptomatic ischemia is inversely related to exercise capacity, left ventricular ejection fraction does not correlate well with exercise tolerance.[2,3]

The objective of exercise testing is to evaluate quantitatively and accurately the following variables. Each is described in the following sections and summarized in Box 6-1:

- Hemodynamics: assessed by the heart rate (HR) and systolic/diastolic blood pressure (SBP/DBP) responses
- ECG waveforms: especially ST-segment displacement and supraventricular and ventricular dysrhythmias
- Limiting clinical signs or symptoms
- Gas exchange and ventilatory responses (e.g., $\dot{V}O_{2max}$, $\dot{V}_E$)
- Responses to exercise tests are useful in evaluating the need for and effectiveness of various types of therapeutic interventions.

HEART RATE RESPONSE

Maximal heart rate (HR_{max}) may be predicted from age using any of several published equations.[4] The relationship between age and HR_{max} for a large sample of subjects is well established; however, interindividual variability is high (standard deviation, 10–12 beats·min^{-1}). As a result, there is potential for considerable error in the use of methods that extrapolate submaximal test data to an age-predicted HR_{max}. Aerobic capacity, anthropometric measures such as height and weight, and body composition do not independently influence HR_{max}. The inabil-

BOX 6-1	**Electrocardiographic, Cardiorespiratory, and Hemodynamic Responses to Exercise Testing and Their Clinical Significance**

Variable	**Clinical Significance**
ST-segment depression (ST ↓)	An abnormal ECG response is defined as ≥1.0 mm of horizontal or downsloping ST ↓ at 80 msec beyond the J point, suggesting myocardial ischemia.
ST-segment elevation (ST ↑)	ST ↑ in leads displaying a previous Q-wave MI almost always reflects an aneurysm or wall motion abnormality. In the absence of significant Q waves, exercise-induced ST ↑ often is associated with a fixed high-grade coronary stenosis.
Supraventricular dysrhythmias	Isolated atrial ectopic beats or short runs of SVT commonly occur during exercise testing and do not appear to have any diagnostic or prognostic significance for CAD.
Ventricular dysrhythmias	The suppression of resting ventricular dysrhythmias during exercise *does not* exclude the presence of underlying CAD; conversely, PVCs that increase in frequency, complexity, or both do not necessarily signify underlying ischemic heart disease. Complex ventricular ectopy, including paired or multiform PVCs, and runs of ventricular tachycardia (≥3 successive beats), are likely to be associated with significant CAD and/or a poor prognosis if they occur in conjunction with signs and/or symptoms of myocardial ischemia, or in patients with a history of sudden cardiac death, cardiomyopathy, or valvular heart disease. Frequent ventricular ectopy during recovery has been found to be a better predictor of mortality than ventricular ectopy that occurs only during exercise.
Heart rate (HR)	The normal HR response to progressive exercise is a relatively linear increase, corresponding to 10 ± 2 beats·MET^{-1} for inactive subjects. Chronotropic incompetence may be signified by:

1. A peak exercise HR that is >2 SD (>20 beats·min^{-1}) below the age-predicted maximal HR for subjects who are limited by volitional fatigue and are not taking β-blockers

2. A chronotropic index (CI) <0.8;[39] where CI is calculated as the percent of heart rate reserve to percent metabolic reserve achieved at any test stage ▶

▶ **Box 6-1, continued**

Systolic blood pressure (SBP)	The normal response to exercise is a progressive increase in SBP, typically 10 ± 2 mm Hg·MET^{-1}, with a possible plateau at peak exercise. Exercise testing-should be discontinued with SBP values of >250 mm Hg. Exertional hypotension (SBP that fails to rise or falls [>10 mm Hg]) may signify myocardial ischemia and/or LV dysfunction. Maximal exercise SBP of <140 mm Hg suggests a poor prognosis.
Diastolic blood pressure (DBP)	The normal response to exercise is no change or a decrease in DBP. A DBP of >115 mm Hg is considered an endpoint for exercise testing.
Anginal symptoms	Can be graded on a scale of 1 to 4, corresponding to perceptible but mild, moderate, moderately severe, and severe, respectively. A rating of 3 (moderately severe) generally should be used as an endpoint for exercise testing.
Aerobic fitness	Average values of $\dot{V}O_{2max}$, expressed as METs, expected in healthy sedentary men and women can be predicted from the following regressions:[40] Men = (57.8–0.445 [age])/3.5; Women = (41.2–0.343 [age])/3.5. Also, see Table 4-8 for age-specific $\dot{V}O_{2max}$ norms.

Abbreviations: ECG, electrocardiographic; MI, myocardial infarction; SVT, supraventricular tachycardia; PVC, premature ventricular contraction; CAD, coronary artery disease; VT, ventricular tachycardia; HR, heart rate; MET, metabolic equivalent; SD, standard deviation; LV, left ventricular; SBP, systolic blood pressure; DBP, diastolic blood pressure; $\dot{V}O_{2max}$, maximal oxygen uptake.

ity to appropriately increase heart rate during exercise (chronotropic incompetence) is associated with the presence of heart disease and increased mortality.[5,6] A delayed decrease in the heart rate during the first minute of recovery (<12 bpm decrease) after a symptom-limited maximal exercise test is also a powerful predictor of overall mortality.[7]

Achievement of age-predicted maximal heart rate should not be used as an absolute test endpoint or as an indication that effort has been maximal, because of its high intersubject variability. The clinical indications for stopping an exercise test are presented in Box 5-2. Good judgment on the part of the physician and/or supervising staff remains the most important criteria for terminating an exercise test.

BLOOD PRESSURE RESPONSE

The normal blood pressure response to dynamic upright exercise consists of a progressive increase in SBP, no change or a slight decrease in DBP, and a widening of the pulse pressure. The following are key points concerning interpretation of the blood pressure response to progressive dynamic exercise:

- A drop in SBP (>10 mm Hg from baseline SBP despite an increase in workload), or failure of SBP to increase with increased workload, is considered an abnormal test response. Exercise-induced decreases in SBP (exertional hypotension) may occur in patients with CAD, valvular heart disease, cardiomyopathies, and serious dysrhythmias. Occasionally, patients without clinically significant heart disease demonstrate exertional hypotension caused by antihypertensive therapy, prolonged strenuous exercise, and vasovagal responses. However, exertional hypotension has been shown to correlate with myocardial ischemia, left ventricular dysfunction, and an increased risk of subsequent cardiac events.[8,9] In some cases this response is improved after coronary bypass surgery.[10]
- The normal postexercise response is a progressive decline in SBP. During passive recovery in an upright posture, SBP may decrease abruptly because of peripheral pooling (and usually normalizes on resuming the supine position). SBP may remain below pretest resting values for several hours after the test. DBP also may drop during the postexercise period.
- In patients on vasodilators, calcium channel blockers, angiotensin-converting enzyme inhibitors, and α- and β-adrenergic blockers, the blood pressure response to exercise is variably attenuated and cannot be accurately predicted in the absence of clinical test data.
- Although maximal heart rates are comparable for men and women, men generally have higher systolic blood pressures (~20 ± 5 mm Hg) during maximal treadmill testing. However, the gender difference is no longer apparent after 70 years of age. A systolic blood pressure >250 mm Hg or a diastolic blood pressure >115 mm Hg should result in test termination.
- The rate-pressure product or double product (SBP × HR) is an indicator of myocardial oxygen demand.[11] Signs and symptoms of ischemia generally occur at a reproducible double product.

ELECTROCARDIOGRAPH WAVEFORMS

Appendix C provides information to aid in the interpretation of resting and exercise electrocardiograms. Additional information is provided here with respect to common exercise-induced changes in ECG variables. The normal ECG response to exercise includes the following:

- Minor and insignificant changes in P wave morphology
- Superimposition of the P and T waves of successive beats
- Increases in septal Q wave amplitude
- Slight decreases in R wave amplitude
- Increases in T wave amplitude (although wide variability exists among subjects)
- Minimal shortening of the QRS duration

- Depression of the J point
- Rate-related shortening of the QT interval

However, some changes in ECG wave morphology may be indicative of underlying pathology. For example, although QRS duration tends to decrease slightly with exercise (and increasing HR) in normal subjects, it may increase in patients with either angina or left ventricular dysfunction. Exercise-induced P wave changes are rarely seen and are of questionable significance. Many factors affect R-wave amplitude; consequently, such changes during exercise have no independent predictive power.[12]

ST-Segment Displacement

ST-segment changes are widely accepted criteria for myocardial ischemia and injury. The interpretation of ST segments may be affected by the resting ECG configuration (e.g., bundle-branch blocks, left ventricular hypertrophy) and pharmacologic agents (e.g., digitalis therapy). There may be J-point depression and tall peaked T-waves at high exercise intensities and during recovery in normal subjects. Depression of the J point that leads to marked ST-segment upsloping is caused by competition between normal repolarization and delayed terminal depolarization forces rather than to ischemia.[13] Exercise-induced myocardial ischemia may be manifested by different types of ST-segment changes on the ECG, as shown in Figure 6-1.

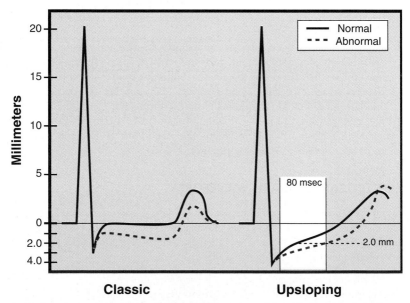

FIGURE 6-1. ST segment changes during exercise. Classic ST segment depression (first complex) is defined as a horizontal of downsloping ST segment that is ≥1 mm below the baseline at 80 msec past the J point. Slowly upsloping ST-segment depression (second complex) should be considered a borderline response, and added emphasis should be placed on other clinical and exercise variables.

ST-Segment Elevation

- ST-segment elevation (early repolarization) may be seen in the normal resting ECG. Increasing HR may cause these elevated ST segments to return to the isoelectric line.
- Exercise-induced ST-segment elevation in leads displaying a previous Q wave infarction may be indicative of wall motion abnormalities or ventricular aneurysm.[14]
- Exercise-induced ST-segment elevation on an otherwise normal ECG (except in aVR or V_{1-2}) generally indicates significant myocardial ischemia, and localizes the ischemia to a specific area of myocardium.[15]
- ST-segment elevation indicates myocardial injury (i.e., an acute transmural infarction) when followed by the evolution of significant Q-waves.

ST-Segment Depression

- ST-segment depression (depression of the J point and the slope at 80 msec past the J point) is the most common manifestation of exercise-induced myocardial ischemia.
- Horizontal or downsloping ST-segment depression is more indicative of myocardial ischemia than is upsloping depression.
- The standard criterion for a positive test is ≥1.0 mm (1 mV) of horizontal or downsloping ST segment 80 msec after the J point.
- Slowly upsloping ST-segment depression should be considered a borderline response, and added emphasis should be placed on other clinical and exercise variables.
- ST-segment depression does not localize ischemia to a specific area of myocardium.
- The more leads with (apparent) ischemic ST-segment shifts, the more severe the disease.
- Significant ST-segment depression occurring only in recovery likely represents a true positive response, and should be considered an important diagnostic finding.[16]
- In the presence of baseline ST abnormalities on the resting ECG, additional ST segment depression during exercise is less specific for myocardial ischemia. In patients with left bundle-branch block, ST-segment abnormalities that develop during exercise are uninterpretable with respect to evidence of myocardial ischemia.[17] In right bundle-branch block, exercise-induced ST-segment depression in the anterior precordial leads (V_1, V_2, and V_3) should not be used to diagnose ischemia; however, ST-segment changes in the lateral leads (V_4, V_5, and V_6) may be indicative of ischemia even in the presence of this conduction abnormality.[17]
- Adjustment of the ST segment relative to the HR may provide additional diagnostic information. The ST/HR index is the ratio of the maximal ST segment change to the maximal change in HR from rest to peak exercise. An ST/HR index of ≥1.6 is defined as abnormal. The ST/HR slope evaluates the maximal slope relating the amount of the ST segment depression to HR during exercise. An ST/HR slope of >2.4 mV/beat/min is defined as abnormal. Several studies have addressed the diagnostic value of these ST/HR variables,[18–20] but

the findings have been inconsistent and preclude a strong recommendation regarding their utility.

ST-Segment Normalization or Absence of Change

- Ischemia may be manifested by normalization of resting ST segments. ECG abnormalities at rest, including T-wave inversion and ST-segment depression, may return to normal during anginal symptoms and during exercise in some patients.[3,21]

Dysrhythmias

Exercise-associated dysrhythmias occur in healthy subjects as well as patients with cardiac disease. Increased sympathetic drive and changes in extracellular and intracellular electrolytes, pH, and oxygen tension contribute to disturbances in myocardial and conducting tissue automaticity and reentry, which are major mechanisms of dysrhythmias.

Supraventricular Dysrhythmias

Isolated premature atrial contractions are common and require no special precautions. Atrial flutter or atrial fibrillation may occur in organic heart disease or may reflect endocrine, metabolic, or drug effects. Sustained supraventricular tachycardia occasionally is induced by exercise and may require pharmacologic treatment or electroconversion if discontinuation of exercise fails to abolish the rhythm. Patients who experience paroxysmal atrial tachycardia may be evaluated by repeating the exercise test after appropriate treatment.

Ventricular Dysrhythmias

Isolated premature ventricular complexes or contractions (PVCs) occur during exercise in 30% to 40% of healthy subjects and in 50% to 60% of patients with CAD. The presence of ventricular ectopy during exercise testing was observed in a large series of patients undergoing exercise testing in a single clinical laboratory. Among 29,244 patients, 3% had frequent ventricular ectopy (>7 PVCs/minute) only during exercise, 2% during exercise and recovery, and 2% only during recovery. Frequent isolated PVCs were observed in 3%, ventricular bigeminy in 1%, each of ventricular trigeminy, couplets and triplet in <1%, nonsustained ventricular tachycardia (<30 seconds in duration) in 0.6%, and sustained ventricular tachycardia (>30 seconds in duration) in 0.01%[24]. In some individuals, graded exercise induces PVCs, whereas in others it reduces their occurrence. Criteria for terminating exercise tests based on ventricular ectopy include sustained ventricular tachycardia, as well as multifocal PVCs, and triplets of PVCs. The decision to terminate an exercise test should also be influenced by simultaneous evidence of myocardial ischemia and/or adverse signs or symptoms (see Box 5-2).

LIMITING SIGNS AND SYMPTOMS

Although patients with exercise-induced ST-segment depression can be asymptomatic, when concomitant angina occurs, the likelihood that the ECG changes result from CAD is significantly increased.[22] In addition, angina pectoris *without* ischemic ECG changes may be as predictive of CAD as ST-segment changes alone.[23] Both are currently considered independent variables that identify patients at increased risk for subsequent coronary events.

GAS EXCHANGE AND VENTILATORY RESPONSES

Gas exchange and ventilatory responses should be used to assess patient effort during an exercise test, especially when a reduction in maximal exercise capacity is suspected. Submaximal efforts from the patient can interfere with the interpretation of the test results and subsequent patient management. In the absence of untoward signs or symptoms, patients should be encouraged to give their best effort so that maximal exercise tolerance can be determined. Maximal or peak oxygen uptake ($\dot{V}O_{2peak}$) provides important information about cardiovascular fitness and prognosis. Population-specific nomograms (see Fig. 5-1) and/or population norms (see Table 4-8) may be used to compare $\dot{V}O_{2peak}$ with the expected value for a given age, gender, and activity status.

Various objective and subjective indicators can be used to confirm that a maximal effort has been elicited during graded exercise testing:

- Failure of HR to increase with further increases in exercise intensity.
- A plateau in oxygen uptake (or failure to increase oxygen uptake by 150 mL·min^1) with increased workload.[24] This criterion has fallen into some disfavor because a plateau is inconsistently seen during continuous graded exercise tests and is confused by various definitions and how data are sampled during exercise.[25]
- A respiratory exchange ratio >1.1; however, there is considerable interindividual variability in this response.
- A postexercise venous lactic acid concentration of >8 mmol also has been used; however, there is great interindividual variability in this response.
- A rating of perceived exertion >17 on the 6 to 20 scale or >9 on the 0 to 10 scale.

Gas exchange and ventilatory responses often are used in clinical settings as an estimation of the point where lactate accumulation in the blood occurs, sometimes referred to as the lactate or anaerobic threshold. Several different methods using both gas exchange and ventilatory responses have been proposed for the estimation of this point. These include the ventilatory equivalents method[26,27] and the V slope method.[28] Whichever method is used, it should be remembered that the use of any of these methods provides only an estimation and the use of these methods is controversial.[29,30] Because exercise beyond the lactate threshold is associated with metabolic acidosis, hyperventilation, and a reduced capacity to perform work, its estimation has evolved into a useful physiologic measurement when evaluating interventions in patients with heart and pulmonary disease as well as studying the limits of performance in healthy individuals.

In addition to estimating when blood lactate values begin to increase, maximal minute ventilation (VE_{max}) can be used in conjunction with the maximal voluntary ventilation (MVV) to determine if there is a ventilatory limitation to maximal exercise. A comparison between the VE_{max} and the MVV can be used when evaluating responses to a graded exercise test. The relationship between these measures, typically referred to as the ventilatory reserve, traditionally has been defined as the percentage of the MVV achieved at maximal exercise (i.e., the VE_{max}/MVV ratio). In most normal subjects this ratio ranges from 50% to 85%.[31] Patients with pulmonary disease typically have values >85%, indicative of a reduced ventilatory reserve and a possible pulmonary limitation to exercise.

Diagnostic Value of Exercise Testing

The diagnostic value of conventional exercise testing for the detection of CAD is influenced by the principles of conditional probability (Box 6-2). The factors that determine the predictive outcome of exercise testing (and other diagnostic tests) are the sensitivity and specificity of the test procedure and the prevalence of CAD in the population tested. Sensitivity and specificity determine how effective the test is in making correct diagnoses in individuals with and without disease, respectively. Disease prevalence is an important determinant of the predictive value of the test. Moreover, non-ECG criteria (e.g., duration of exercise or maximal MET level, hemodynamic responses, symptoms of angina or dyspnea) should be considered in the overall interpretation of exercise test results.

SENSITIVITY

Sensitivity refers to the percentage of patients tested with known CAD who demonstrate significant ST segment (i.e., positive) changes. Exercise ECG sensitivity for the detection of CAD usually is based on subsequent angiographically

---

BOX 6-2	**Sensitivity, Specificity, and Predictive Value of Diagnostic Graded Exercise Testing**

Sensitivity = TP/(TP + FN) = the percentage of patients with CAD who have a positive test

Specificity = TN/(TN + FP) = the percentage of patients without CAD who have a negative test

Predictive Value (positive test) = TP/(TP + FP) = the percentage of patients with a positive test result who have CAD

Predictive Value (negative test) = TN/(TN + FN) = the percentage of patients with a negative test who do not have CAD

Abbreviations: TP, true positive (positive exercise test and coronary artery disease [CAD]); FP, false positive (positive exercise test and no CAD); TN, true negative (negative exercise test and no CAD); FN, false negative (negative exercise test and CAD).

BOX 6-3	Causes of False-Negative Test Results

- Failure to reach an ischemic threshold
- Monitoring an insufficient number of leads to detect ECG changes
- Failure to recognize non-ECG signs and symptoms that may be associated with underlying coronary artery disease (CAD) (e.g., exertional hypotension)
- Angiographically significant CAD compensated by collateral circulation
- Musculoskeletal limitations to exercise preceding cardiac abnormalities
- Technical or observer error

determined coronary artery stenosis of 70% or more in at least one vessel. A true positive exercise test reveals ST-segment depression of 1.0 mm or more and correctly identifies a patient with CAD. False-negative test results show no or nondiagnostic ECG changes and fails to identify patients with underlying CAD.

Common factors that contribute to false-negative exercise tests are summarized in Box 6-3. Test sensitivity is decreased by inadequate myocardial stress, drugs that attenuate cardiac demands to exercise or reduce myocardial ischemia (e.g., β-blockers, nitrates, calcium channel blocking agents), and insufficient ECG lead monitoring. The use of right precordial leads along with the standard six left precordial leads during exercise electrocardiography may improve the sensitivity of exercise testing in the detection of CAD,[32] although this has not been demonstrated consistently. Preexisting ECG changes, such as left ventricular hypertrophy, left bundle-branch block, or the preexcitation syndrome (Wolff-Parkinson-White syndrome), limit the ability to interpret exercise-induced ST-segment changes as ischemic ECG responses.

SPECIFICITY

The specificity of exercise tests refers to the percentage of patients without CAD who demonstrate nonsignificant (i.e., negative) ST segment changes. A true negative test correctly identifies a person without CAD. Many conditions may cause abnormal exercise ECG responses in the absence of significant obstructive coronary artery disease (Box 6-4). Reported values for the specificity and sensitivity of exercise ECG testing vary because of differences in patient selection, test protocols, ECG criteria for a positive test, and the angiographic definition of CAD. In studies that controlled for these variables, the pooled results show a sensitivity of 68% and a specificity of 77%.[1]

PREDICTIVE VALUE

The predictive value of exercise testing is a measure of how accurately a test result (positive or negative) correctly identifies the presence or absence of CAD in tested patients. For example, the predictive value of a positive test is the percentage of those persons with an abnormal test who have CAD. Nevertheless, a test should not be classified as "negative" unless the patient has attained an ade-

BOX 6-4	Causes of Abnormal ST Changes in the Absence of Obstructive Coronary Artery Disease*

- Resting repolarization abnormalities (e.g., left bundle-branch block)
- Cardiac hypertrophy
- Accelerated conduction defects (e.g., Wolff-Parkinson-White syndrome)
- Digitalis
- Nonischemic cardiomyopathy
- Hypokalemia
- Vasoregulatory abnormalities
- Mitral valve prolapse
- Pericardial disorders
- Technical or observer error
- Coronary spasm in the absence of significant coronary artery disease
- Anemia
- Female gender

*Selected variables simply may be associated with rather than be causes of abnormal test results.

quate level of myocardial stress, generally defined as having achieved 85% or more of predicted maximal heart rate during the test. Predictive value cannot be estimated directly from a test's specificity or sensitivity because it depends on the prevalence of disease in the population being tested.

COMPARISON WITH IMAGING STRESS TESTS

The overall sensitivity and specificity of exercise echocardiography ranges from 74% to 97% and 64% to 94%, respectively, with higher sensitivities observed in patients with multivessel disease.[33] Exercise with concomitant nuclear imaging using technetium (Tc99m) agents has shown similar accuracy to those using thallous (thallium) chloride-201 agents in the detection of myocardial ischemia. For planar imaging, the sensitivity and specificity of technetium agents have been measured at 84% and 83%, compared with 83% and 88% for thallium agents. In single photon emission computed tomography (SPECT) imaging, the sensitivities and specificities were 90% and 93% for technetium agents, compared with 89% and 76% for thallium agents. In addition, when normal, reversible, and nonreversible segments scanned with technetium and thallium agents are compared, there is 88% agreement with planar and 92% agreement with SPECT imaging. The sensitivity and specificity are similar for planar and tomographic nuclear imaging.[34,35]

PROGNOSTIC APPLICATIONS OF THE EXERCISE TEST

Risk or prognostic evaluation is an important activity in medical practice on which many patient management decisions are based. In patients with CAD, several clinical factors contribute to patient outcome, including severity and stability of symptoms; left ventricular function; angiographic extent and severity of CAD; electrical stability of the myocardium; and the presence of other comorbid conditions. Unless cardiac catheterization and immediate coronary revascularization are indicated, an exercise test should be performed in persons with known or suspected CAD to assess risk of future cardiac events, and to assist in subsequent management decisions. As stated in Chapter 5, data derived from the exercise test are most useful when considered in the context of other clinical information. Important prognostic variables that can be derived from the exercise test are summarized in Box 6-1.

Use of the Veteran's Administration score[36] (validated for the male veteran population) and the Duke nomogram[37] (validated for the general population, including women) (Fig. 6-2) can be helpful when applied appropriately. The Duke nomogram does not appear to be valid in patients more than 75 years old.[38] Patients who recently have suffered an acute myocardial infarction and received thrombolytic

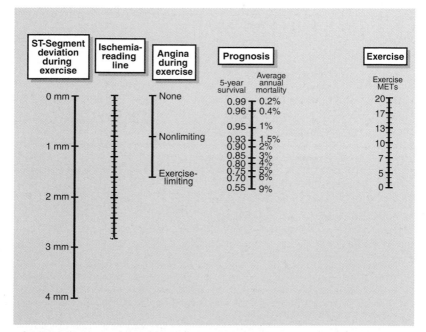

FIGURE 6-2. Duke Nomogram uses five steps to estimate prognosis for a given individual from the parameters of the Duke score. First, the observed amount of ST-depression is marked on the ST-segment deviation line. Second, the observed degree of angina is marked on the line for angina, and these two points are connected. Third, the point where this line intersects the ischemia reading line is noted. Fourth, the observed exercise tolerance is marked on the line for exercise capacity. Finally, the mark on the ischemia reading line is connected to the mark on the exercise capacity line, and the estimated 5-year survival or average annual mortality rate is read from the point at which this line intersects the prognosis scale.

therapy and/or have undergone coronary revascularization generally have a low subsequent cardiac event rate. Exercise testing still can provide prognostic information in this population, as well as assist in activity counseling and exercise prescription.

REFERENCES

1. Gibbons RJ, Balady GJ, Bricker J, et al. ACC/AHA 2002 guideline update for exercise testing: a report of the American College of Cardiology/American Heart Association Task Force on Practice Guidelines (Committee on Exercise Testing). 2002. American College of Cardiology web site. available at: www.acc.org/clinical/guidelines/exercise/dirIndex.htm.
2. Myers J, Froelicher VF. Hemodynamic determinants of exercise capacity in chronic heart failure. Ann Intern Med 1991;115:377–386.
3. McKirnan MD, Sullivan M, Jensen D, et al. Treadmill performance and cardiac function in selected patients with coronary heart disease. J Am Coll Cardiol 1984;3:253–261.
4. Londeree BR, Moeschberger ML. Influence of age and other factors on maximal heart rate. J Cardiac Rehab 1984;(4)44–49.
5. Ellestad MH. Chronotropic incompetence. The implications of heart rate response to exercise (compensatory parasympathetic hyperactivity?). Circulation 1996;93:1485–1487.
6. Lauer MS, Francis GS, Okin PM, et al. Impaired chronotropic response to exercise stress testing as a predictor of mortality. JAMA 1999;281:524–529.
7. Cole CR, Blackstone EH, Pashkow FJ, et al. Heart-rate recovery immediately after exercise as a predictor of mortality. N Engl J Med 1999;341:1351–1357.
8. Comess KA, Fenster PE. Clinical implications of the blood pressure response to exercise. Cardiology 1981;68:233–244.
9. Irving JB, Bruce RA, DeRouen TA. Variations in and significance of systolic pressure during maximal exercise (treadmill) testing. Am J Cardiol 1977;39:841–848.
10. Weiner DA, McCabe CH, Cutler SS, et al. Decrease in systolic blood pressure during exercise testing: reproducibility, response to coronary bypass surgery and prognostic significance. Am J Cardiol 1982;49:1627–1631.
11. Kitamura K, Jorgensen CR, Gobel FL, et al. Hemodynamic correlates of myocardial oxygen consumption during upright exercise. J Appl Physiol 1972;32:516–522.
12. Myers J, Ahnve S, Froelicher V, et al. Spatial R wave amplitude changes during exercise: relation with left ventricular ischemia and function. J Am Coll Cardiol 1985;6:603–608.
13. Mirvis DM, Ramanathan KB, Wilson JL. Regional blood flow correlates of ST segment depression in tachycardia-induced myocardial ischemia. Circulation 1986;73:365–373.
14. Bruce RA, Fisher LD, Pettinger M, et al. ST segment elevation with exercise: a marker for poor ventricular function and poor prognosis. Coronary Artery Surgery Study (CASS) confirmation of Seattle Heart Watch results. Circulation 1988;77:897–905.
15. Nostratian F, Froelicher VF. ST elevation during exercise testing: a review. Am J Cardiol 1989; 63:986–988.
16. Lachterman B, Lehmann KG, Detrano R, et al. Comparison of ST segment/heart rate index to standard ST criteria for analysis of exercise electrocardiogram. Circulation 1990;82:44–50.
17. Whinnery JE, Froelicher VF Jr, Longo MR Jr, et al. The electrocardiographic response to maximal treadmill exercise of asymptomatic men with right bundle branch block. Chest 1977;71:335–340.
18. Froelicher VF, Fearon WF, Ferguson CM, et al. Lessons learned from studies of the standard exercise ECG test. Chest 1999;116:1442–1451.
19. Okin PM, Kligfield P. Heart rate adjustment of ST segment depression and performance of the exercise electrocardiogram: a critical evaluation. J Am Coll Cardiol 1995;25:1726–1735.
20. Morise AP. Accuracy of heart rate-adjusted ST segments in populations with and without posttest referral bias. Am Heart J 1997;134(4):647–655.
21. Lavie CJ, Oh JK, Mankin HT, et al. Significance of T-wave pseudonormalization during exercise. A radionuclide angiographic study. Chest 1988;94:512–516.
22. Weiner DA, Ryan TJ, McCabe CH, et al. Exercise stress testing. Correlations among history of angina, ST-segment response and prevalence of coronary-artery disease in the Coronary Artery Surgery Study (CASS). N Engl J Med 1979;301:230–235.

23. Cole JP, Ellestad MH. Significance of chest pain during treadmill exercise: correlation with coronary events. Am J Cardiol 1978;41:227–232.
24. Taylor HL, Buskirk ER, Henschel A. Maximal oxygen uptake as an objective measure of cardiorespiratory performance. J Appl Physiol 1955;8:73–80.
25. Noakes TD. Challenging beliefs: ex Africa semper aliquid novi. Med Sci Sports Exerc 1997; 29:571–590.
26. Wasserman K, Whipp BJ, Koyl SN, et al. Anaerobic threshold and respiratory gas exchange during exercise. J Appl Physiol 1973;35:236–243.
27. Caiozzo VJ, Davis JA, Ellis JF, et al. A comparison of gas exchange indices used to detect the anaerobic threshold. J Appl Physiol 1982;53:1184–1189.
28. Beaver WL, Wasserman K, Whipp BJ. A new method for detecting anaerobic threshold by gas exchange. J Appl Physiol 1986;60:2020–2027.
29. Brooks GA. Anaerobic threshold: review of the concept and directions for future research. Med Sci Sports Exerc 1985;17:22–34.
30. Sue DY, Wasserman K, Moricca RB, et al. Metabolic acidosis during exercise in patients with chronic obstructive pulmonary disease. Use of the V-slope method for anaerobic threshold determination. Chest 1988;94:931–938.
31. American Thoracic Society and American College of Chest Physicians. ATS/ACCP Statement on cardiopulmonary exercise testing. Am J Respir Crit Care Med 2003;167:211–277.
32. Michaelides AP, Psomadaki ZD, Dilaveris PE, et al. Improved detection of coronary artery disease by exercise electrocardiography with the use of right precordial leads. N Engl J Med 1999;340: 340–345.
33. Chetlin MD, Alpert JS, Armstrong WF. ACC/AHA guidelines for the clinical application of echocardiography: a report of the American College of Cardiology/American Heart Association Task Force on Practice Guidelines (Committee on Clinical Application of Echocardiography). J Am Coll Cardiol 1997;29:862–879.
34. Berman DS, Kiat H, Leppo J. Technetium-99m myocardial perfusion imaging agents. In: Marcus ML, Schelbert HR, Skorton DJ, eds. Cardiac Imaging: A Companion to Baunwald's Heart Disease. Philadelphia: WB Saunders, 1997:1097–1109.
35. Ritchie JL, Bateman TM, Bonow RO. Guidelines for clinical use of cardiac radionuclide imaging. Report of the American College of Cardiology/American Heart Association Task Force on Assessment of Diagnostic and Therapeutic Cardiovascular Procedures (Committee on Radionuclide Imaging). J Am Coll Cardiol 1995;25(2):521–554.
36. Morrow K, Morris CK, Froelicher VF, et al. Prediction of cardiovascular death in men undergoing noninvasive evaluation for coronary artery disease. Ann Intern Med 1993;118:689–695.
37. Mark DB, Hlatky MA, Harrell FE Jr, et al. Exercise treadmill score for predicting prognosis in coronary artery disease. Ann Intern Med 1987;106:793–800.
38. Kwok JM, Miller TD, Hodge DO, et al. Prognostic value of the Duke treadmill score in the elderly. J Am Coll Cardiol 2002;39:1475–1481.
39. Wilkoff B, Miller R. Exercise testing for chronotropic assessment. Cardiol Clin 1992;10:705–717.
40. Bruce RA, Kusumi F, Hosmer D. Maximal oxygen intake and nomographic assessment of functional aerobic impairment in cardiovascular disease. Am Heart J 1973;85:546–562.

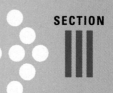

Exercise Prescription

General Principles of Exercise Prescription

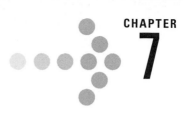

The primary focus on achieving health-related goals has been on prescribing exercise for improvements in cardiorespiratory (CR) fitness, body composition, and muscular fitness. To facilitate change, the Centers for Disease Control (CDC) and American College of Sports Medicine (ACSM) recommended that all adults in the United States should accumulate 30 minutes or more of moderate-intensity physical activity on most, and preferably all, days of the week.[1] The success of exercise implementation is predicated on a willingness and readiness to change behavior. See the latter section of this chapter and Section 12 of the *ACSM's Resource Manual for Guidelines for Exercise Testing and Prescription* (5th ed.) for additional information on behavior modification.

In 1996, the United States Office of the Surgeon General (SGR) issued the first report on physical activity and health. This report concurred with the CDC/ACSM recommendations and concluded that people of all ages benefit from regular physical activity.[1] The SGR indicated that although health benefits improve with moderate amounts of physical activity (15 minutes of running, 30 minutes of brisk walking, or 45 minutes of playing volleyball), greater benefits are obtained with greater amounts of physical activity.[2] In October 2000, an international consensus committee conducted an evidence-based symposium that examined the dose-response of physical activity and health. The proceedings for this symposium indicate ample evidence to support the beneficial effects of regular physical activity on more than a dozen health outcomes.[3] See Table 1-2 for a summary of the dose-response evidence. The panel suggested that, when assessing dose-response, consideration be given to not only the dose that induces the greatest health benefit, but also the potential risk in a particular population. They noted that the greater intensity and volume of exercise, the greater the risk of injury, especially musculoskeletal injury in general, and cardiovascular injury for those with disease.[4] Regular physical activity to enhance health benefits for all populations is supported by numerous organizations and research. The Physical Activity Pyramid has been suggested as one way to facilitate this objective (Fig. 7-1).

Some fitness professionals viewed this recommendation as a major departure from the traditional ACSM exercise programming recommendations published in earlier editions of this text and various ACSM position stands. Others saw the new recommendation as part of a continuum of physical activity recommendations that meets the needs of almost all individuals to improve health status. The lower end of the moderate intensity scale (40%–59% of heart rate reserve) can

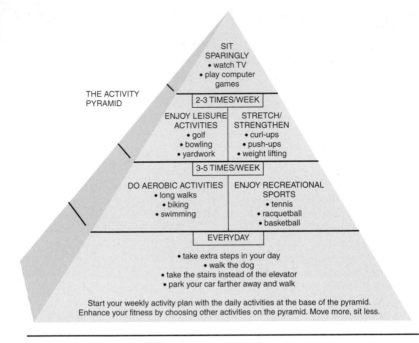

THE ACTIVITY PYRAMID

SIT SPARINGLY
• watch TV
• play computer games

2-3 TIMES/WEEK

ENJOY LEISURE ACTIVITIES
• golf
• bowling
• yardwork

STRETCH/ STRENGTHEN
• curl-ups
• push-ups
• weight lifting

3-5 TIMES/WEEK

DO AEROBIC ACTIVITIES
• long walks
• biking
• swimming

ENJOY RECREATIONAL SPORTS
• tennis
• racquetball
• basketball

EVERYDAY

• take extra steps in your day
• walk the dog
• take the stairs instead of the elevator
• park your car farther away and walk

Start your weekly activity plan with the daily activities at the base of the pyramid. Enhance your fitness by choosing other activities on the pyramid. Move more, sit less.

FIGURE 7-1. The Activity Pyramid, analogous to the USDA's Food Guide Pyramid, has been suggested as a model to facilitate public and patient education for the adoption of a progressively more active lifestyle. (The Activity Pyramid © 2003 Park Nicollet Health Innovations, Minneapolis, U.S.A. 1-888-637-2675. Reprinted with permission.)

improve fitness for many sedentary, overweight, or low-fitness individuals. The combined ACSM/CDC and traditional ACSM recommendations represent a true continuum for one of the primary variables in exercise prescription; that is, the intensity of exercise. Those who follow the more recent recommendation[1] experience many of the health-related benefits of physical activity, and if they are interested in achieving higher levels of fitness, they will be ready to do so. This chapter describes how to structure exercise prescriptions to achieve and maintain health and fitness goals.

Principles of Training

The health-related physical fitness components identified and evaluated in Chapter 4 included body composition, CR fitness ($\dot{V}O_{2max}$), muscular strength, muscular endurance, and flexibility. Improvements in the final four components follow the two major principles of training progression: overload and specificity. The principle of progressive overload states that for a tissue or organ to improve its function, it must be exposed to a stimulus greater than it is normally accustomed to. Repeated exposure is associated with an adaptation by the tissue or organ that leads to improved functional capacity and/or efficiency. An exercise prescription specifies the mode, intensity, duration, and frequency of training;

the interaction of these variables results in the cumulative overload to which the tissue or organ must adapt.

The principle of specificity states that training effects derived from an exercise program are specific to the exercise performed and muscles involved. For example, running improves $\dot{V}O_{2max}$ through both central circulation and peripheral muscle adaptations; however, this results in limited carryover for swim performance.[5] Although numerous modes of aerobic exercise can provide a general adaptation of the myocardium, changes in oxygen extraction and delivery at the muscle site are specific to the muscle recruited and intensity of exercise.[6] The training effect, specific to the muscles recruited, is exemplified by different modes of aerobic exercise that produce different outcomes, despite exercising at the same percentage of $\dot{V}O_{2max}$ or rating of perceived exertion (RPE).[7] Consequently, a fitness program that involves a wide variety of exercises and recruits most of the major muscle groups increases the likelihood that the training effect may transfer to vocational and recreational activities. Conversely, if the goal is to improve one specific activity, the physical activity should focus on that activity.

The individual rate of progression in response to similar stimuli can vary significantly.[8] Genetic characteristics and health status are responsible for the different response rates. Some individuals may be classified as responders versus nonresponders based on different changes to similar stimuli.

Overview of the Exercise Prescription

Exercise prescriptions are designed to enhance physical fitness, promote health by reducing risk factors for chronic disease (e.g., high blood pressure, glucose intolerance), and ensure safety during exercise participation. Based on individual interests, health needs, and clinical status, these common purposes do not carry equal or consistent weight. For the sedentary person at risk for premature chronic disease, adopting a moderately active lifestyle (i.e., the ACSM/CDC recommendation) may provide important health benefits and represent a more attainable goal than achievement of a high $\dot{V}O_{2max}$. However, enhancing physical fitness, whenever possible, is a desirable feature of exercise prescriptions. In all cases, specific outcomes identified for a particular person should be the ultimate target of the exercise prescription.

The essential components of a systematic, individualized exercise prescription include the appropriate mode(s), intensity, duration, frequency, and progression of physical activity. These five components apply when developing exercise prescriptions for people of all ages and fitness levels, regardless of the individual health status. The optimal exercise prescription for an individual is determined from an objective evaluation of that person's response to exercise, including observations of heart rate (HR), blood pressure (BP), subjective response to exercise (RPE), electrocardiogram (ECG) when applicable, and $\dot{V}O_{2max}$ measured directly or estimated during a graded exercise test. As discussed in Chapter 2, a health/medical screening helps determine the necessary or recommended evaluation before beginning a physical conditioning program. However, the exercise prescription should be developed with careful consideration of the individual's health status (including medications), risk factor profile, behavioral characteristics, personal goals, and exercise preferences.

The Art of Exercise Prescription

The guidelines for exercise prescription presented in this book are based on a solid foundation of scientific information. Given the diverse nature and health needs of the population, these guidelines cannot be implemented in an overly rigid fashion by simply applying mathematical calculations to test data. The recommendations presented should be used with careful attention to the goals of the individual. Exercise prescriptions require modification in accordance with observed individual responses and adaptations because of the following:

- Physiologic and perceptual responses to acute exercise vary among individuals and within an individual performing different types of exercise. There is a need to adjust the intensity and duration of exercise and monitor HR, BP, RPE, and, where appropriate, ECG responses to achieve a safe and effective exercise stimulus.
- Adaptations to exercise training vary in terms of magnitude and rate of development, and are dependent on health status and genetic potential. Progress should be monitored by checking HR and RPE responses to allow fine-tuning of the exercise stimulus.
- Desired outcomes based on individual need(s) may be achieved with exercise programs that vary considerably in structure, so one should address individual interests, abilities, and limitations in the design of the program.

A fundamental objective of exercise prescription is to bring about a change in personal health behavior to include habitual physical activity. Thus, the most appropriate exercise prescription for a particular individual is the one that is most helpful in achieving this behavioral change. *The art of exercise prescription is the successful integration of exercise science with behavioral techniques that result in long-term program compliance and attainment of the individual's goals.* As such, knowledge of methods to change health behaviors is essential and is addressed later in this chapter. Although an abundance of literature exists on this topic, an excellent source is Section 5 of the *ACSM's Resource Manual for Guidelines for Exercise Testing and Prescription* (5th ed.).[9]

Components of the Training Session

Once the exercise prescription has been formulated, it is integrated into a comprehensive physical conditioning program, which generally is complemented by an overall health improvement plan. The format for the exercise session should include a warm-up period (approximately 5 to 10 minutes), a stimulus or conditioning phase (CR, flexibility, resistance training) (20 to 60 minutes), an optional recreational game (provides variety), and a cool-down period (5 to 10 minutes) (Fig. 7-2). All training (e.g., CR, resistance, flexibility) should be prescribed in specific terms of intensity (how difficult), duration (how long), frequency (how often), and type of activities.[4] Flexibility training can be included as part of the warm-up or cool-down, or undertaken at a separate time. Resistance training often is performed on alternate days when endurance training is not; however, both activities can be combined into the same workout. Cardiorespiratory, flexibility, and resistance training should be integral parts of a comprehensive training program.

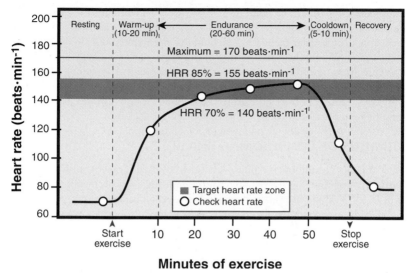

Minutes of exercise

FIGURE 7-2. Format of a typical aerobic exercise session illustrating the warm-up, endurance, and cool-down phases along with a representative heart rate response. At the conclusion of warm-up, heart rate approached the lower limit of the target zone for training, corresponding to 70% to 85% of the peak heart rate reserve achieved during maximal exercise testing.

The sequence of performing endurance or resistance training is a personal preference without a scientific mandate.

WARM-UP

Warm-up facilitates the transition from rest to exercise, stretches postural muscles, augments blood flow, elevates body temperature, dissociates more oxygen, and increases the metabolic rate from the resting level (1 MET) to the aerobic requirements for endurance training.[10] A warm-up may reduce the susceptibility to musculoskeletal injury by increasing connective tissue extensibility, improving joint range of motion and function, and enhancing muscular performance.[11] A preliminary warm-up also may have preventive value, decreasing the occurrence of ischemic ST-segment depression,[12,13] threatening ventricular dysrhythmias, and transient global left ventricular dysfunction following sudden strenuous exertion.[14,15] However, studies in healthy subjects and postmyocardial infarction patients who were taking β-blockers have failed to confirm these cardiovascular abnormalities during sudden strenuous exercise.[16,17]

The exercise session should begin with 5 to 10 minutes of low-intensity large muscle activity (10% to 30% $\dot{V}O_2R$) and progress to an intensity at the lower limit prescribed for endurance training. For example, participants who use brisk walking during the endurance phase might conclude the warm-up period with slow walking. Similarly, brisk walking serves as an ideal warm-up to for participants who jog slowly during the endurance phase. The stretching activities may be conducted after the initial large muscle warm-up and should stretch the major muscle groups using static techniques. Dynamic stretching or modified proprioceptive neuromuscular facilitation techniques or combinations thereof also can be incorporated into the latter portion of the warm-up.[11] Generally low-intensity stretching is preferred before vigorous endurance activity. Stretching (flexibility) exercises performed as part of the warm-up may primarily have an acute effect, whereas flexibility performed during the cool-down may provide a more long-term benefit. Studies to confirm this hypothesis are lacking.

STIMULUS OR CONDITIONING PHASE

The stimulus (conditioning) phase includes CR (endurance), resistance, and flexibility programming. Depending on the individual's goals or outcomes; one, two, or all program areas can be included. A comprehensive program should include all three conditioning components. Figure 7-2 depicts a typical exercise training session with the CR phase exemplified. Later sections of this chapter focus on exercise programming by CR conditioning, resistance training, and flexibility training.

RECREATIONAL ACTIVITIES

Activities like golf are unlikely to elicit a cardiovascular training effect for fit individuals, but are enjoyable, have definite recreational value, and may yield health-related benefits. The inclusion of enjoyable recreational activities during (or immediately after) the endurance phase may enhance adherence. However, game rules may be modified to decrease skill requirements, competition, energy cost, and heart rate responses to play. Game modifications should maximize the experience of successful participation; winning or losing should be of lesser importance.[18] Because of a potential discordance between RPE and HR during game activities, the latter should be monitored periodically to adjust the intensity of play. The imaginative exercise leader may suggest a smaller court size, lowered net height, frequent player-position rotation, intermittent rest periods, minor rule changes, and adjusted scoring. For example, playing volleyball while allowing one bounce of the ball per side facilitates longer rallies, provides additional fun, and reduces the skill required to play the game successfully. Many other team games and individual sports can be modified in a similar fashion.[18]

COOL-DOWN

The cool-down period provides a gradual recovery from the endurance/games phase and includes exercises of diminishing intensities; for example, approximately 5 minutes of slower walking or jogging, cycling and approximately 5 minutes of stretching exercises, and in some cases, alternate activities (e.g., yoga, tai chi, relaxation training). The cool-down is critical to attenuate the exercise-induced circulatory responses and return HR and BP to near resting values; maintain adequate venous return, thereby reducing the potential for postexercise hypotension and dizziness; facilitate the dissipation of body heat; promote more rapid removal of lactic acid than stationary recovery; and combat the potential, deleterious effects of the postexercise rise in plasma catecholamines.[19] The attenuation of the catecholamine response, especially in patients with heart disease, may reduce the likelihood of threatening ventricular dysrhythmias, which are potential harbingers of sudden cardiac death.

Omission of a cool-down in the immediate postexercise period theoretically increases the opportunity for cardiovascular complications. Presumably, the sudden termination of exercise results in a transient decrease in venous return, possibly reducing coronary blood flow when HR and myocardial oxygen demands still may be high. Consequences may include ischemic ST-segment depression, with or without anginal symptoms (e.g., back pain, diffuse arm pain, throat pain), serious ventricular dysrhythmias, or combinations thereof. Cool-down is a critical ingredient of a comprehensive, safe program for both healthy participants, as well as patients with disease.

Cardiorespiratory Exercise Prescription

This phase develops CR and local muscle fitness. Cardiorespiratory fitness, $\dot{V}O_{2max}$, aerobic capacity, and cardiovascular fitness are used synonymously. These terms refer to the maximal capacity to produce energy aerobically and usually are expressed in METs or mL $O_2 \cdot kg^{-1} \cdot min^{-1}$. Cardiorespiratory endurance, aerobic endurance, or cardiovascular endurance refers to the ability to persist or continue in strenuous activity requiring large-muscle groups for prolonged time.

Improvements in the ability of the heart to deliver oxygen (O_2) to the working muscles and in the muscle's ability to generate energy with O_2 result in increased CR fitness. Alteration in CR fitness is measured by assessing the change in $\dot{V}O_{2max}$, which is related to a minimal threshold of frequency, duration, intensity, and volume of exercise.[11,20,21] Because of heterogeneity in the response to an exercise stimulus, aerobic endurance training below a minimal threshold (20% HRR or 50% max HR) may be sufficient for developing aerobic fitness in healthy adults, who have a low $\dot{V}O_{2max}$ (<30 mL$\cdot kg^{-1} \cdot min^{-1}$).[22] The training-induced increase in $\dot{V}O_{2max}$, which generally ranges from 5% to 30%, may be proportional to the quality of the stimulus above the minimal threshold. Genetics also influence the magnitude and rate of change. Individuals with low initial levels of fitness, such as cardiac patients and those experiencing concomitant reductions in body weight and fat stores, generally demonstrate the greatest percent increase in $\dot{V}O_{2max}$. In contrast, more modest increases occur in healthy individuals with high initial levels of fitness and in those whose body weight remains unchanged.[11]

MODE OF EXERCISE

Exercises for the endurance phase employ large muscle groups in activities that are rhythmic or dynamic in nature. Sports such as tennis, racquetball, handball, and basketball also have aerobic conditioning potential if they are pursued for a sufficient duration and intensity. Using a constant mode (type) of exercise for both testing and training provides ideal specificity, and is the most accurate measure of change in oxygen consumption. The greatest improvement in $\dot{V}O_{2max}$ occurs when exercise involves the use of large muscle groups over prolonged periods in activities that are rhythmic and aerobic in nature (e.g., walking, hiking, running, machine-based stair climbing, swimming, elliptical activity, cycling, rowing, combined upper and lower body ergometry, dancing, skating, cross-country skiing, endurance games). Clearly, this wide range of activities provides for individual variability relative to skill and enjoyment, factors that influence compliance to the exercise program and thus desired outcomes. Box 7-1 groups commonly prescribed activities by the consistency of the exercise intensity. In the development of the exercise prescription for the novice exerciser, it may be useful to begin with group 1 activities and progress depending on the individual's interest, adaptation, and clinical status.

Walking may be the activity of choice for many individuals because it is readily accessible, offers tolerable exercise intensity, and is an easily regulated exercise for improving health outcomes and CR fitness. Even extremely slow walking (<2 mph) approximates 2 METs and may impose metabolic loads sufficient for exercise training in lower-fit subjects.[23] Brisk walk training programs provide an activity intense enough to increase aerobic capacity and decrease body weight and fat stores in previously sedentary, middle-aged men.[24] Variations of conventional walking training, including walking with a 3- to 6-kg backpack load[25] and swimming pool walking[26] offer additional options for those who wish to reduce body weight and fat stores, improve CR fitness, or both. Brisk walking (2.9 to 3.9 mph), which can be attained by healthy, habitual walkers can elicit an aerobic training stimulus comparable to

---

BOX 7-1   Grouping of Cardiorespiratory Endurance Activities

Group 1
Activities that can be readily maintained at a constant intensity and interindividual variation in energy expenditure is relatively low. Desirable for more precise control of exercise intensity, as in the early stages of a rehabilitation program. Examples of these activities are walking and cycling, especially treadmill and cycle ergometry.

Group 2
Activities in which the rate of energy expenditure is highly related to skill, but can provide a constant intensity for a given individual. Such activities also may be useful in the early stages of conditioning, but individual skill levels must be considered. Examples include swimming and cross-country skiing.

Group 3
Activities where both skill and intensity of exercise are highly variable. Such activities can be very useful to provide group interaction and variety in exercise, but must be employed cautiously for high-risk, low-fit, and/or symptomatic individuals. Competitive factors also must be considered and minimized. Examples of these activities are racquet sports and basketball.

50% HRR or 70% HR max in older adults (>50 years of age).[27,28] Many individuals might logically progress through walking and jogging programs before engaging in group 2 and 3 activities.

The risk of injury associated with high-impact activities or highly repetitive training also must be considered when prescribing exercise modalities, especially for the overweight or novice exerciser. It may be desirable to have the individual cross train (engage in several different activities) to reduce repetitive orthopedic stresses and involve the greatest number of muscle groups. Because improvement in muscular function is largely specific to the muscles involved in exercise, it is important to consider unique vocational or recreational objectives of the exercise program when recommending activities. Finally, if possible, one should design programs to eliminate or attenuate barriers that might decrease the likelihood of compliance with, or adherence to, the exercise program.

EXERCISE INTENSITY

Intensity and duration of exercise determine the total caloric expenditure during a training session, and are inversely related. For example, improvements in health related benefits may be achieved by a low-intensity, longer-duration regimen, whereas improvements in CR fitness ($\dot{V}O_{2max}$) are associated with a higher-intensity, shorter-duration program.[12] The risk of orthopedic injury is purported to be increased with the latter; however, programs emphasizing moderate to vigorous exercise with a longer training duration (>20 minutes) are recommended for most individuals.[11] Improvements in $\dot{V}O_{2max}$ can occur with a high-intensity stimulus and low duration (<10 minutes),[20-21] but this training should be reserved for asymptomatic, apparently healthy, and highly motivated individuals. The ACSM recommends an intensity of exercise corresponding to 40% and 50% (40%/50%) to 85% of oxygen uptake reserve ($\dot{V}O_2R$) or heart rate reserve (HRR), or 64% and 70% (64%/70%) to 94% of maximum heart rate (HR_{max}).[11,29] The $\dot{V}O_2R$ is the difference between $\dot{V}O_{2max}$ and resting $\dot{V}O_2$. Similarly, the HRR is the difference between HR_{max} and resting HR. When exercise intensities are set according to $\dot{V}O_2R$, the percent values are approximately equal to the percent values for the HRR.[11,30] Consequently, use of the $\dot{V}O_2R$ improves the accuracy of calculating a target $\dot{V}O_2$ from a HRR prescription, especially for low-fit clients, but does not alter the current methods of calculating target heart rates.

The intensity range to increase and maintain CR fitness is intentionally broad and reflects the fact that low-fit or deconditioned individuals may demonstrate increases in CR fitness with exercise intensities of only 40% to 49% HRR or 64% to 70% HR_{max}. For individuals with $\dot{V}O_{2max}$ below 40 mL·kg^{-1}·min^{-1}, a minimal intensity of 30% $\dot{V}O_2R$ can elicit improvement in $\dot{V}O_{2max}$. In contrast, individuals with greater CR fitness (>40 mL·kg^{-1}·min^{-1}) require a minimal threshold of 45% $\dot{V}O_2R$.[22] Those who are already physically active (in aerobic activity) require exercise intensities at the high end of the continuum to further augment their CR fitness. For most individuals, intensities within the range of 60% to 80% HRR or 77% to 90% HR_{max} are sufficient to achieve improvements in CR fitness when combined with an appropriate frequency and duration of training. These ranges of exercise intensities have been successful for increasing $\dot{V}O_{2max}$ in participants in primary and secondary prevention programs.[31-33]

Factors to consider before determining the level of exercise intensity include the following:

- Low-fit, sedentary, and clinical populations can improve fitness with lower-intensity, longer-duration exercise sessions. Higher fit individuals need to work at the higher end of the intensity continuum to improve and maintain their fitness. Athletes may frequently train at intensities in excess of 90% $\dot{V}O_2R$ to achieve improvements in performance.
- Medical conditions, such as musculoskeletal disorders, asthma, or metabolic conditions.
- Medications (see Appendix A) that may influence HR require special attention when defining the initial target HR range and when the dose or timing of medication is changed.
- Risk of cardiovascular and orthopedic injuries is higher and adherence is lower with higher-intensity exercise programs.
- Individual preferences for exercise must be considered to improve the likelihood that the individual will adhere to the exercise program.
- Individual program objectives (lower BP; lower body fatness; increased $\dot{V}O_{2max}$) help define the characteristics of the exercise prescription.

Intensity Prescription by $\dot{V}O_2$

Traditionally, the range of exercise training intensities ($mL \cdot kg^{-1} \cdot min^{-1}$ or in METs) has been based on a straight percentage of $\dot{V}O_{2max}$. For example, if an individual had a measured $\dot{V}O_{2max}$ of 40 $mL \cdot kg^{-1} \cdot min^{-1}$, the prescribed intensity could be set at 24 to 32 $mL \cdot kg^{-1} \cdot min^{-1}$, corresponding to 60% and 80% of $\dot{V}O_{2max}$, respectively. In the ACSM position stand, the exercise intensity has been expressed as a percentage of oxygen uptake reserve (%$\dot{V}O_2R$).[11] To calculate the target $\dot{V}O_2$ based on VO_2R, the following equation is used:

$$\text{Target } \dot{V}O_2 = (\dot{V}O_{2max} - \dot{V}O_{2rest}) \text{ (exercise intensity)} + \dot{V}O_{2rest}$$

This equation has the same form as the heart rate reserve (HRR) calculation of target heart rate (see the following). In the target $\dot{V}O_2$ equation, $\dot{V}O_{2rest}$ is 3.5 $mL \cdot kg^{-1} \cdot min^{-1}$ (1 MET) and the exercise intensity is 50% to 85% (or as low as 40% for very deconditioned individuals). Intensity is expressed as a fraction in the equation. For example, what is the target $\dot{V}O_2$ at 40% of $\dot{V}O_2R$ for a person with a $\dot{V}O_{2max}$ of 17.5 $mL \cdot kg^{-1} \cdot min^{-1}$ (5 METs)?

$$\text{Target } \dot{V}O_2 \text{ } mL \cdot kg^{-1} \cdot min^{-1} = (17.5 - 3.5) \text{ } (0.40) + 3.5$$
$$\text{Target } \dot{V}O_2 \text{ } mL \cdot kg^{-1} \cdot min^{-1} = (14.0) \text{ } (0.40) + 3.5$$
$$\text{Target } \dot{V}O_2 \text{ } mL \cdot kg^{-1} \cdot min^{-1} = 5.6 + 3.5$$
$$\text{Target } \dot{V}O_2 \text{ } mL \cdot kg^{-1} \cdot min^{-1} = 9.1 \text{ } mL \cdot kg^{-1} \cdot min^{-1}$$

Once a $\dot{V}O_2$ (MET) target level is identified, a corresponding work rate may be calculated through the use of metabolic equations (see Appendix D) or by selecting an activity with a corresponding MET level from published tables.[34] However, there are limitations to the use of $\dot{V}O_2$ in prescribing exercise:

- The caloric cost for activities in groups 2 and 3 (see Box 7-1) are quite variable and depend on the skill of the participant and/or the level of competition.

- The caloric cost of activities can provide a starting point for prescribing exercise intensity for individuals with cardiac and/or pulmonary disease, and for individuals with low functional capacities, but the load should be titrated depending on the physiologic responses, perceived exertion, and symptoms.
- The caloric cost of an activity does not take into consideration the effect of environment (e.g., heat, humidity, altitude, pollution), level of hydration, and other variables that can alter the HR and RPE responses to exercise. The ability of individuals to undertake exercise successfully at a given absolute intensity is directly related to their relative effort as reflected by HR and RPE.

Consequently, the most common methods of setting the intensity of exercise to improve or maintain CR fitness use HR and RPE.

Heart Rate Methods

Heart rate is used as a guide to set exercise intensity because of the relatively linear relationship between HR and VO_2. It is best to measure maximal HR (HR_{max}) during a progressive maximal exercise test whenever possible because HR_{max} declines with age (e.g., estimated HR_{max} = 220–age) and the variance for any given age is considerable (1 SD $\pm$ 10–12 beats·min^{-1}) (Fig. 7-3). Currently, all

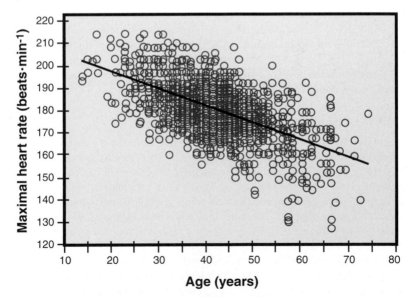

FIGURE 7-3. The relationship between age and maximal heart rate for men demonstrates a high SEE, which is similar for women. Note: y = 213.6–0.789 (age); r =–0.603; SEE = 10.7; P <.0001. (Reproduced with permission from Whaley MH, Kaminsky LA, Dwyer GB. Predictions of over- and underachievement of age-predicted maximal heart rate. Med Sci Sports Exerc 1992;24(10):1173–1179.)

prediction formulae for maximal heart rate contain large standard errors of estimate, which may result in inaccuracy when applied to general populations.[35] Prediction equations, which are population specific (e.g., smokers, obese, aged, those with elevated resting HR), may provide more accurate estimates of maximal HR.[36,37] Specific medications (β-blockers) preclude the use of a predicted maximal HR; thus other methods of monitoring intensity are necessary (e.g., RPE, METs).

The actual maximal HR is specific to the mode of exercise and may differ within populations of the same age and sex. Until a multivariate regression equation is developed that accurately predicts maximal HR, obtaining the actual maximal HR through a maximal exercise test is preferred. In the absence of a true determination of maximal HR, the traditional, empirically based, easy-to-use (220-age) is still viable, despite the large standard error. During an exercise session, the assumption is that the individual will achieve a steady-state HR response in the prescribed range; in reality (and certainly during discontinuous exercise) HR is likely to be both above and below the prescribed intensity. The goal should be to maintain an average HR close to the midpoint of the prescribed range. There are several approaches to determining a target HR range for prescriptive purposes.

Direct Method

The direct method of obtaining the target HR range involves plotting measured HR against either measured $\dot{V}O_2$ (Fig. 7-4) or exercise intensity (as discussed in Chapter 4). If RPE data are available, the HR–$\dot{V}O_2$ relationship can be evaluated further in relation to the individual's RPE, which is helpful in monitoring the exercise intensity. This method is appropriate for setting exercise intensity for persons with low fitness levels, those with cardiovascular and/or pulmonary disease, and those taking medications (e.g., β-blockers) that affect the HR response to exercise. The direct method allows one to prescribe an appropriate training HR range below the point of adverse signs or symptoms experienced by the individual during exercise testing.

Percent of HR$_{max}$ (Zero to Peak Method)

One of the oldest methods of setting the target HR range uses a straight percentage of the HR$_{max}$. Early researchers and clinicians used 70% to 85% of an individual's HR$_{max}$ as the prescribed exercise intensity. This range of exercise intensities approximates 50% to 70% $\dot{V}O_{2max}$[38] and provides the stimulus needed to improve or maintain $\dot{V}O_{2max}$ in individuals exercising in clinical and adult fitness settings.[31-33] It is also simple to compute. If an individual's HR$_{max}$ is 180 beats·min^{-1}, the target HR range is 126 to 153 beats·min^{-1}. This is a conservative approach that is very inaccurate at low intensity target zones. For example, prescribing a cool down intensity of 30% HR$_{max}$ for an individual with a maximal HR of 180 yields a target HR of 54 (.30 × 180 = 54), which is often below the resting HR.

HR Reserve Method (Karvonen)

The HR reserve (HRR) method is also known as the Karvonen method.[39] In this method, resting heart rate (HR$_{rest}$) is subtracted from the maximal heart rate (HR$_{max}$) to obtain HRR. For example, if the resting HR is 60 and the maximal

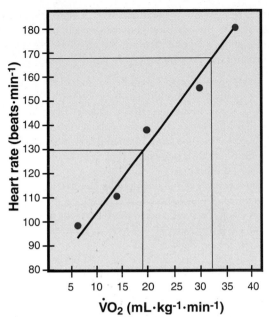

FIGURE 7-4. A line of best fit has been drawn through the data points on this plot of heart rate and oxygen consumption data observed during a hypothetical maximal exercise test in which $\dot{V}O_{2max}$ was observed to be 38 mL·kg^{-1}·min^{-1} and maximal heart rate was 184 bpm^{-1}. A target heart rate range was determined by finding the heart rates that correspond to 50% and 85% of $\dot{V}O_{2max}$. For this individual, 50% of $\dot{V}O_{2max}$ was approximately 19 mL·kg^{-1}·min^{-1}, and 85% of $\dot{V}O_{2max}$ was approximately 32 mL·kg^{-1}·min^{-1}. The corresponding target heart rates are approximately 130 and 168 beats·min^{-1}.

HR is 180, then: 180 beats·min^{-1} minus 60 beats·min^{-1} = 120 beats·min^{-1}. One then takes 60% and 80% of the HRR and adds each of these values to resting HR to obtain the target HR range:

$$\text{Target HR range} = ([HR_{max}-HR_{rest}] \times \text{percent intensity}) + HR_{rest}$$

$$\text{Target HR range of 60\% intensity} = ([180 - 60] \times 0.60) + 60 = 132 \text{ beats·min}^{-1}$$

$$\text{Target HR range of 80\% intensity} = ([180 - 60] \times 0.80) + 60 = 156 \text{ beats·min}^{-1}$$

The HRR method yields a target HR range of 132 to 156 beats·min^{-1} for this subject, similar to the target HR range calculated by the percent of maximal HR method. Sixty to eighty percent of the HRR is equal to about 60% to 80% of $\dot{V}O_{2max}$ for most fit individuals, but is more closely linked to the %$\dot{V}O_2$R across the entire range of fitness levels. The latter point is most important when working with low-fit clients.

The target HR range for the %HR$_{max}$ and the HRR methods are different because different resting heart rates are used in the target HR calculation. The systematic difference between the two HR methods is reduced as the intensity increases. Either method can be used to approximate the range of exercise intensities known to increase or maintain $\dot{V}O_{2max}$; however, the HRR method more accurately depicts the intensity relative to oxygen consumption. As "the art of exercise prescription" suggested earlier, the target HR range is only a *guideline* used in setting the exercise intensity:

- Some individuals prefer to exercise at the low end of the target HR range and focus on long duration (>40 minutes) to accomplish fitness goals, although the evidence is weak to suggest that a longer duration further enhances $\dot{V}O_{2max}$. As the duration increases the opportunity for cardiovascular drift (e.g., a rise in HR over time from increased core temperature, dehydration, and blood redistribution) is increased; thus, a reduction in the workload may maintain the target HR range.
- Because of the specificity of training and the fact that *measured* maximal heart rate is different for different modes of exercise, an individual's perception of effort will vary among exercise modes when exercising at exactly same HR.[7]
- Conversion of a $\%HR_{max}$ value to a $\%\dot{V}O_{2max}$ value carries with it a standard error of estimate of $\pm 5.7\% \dot{V}O_{2max}$.[38]
- If an estimate of HR_{max} (e.g., 220–age) is used in the preceding calculations rather than measured HR, the error inherent in that estimate is carried over to the calculated target HR range (see Fig. 7-3). This must be considered when an individual begins an exercise program. The RPE can be helpful in adjusting the exercise intensity in such situations.[39]

Rating of Perceived Exertion

Commonly used RPE scales are found in Chapter 4. Use of RPE is considered an adjunct to monitoring HR because RPE determined during a graded exercise test may not consistently translate to the same intensity during an exercise session or for different modes of exercise.[7,40,41] However, the RPE has proved to be a valuable aid in prescribing exercise for individuals who have difficulty with HR palpation, and in cases where the HR response to exercise may have been altered because of a change in medication. The average RPE range associated with physiologic adaptation to exercise is 12 to 16 (in the range of "somewhat hard" to "hard") on the Borg scale (see Chapter 4). However, because of significant interindividual variability in the psychophysiologic relationship, one should suit the RPE to the individual on a specific mode of exercise and not expect an exact matching of the RPE to a $\%HR_{max}$ or $\%HRR$.[42] Consequently, the RPE should be used as a *guideline* in setting the exercise intensity. It is important to establish the target RPE within the training environment.

In the final analysis, the appropriate exercise intensity is one that is safe, enhances aerobic capacity ($\dot{V}O_{2max}$), compatible with a long-term active lifestyle for that individual, and achieves the desired caloric output given the time constraints of the exercise session.

EXERCISE DURATION

The duration of an exercise session interacts with the intensity to result in the expenditure of a sufficient number of calories to achieve health and fitness goals such as improved body composition. The CR phase usually includes 20 to

60 minutes of continuous or intermittent activity (10-minute bouts accumulated throughout the day). The ACSM position stand recommends a minimum of 20 minutes of cardiovascular exercise for improvement in aerobic capacity.[11] Significant improvement in $\dot{V}O_{2max}$ has been demonstrated with multiple short bouts (10 minutes) of exercise equivalent to the total duration of a single long bout (30 minutes) of exercise.[43–45] People training at low intensity should conduct the exercise sessions over a longer period of time (30 minutes or more), and, conversely, individuals training at higher levels of intensity may train for 20 minutes or less. Consequently, exercising at 60% to 80% HRR or 77% to 90% HR_{max} for 20 to 30 minutes, excluding time spent warming up and cooling down, enables most individuals to fulfill their goals.[4]

In addition, limited data on short bouts (12 minutes at high intensity)[20] or interval training (six to seven bouts of 20 seconds at >170% $\dot{V}O_{2max}$)[21] have demonstrated improvements in $\dot{V}O_{2max}$. Although fitness may improve through short duration, high -intensity exercise, scientific evidence to support the health benefits of short duration exercise is lacking. High-intensity exercise is associated with an increased risk of orthopedic injury, cardiovascular incidence, and lower compliance.[46] Therefore, moderate intensity, moderate duration (20 to 30 minutes) exercise is recommended for improving aerobic capacity ($\dot{V}O_{2max}$) of most adults. Duration is inversely related to the intensity of the activity. Lower-intensity activity should be done for a longer period of time (30 minutes or more).

Consistent with the manner in which the intensity of a session is gradually increased over weeks of training, the duration (e.g., 30 minutes) can begin with as little as multiple (4 to 10), 2-to 5-minute bouts with rest periods between bouts for those with low levels of CR fitness. The duration of the exercise bout can be extended until the goal is achieved. Increases in exercise duration should be made as the individual adapts to training without evidence of undue fatigue or injury.

Exercise Frequency

The ACSM recommends an exercise frequency of 3 to 5 $d \cdot wk^{-1}$. For those exercising at 60% to 80% HRR or 77% to 90% HR_{max}, an exercise frequency of 3 $d \cdot wk^{-1}$ is sufficient to improve or maintain $\dot{V}O_{2max}$. For those exercising at the lower end of the intensity continuum, exercising more than 3 $d \cdot wk^{-1}$ may be needed to achieve the caloric expenditure associated with weight loss and fitness goals. Patients with functional capacities of fewer than 3 METs may benefit from multiple brief daily exercise sessions; one to two short sessions per day are appropriate for those with 3 to 5 MET capacities; and three to five sessions per week are recommended for individuals with a functional capacity of >5 METs.

Although deconditioned persons may improve CR fitness with only twice-weekly exercise, greater improvement is achieved with a frequency of three to five sessions per week, but improvements generally plateau within the 3 to 5 $d \cdot wk^{-1}$ frequency.[47] Additional benefits of training 6 or more $d \cdot wk^{-1}$ appear to be minimal, and should be reserved for the performance oriented individuals or competitive athletes. The risk of musculoskeletal injury increases abruptly with increased frequency of training beyond 6 $d \cdot wk^{-1}$. Vigorous training 7 $d \cdot wk^{-1}$ is not recommended; however, 30 minutes or more of moderate intensity physical activity is preferable on most days of the week for health-related benefits. Clearly, the number of exercise sessions per week varies depending on the caloric goals, participant preferences, and limitations imposed by the participant's lifestyle. The optimal training frequency is still elusive.

Energy Expenditure Goals

The interaction of physical activity intensity, duration, and frequency determines net caloric expenditure from the activity. It is generally accepted that many of the health benefits and training adaptations associated with increased physical activity are related to the total amount of work (volume) accomplished during training.[1,2,48] However, the caloric thresholds necessary to elicit significant improvements in $\dot{V}O_{2max}$, weight loss, or a reduced risk of premature chronic disease may be different. Therefore, individualized exercise prescriptions should be designed with energy expenditure goals in mind.

The ACSM recommends a target range of 150 to 400 kcal of physical activity and/or exercise energy expenditure per day.[2,48] The lower end of this range represents a minimal caloric threshold of ~1,000 kcal·wk^{-1} from physical activity, which is associated with a significant 20% to 30% reduction in risk of all-cause mortality,[2,48,49] and this should be the initial goal for previously sedentary individuals. Based on the dose-response relationships between physical activity and health and fitness, individuals should be encouraged to move toward attainment of the upper end of the recommended range (e.g., 300 to 400 kcal·day^{-1} from activity) as their fitness levels improve during the training program. The application of the 1,000 kcal threshold (150 kcal·day^{-1} × 7 d·wk^{-1}) for weight loss and weight loss maintenance may be insufficient for effective control.[50,51] Recent reports suggest that 60 minutes or more per day may be necessary for weight loss and maintenance, which is double the current recommendation for health-related physical activity.[50-52] Physical activity and/or exercise energy expenditure in excess of 2,000 kcal·wk^{-1} have been successful for both short- and long-term weight control.[53]

Estimating caloric expenditure during exercise has been problematic for exercise professionals, and developing an exercise plan based on caloric thresholds should not be viewed as an exact science. Interindividual differences in skill, coordination, and exercise economy (the $\dot{V}O_2$ at a given submaximal work rate) and the variable intensities within each available activity strongly influence estimation of caloric expenditure during exercise. Accelerometers have been used to estimate caloric expenditure during various recreational and household activities. The energy expenditure associated with walking can be predicted with reasonable accuracy, but other activities, such as golf and household activities may be underestimated by 30% to 60%.[54] Accelerometers provide a general estimate of caloric expenditure and may be more valuable on a relative (pre-, post-) comparison within the same individual. Any attempt to quantify energy expenditure by accelerometry must be viewed cautiously.[55] Another useful method to approximate the caloric cost of exercise is by using the following equation based on the MET level of the activity:

$$(\text{METs} \times 3.5 \times \text{body weight in kg})/200 = \text{kcal·min}^{-1}$$

This formula helps an individual understand the components of the exercise prescription and the volume of exercise necessary to achieve the caloric goals of the program. Consider the following example. The weekly goal of the exercise program has been set at a net caloric expenditure of 1,000 kilocalories for an individual who weighs 70 kg, and the MET level of the prescribed activity is 6 METs. In this example, the *net* caloric expenditure from the exercise is 5 METs because 1 MET of the activity represents resting metabolic rate. Therefore, the *net* caloric expenditure from the exercise is 6 kcal·min^{-1}, which requires 167 minutes per week to attain the 1,000 kilocalorie threshold. Given a 4 d·wk^{-1} program, the individual would require approximately 42 minutes per day to achieve the 1,000 kcal goal (or 33 minutes per day, 5 d·wk^{-1}). Working backward from the caloric goal to determine the volume of exercise needed to reach the goal is useful in determining the appropriate exercise prescription components. If the goal was a more aggressive 2,000 kcal·wk^{-1} for long-term weight control, the net caloric expenditure of 6 kcal·min^{-1} would require 333 minutes per week or ~48 minutes per day on all days of the week. For information on MET values for over 500 physical activities, see Ainsworth et al.[34] or the *ACSM's Resource Manual for Exercise Testing and Prescription* (5th ed.).

Rate of Progression

The recommended rate of progression in an exercise program depends on functional capacity, medical and health status, age, individual activity preferences and goals, and tolerance to the current level of training. For healthy adults, the endurance aspect of the exercise prescription has three stages of progression: initial, improvement, and maintenance (Table 7-1). Exercise professionals should

TABLE 7-1. Training Progression for the Sedentary Low-Risk* Participants

Program Stage	Week	Exercise Frequency (sessions·wk^{-1})	Exercise Intensity (%HRR)	Exercise Duration (min)
Initial stage	1	3	40–50	15–20
	2	3–4	40–50	20–25
	3	3–4	50–60	20–25
	4	3–4	50–60	25–30
Improvement stage	5–7	3–4	60–70	25–30
	8–10	3–4	60–70	30–35
	11–13	3–4	65–75	30–35
	14–16	3–5	65–75	30–35
	17–20	3–5	70–85	35–40
	21–24	3–5	70–85	35–40
Maintenance Stage†	24+	3–5	70–85	20–60

*Defined as the lowest risk categories in Table 2-4 and Boxes 2-1 and 2-2.

†Depending on long-term goals of program, the intensity, frequency, and duration may vary.

Abbreviations: HRR, heart rate reserve; it is recommended that low-risk cardiac patients train at the lower end of these ranges.

recognize that recent physical activity recommendations from the ACSM/CDC[1] and the Surgeon General[2] include 30 minutes of *moderate* intensity physical activity on most, if not all, days of the week for health-related benefits. Although some apparently healthy but sedentary individuals may not be able to attain this initial level of activity, they should be encouraged to progress to this goal during the first few weeks of the training program.

INITIAL CONDITIONING STAGE

The initial stage should include an extended warm-up (10 to 15 minutes), moderate intensity aerobic activities (40% to 60% of HRR) in an interval format; low-intensity muscular fitness exercises that are compatible with minimal muscle soreness, discomfort, and injury; and an extended cool-down (10 to 15 minutes) with the majority of cool-down time devoted to stretching. Exercise adherence may decrease if the program is initiated too aggressively. This stage may last 1 to 6 weeks, but the length depends on the adaptation of the individual to the exercise program. The duration of the exercise session during the initial stage may begin with approximately 15 minutes of the cardiovascular stimulus phase and progress to 30 minutes. It is recommended that individuals who are starting a moderate-intensity conditioning program should exercise three to four times per week. This initial conditioning stage should prepare the participant for the novel activities and develop an orthopedic tolerance to the exercise stress. Individual goals should be established early in the exercise program and must be realistic, with a system of rewards.

IMPROVEMENT STAGE

The goal of this stage of training is to provide a gradual increase in the overall exercise stimulus to allow for significant improvements and adaptations in CR fitness. The improvement stage of the conditioning program differs from the initial stage in that the participant is progressed at a more rapid rate. This stage typically lasts 4 to 8 months, during which intensity is progressively increased within the upper portion of the target range of 50% to 85% of HRR. Duration is increased consistently, with increments of no more than 20% each week until participants are able to exercise at a moderate to vigorous intensity continuously for 20 to 30 minutes. The frequency and magnitude of the increments are dictated by the rate at which the participant adapts to the conditioning program. Increases of duration and/or frequency usually precede increases in intensity. Once the target duration and frequency are achieved, adjustments in intensity of no more than 5% of HRR every sixth exercise session are well tolerated. The progression of intensity also can be achieved through interval training incorporating extended higher-intensity work intervals or by adding one higher-intensity exercise session each week until the target intensity is achieved. Deconditioned individuals should be permitted more time for adaptation at each stage of conditioning. Age also should be taken into consideration when progressions are recommended; experience suggests that adaptation to conditioning may take longer in older individuals.[11]

MAINTENANCE STAGE

The goal of this stage of training is the long-term maintenance of CR fitness developed during the improvement stage. This stage of the exercise program usually begins after the participant has reached preestablished fitness goals. During this stage, the participant may no longer be interested in further increasing the conditioning stimulus. Further improvement may be minimal, but continuing the same workout routine enables individuals to maintain their fitness levels. At this point, the goals of the program should be reviewed and new goals set. The goal of each participant should be to reach a minimum of the 50th percentile in all health-related fitness parameters. To maintain CR fitness, an exercise prescription should incorporate an intensity, frequency, and duration consistent with the participant's long-term goals, and should also meet, and preferably exceed, the minimal caloric thresholds identified earlier in the chapter. If there is the need for further weight loss during this phase of the program, a caloric restriction combined with a moderate intensity exercise program that results in a significant negative caloric balance (500 to 800 kcal·day^{-1}) is recommended. However, such programs usually are associated with increased exercise duration, frequency, or both. It is important to include exercises and recreational activities (see Box 7-1, group 3 activities) that the individual finds enjoyable. It is also helpful to provide variety within and between each exercise session to maintain participant interest.

Training Specificity

Numerous studies have investigated the CR and metabolic responses of trained versus untrained muscles to chronic aerobic conditioning. For example, upper extremity or lower extremity training resulted in only minor improvements in submaximal and maximal lower extremity or upper extremity exercise responses, respectively. Thus, subjects trained by lower extremity exercise failed to demonstrate a conditioning bradycardia during upper extremity work, and vice versa (Fig. 7-5).[57] Similar differences in muscle-specific adaptations have been shown for blood lactate[58] and pulmonary ventilation.[59] The use of arm training during a detraining phase failed to maintain the gains accrued during leg training, thus confirming the specificity of training.[60] These findings suggest that a substantial portion of the training effect derives from peripheral rather than central changes, including cellular and enzymatic adaptations that increase the oxidative capacity of chronically exercised skeletal muscle.[61]

Some *transfer-of-training effects* have been reported, including increased $\dot{V}O_{2max}$ or reduced submaximal heart rate with untrained limbs, thus providing evidence for central circulatory adaptations to chronic endurance exercise.[62,63] It has been suggested that approximately half of the increase in trained limb performance results from a centralized training effect and half from peripheral adaptations, specifically alterations in trained skeletal muscle.[64] However, the peripheral adaptations may predominate in some patient subsets, for example, cardiac patients with left ventricular dysfunction.[65] Although the conditions under which the interchangeability of arm and leg training effects may vary, there is evidence to suggest that the initial fitness of the subjects as well as the

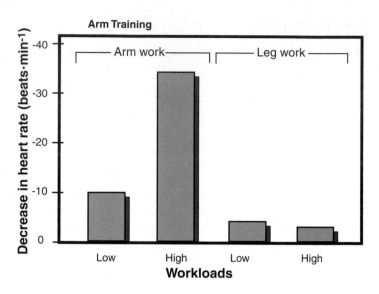

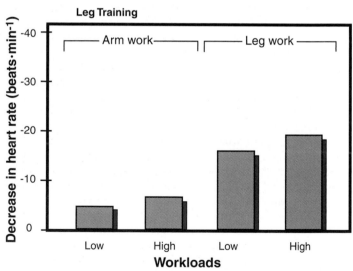

FIGURE 7-5. Importance of peripheral adaptation to training of the arms (**top**) and legs (**bottom**). Arm training on the cycle ergometer reduced the heart rate during arm work but not during leg work. Similarly, leg training was associated with a lower heart rate response during leg exercise but not during arm exercise. (Adapted from Clausen JP, Trap-Jensen J, Lassen NA. The effects of training on the heart rate during arm and leg exercise. Scand J Clin Lab Invest 1970;26:295–301.)

intensity, frequency, and duration of training may be important variables in determining the extent of cross-training benefits.[66]

The limited degree of cardiovascular and metabolic crossover benefits of training from one set of limbs to another appears to discredit the general practice of limiting exercise training to the lower extremity alone. Many recreational and occupational activities require sustained arm work to a greater extent than leg work. Consequently, individuals who rely on their upper extremities should be advised to train the upper as well as the lower extremities, with the expectation of improved CR, and hemodynamic and perceived exertion responses to both forms of effort. Such programs should serve to maximize the conditioning response through increased crossover of training benefits to real-life situations.

SUMMARY OF GUIDELINES FOR CARDIOVASCULAR STIMULUS PHASE

- The goal of each participant should be to reach a minimum of the 50th percentile in all health-related fitness parameters.
- The ACSM recommends an intensity of exercise corresponding to 40% and 50% (40%/50%) to 85% of oxygen uptake reserve ($\dot{V}O_2R$) or heart rate reserve (HRR), or 64% and 70% (64%/70%) to 94% of maximum heart rate. HRR and $\dot{V}O_2R$ can be used interchangeably.
- Aerobic endurance training below a minimal threshold (20% HRR or 50% HR_{max}) may be sufficient for developing aerobic fitness in healthy adults, who have a low $\dot{V}O_{2max}$ (<30 mL·kg^{-1}·min^{-1}).
- For people with $\dot{V}O_{2max}$ below 40 mL·kg^{-1}·min^{-1}, a minimal intensity of 30% $\dot{V}O_2R$ can provide for improvement in $\dot{V}O_{2max}$.
- For most individuals, intensities within the range of 60% to 80% HRR or 77 to 90% HR_{max} are sufficient to achieve improvements in CR fitness, when combined with an appropriate frequency and duration of training.
- Athletes may frequently train at intensities in excess of 90% $\dot{V}O_2R$ to achieve improvements in performance.
- The HRR method is recommended for prescribing exercise intensity rather than the HR_{max} method because the HRR method more accurately depicts the intensity relative to oxygen consumption.
- The CR phase usually includes 20 to 60 minutes of continuous or intermittent (10-minute bouts accumulated throughout the day) activity.
- Although deconditioned persons may improve CR fitness with only twice-weekly exercise, greater improvement is achieved with a frequency of 3 to 5 d·wk^{-1}, but improvements generally plateau within the 3 to 5 d·wk^{-1} frequency.
- Progression of the CR stimulus: Duration is increased consistently, with increments of no more than 20% each week until participants are able to exercise at a moderate to vigorous intensity for 20 to 30 minutes continuously. Increases of duration and/or frequency usually precede increases in intensity. Once the target duration and frequency are achieved, adjustments in intensity of no more than 5% of HRR every sixth exercise session are well tolerated.

- A target range of 150 to 400 kcal of physical activity and/or exercise energy expenditure per day or a minimal caloric threshold of approximately 1,000 $kcal \cdot wk^{-1}$ from physical activity is recommended.
- Physical activity and/or exercise energy expenditure in excess of 2000 $kcal \cdot wk^{-1}$ have been successful for both short- and long-term weight control.

Resistance Exercise Prescription

Muscular strength and muscular endurance directly impact on activities of daily living (ADLs) because daily living activity requires a given percentage of one's muscular capacity to perform common tasks. The enhancement of muscular strength and endurance enables an individual to perform such tasks with less physiologic stress and aids in maintaining functional independence throughout the life span. Even the cardiovascular stress of lifting or holding a given weight (object) is proportional to the percentage of maximal strength involved. Improving muscular function through resistance training (weight training) may accrue health-related benefits.[67] A reduction in the risk of osteoporosis, low back pain, hypertension, and diabetes are associated with resistance training.[68–70] In addition, the benefits of increased muscular strength and endurance, bone density, enhanced strength of connective tissue, and the increase or maintenance of lean body weight also may occur. These adaptations are beneficial for all ages, including middle-aged and older adults, and, in particular, postmenopausal women who may experience a more rapid loss of bone mineral density.[71]

Although resistance training may elevate heart rate because of sympathetic activity and catecholamine responses, the heart rate is disproportionate to oxygen consumption.[72,73] Heart rate should not be used as a measure of intensity during resistance training. Resistance training does little to increase the $\dot{V}O_{2max}$,[70] although resistance training may improve cardiovascular endurance. For example, when cardiovascular endurance is defined as the length of time a person can walk on a treadmill during a graded exercise test protocol, resistance training may permit one to extend the duration of the exercise because of increased muscular strength and muscular endurance without increasing $\dot{V}O_{2max}$.[74] Circuit weight training (a series of resistance exercises, performed one after another, with little rest between exercises) results in an average improvement in $\dot{V}O_{2max}$ of about 6%. Thus, it is not generally recommended as an activity for improving CR endurance.[11]

The use of resistance training as a primary mode for weight and body fat loss is controversial. Although successful fat loss is associated with a caloric deficit achieved through a combination of dietary restriction and caloric expenditure, resistance training per se expends only moderate amounts of calories. Energy expenditure estimates range from 4 to 10 $kcal \cdot min^{-1}$ while engaged in actual resistance training.[72,73,75] This does not include rest intervals and is proportional to the amount of muscle mass involved. Moderate aerobic exercise exceeds the energy expenditure of resistance exercise and a cardiovascular stimulus can be maintained for a longer duration. Thus, for a given length of time, more calories can be expended in aerobic exercise compared to resistance training. For example, a 70-kg person jogging for 30 minutes at 6.0 mph (161 $m \cdot min^{-1}$) would typically demonstrate a net caloric expenditure of 338 kcal; whereas a half hour resistance training session, of which 15 minutes is lifting and 15 minutes is recovery, accounts for a net caloric expenditure of 60 to 150 kcal.

A small increase in caloric expenditure occurs during recovery from both aerobic and resistance training but it is transient and usually dissipates within 2 hours postexercise.[76,77] Reports of elevations in resting metabolic rate (RMR) following a bout of resistance training have generally accounted for less than 100 net calories over 24 hours,[78] with several studies reporting a net expenditure of only 19 to 50 kcal in the 2-hour postexercise period.[78–81]

Resting metabolic rate may be influenced by a greater amount of fat-free mass;[82] however, resistance training studies suggest that the relative metabolic rate (kcal·kg FFM^{-1}) does not change.[83,84] One study even revealed no alteration of sleeping metabolic rate despite a 1.1-kg increase in fat-free mass after 12 weeks of resistance training.[85] To raise the resting metabolic rate through resistance training requires increases in the quantity of lean tissue. Typical increases in lean body mass (LBM) in up to 6 months of resistance training range from 0.3 to 2.0 kg, with the greatest improvement in males.[83,86] Increases in LBM that were similar between resistance training programs lasting 12 to 24 weeks, suggest that additional increase in LBM after 12 weeks of training may be somewhat limited for the general population.[86] Although not well studied, the ability to increase LBM is linked to genetic factors.[87] Responses to resistance training may be subject to individual heterogeneity[87] similar to responses to cardiovascular exercise training.[8] The ability to demonstrate large increases in LBM appears limited in the general population.

Resistance training (i.e., sufficient to develop and maintain muscular fitness and fat-free mass or reduce the normal decrease in fat-free mass associated with aging) should be an integral part of primary and secondary prevention programs. Unlike cardiovascular activity, intensity for resistance exercise is not easily determined. The common use of a percentage of the 1 RM (repetition maximum) to estimate intensity does not portray a true intensity and is only used as a general guideline. The number of repetitions performed at a given percentage of 1 RM differs between muscle groups (e.g., bench press versus leg curl) as well as between individuals.[88,89] This variability in the number of repetitions performed at a percentage of 1 RM precludes its use as an accurate measure of intensity. Intensity can be defined as the *effort* or how difficult the training stimulus or exercise is. A resting muscle represents minimal intensity, whereas momentary muscular fatigue (failure) in the concentric portion of an exercise performed in strict form represents high intensity. All other levels of muscle activity are somewhere between these two extremes. A 3 RM, 10 RM, and 15 RM result in a similar intensity as defined by the repetition maximum. The RM indicates that the muscle has reached a point of fatigue or failure in which the force-generating capacity falls below the required force to shorten the muscle against the imposed resistance. At this point, the progressive recruitment of muscle fiber motor units has occurred and the muscle is at high intensity.[90] With each repetition, there is a progressive increase in active muscle mass, until a maximal voluntary contraction is achieved. Thus, high intensity can be reached by performing a few repetitions (e.g., three to six) with a heavier resistance or several repetitions (e.g., 8 to 12) with a lighter resistance.

The progressive increase in muscle fiber recruitment parallels increases in blood pressure, regardless of the size of the muscle mass involved.[91,92] The magnitude of the blood pressure response depends on the degree of effort (intensity), not the absolute force of contraction.[91,92] A similar blood pressure is evident at the same relative degree of effort despite significant differences in absolute force production.[91,92] If high intensity is achieved (momentary muscular fatigue), whether by small versus large muscle groups, or few versus several repetitions, the results are similar; the muscle has been stimulated to a high degree. The elevation in blood pressure associated with this high intensity is extreme even when recruiting a small muscle mass.[92] For a healthy, asymptomatic population, the brief exposure to these high blood pressures is considered inconsequential. Individuals with hypertension, diabetes, at risk for stroke, or at other medical risk from exposure to high blood pressures should avoid high-intensity resistance training. They can engage in lower-intensity resistance training, by terminating lifting before fatigue. Although undefined, a threshold for improvements in muscle strength and endurance is evident below momentary muscular fatigue (high intensity).[69,93,94] Submaximal training can occur by terminating the exercise when the participant demonstrates an obvious unintentional increase in concentric repetition duration (e.g., slower speed of movement), or when one to three more repetitions could still be performed or by using the RPE scale as an index of intensity. An initial goal of 12 to 13 and a final goal of 15 to 16 on the RPE scale has been recommended for submaximal training.[95–97] A target of 19 to 20 on the RPE scale is synonymous with high-intensity strength stimuli for healthy populations.

The theory of a strength–endurance continuum producing specific adaptations related to the number of repetitions has limited scientific support.[98] Muscular strength and endurance can be developed simultaneously within a reasonable range of repetitions (3 to 6, 6 to 10, 10 to 12, etc.).[69,94,99–103] If the resistance training stimulus is generally less than 90 seconds to fatigue per exercise, both muscular strength and absolute muscular endurance (number of repetitions performed at a specific amount of resistance) increase, but not necessarily to the same degree. For example, doubling the number of repetitions performed at a given resistance does not mandate the performance of twice the resistance for 1 RM. Successful resistance training typically increases strength and absolute muscular endurance, yet relative muscular endurance (a specific percentage of the 1 RM adjusted for both pre- and post-training) remains stable.[86,104]

Thus, for any common range of repetitions (3 to 6, 6 to 10, 10 to 12, etc.) there is little evidence to suggest a specific number of repetitions will provide a superior response relative to muscular strength, hypertrophy, or absolute muscular endurance. However improvements in bone mineral density have been associated with lower (7 to 10) repetitions versus higher (14 to 18) repetitions in older populations.[68,105,106] This may provide insight for training individuals prone to osteopenia or osteoporosis. Women who may have a predisposition to osteoporosis should be advised to resistance train with higher resistance with fewer repetitions and a variety of exercises to benefit from site-specific bone improvement, without a fear of muscular hypertrophy. To elicit improvement in both muscular strength and endurance, 8 to 12 repetitions at a high intensity (approximate momentary muscular fatigue) is recommended for healthy populations.

Any overload beyond a minimal threshold results in strength development. A higher-intensity effort at or near maximal effort produces the greatest stimulus, but may not produce any greater adaptation. The increase of intensity of resistance training can be manipulated by varying any one of the following variables, while keeping all the other variables constant:

- The weight (resistance)
- The number of repetitions
- Reducing momentum by increasing the repetition duration (reducing speed of movement)
- Maintaining muscular tension versus "locking out" the joint when performing multiple joint exercise (e.g., bench press, military press, leg press, squat)

An overload or progression can occur with any exercise by requiring an increased intensity with controlled repetition duration (movement speed). The initial repetition is typically least difficult and each subsequent repetition progresses in intensity until the terminal repetition. All muscle groups can be trained through a variety of exercises, which can provide novel or different stimuli to the muscle and bone. A variety of exercises for each muscle group also may maintain participant adherence and interest in the exercise program. Develop a menu of exercises for each muscle group and choose one for each exercise session. There is no evidence to suggest there is an absolute best exercise for any specific muscle group, but each is specific in its purpose. Some exercises may be more difficult to perform (stability ball activity) because of increased neuromuscular coordination or balance, but there is no evidence to indicate these activities are *better* in terms of muscle strength or endurance. They are simply different. For example, performing a bench press exercise on a flat bench versus a stability ball is different. There is no evidence to show one form of bench press is superior to the other. Modifications such as a change in the length of the external moment arm (e.g., bicep curl move from a position of the upper arm vertical to a preacher curl position) or the base of support (e.g., stability ball) or other variables (e.g., standing curl versus machine curl) can change the difficulty of the exercise; therefore, the exercise activity has been changed.

A few researchers report a superior response from multiple set resistance training.[107–111] However, the preponderance of evidence reports similar responses of muscular strength, hypertrophy, and muscular endurance between single and multiple set resistance training programs.[11,95–97,102,112–123] Single set programs require less time and are efficient.[11,97,122] In addition, an effective resistance training program conducted within a limited time commitment may improve exercise compliance. Caution is advised for training that emphasizes accentuated lengthening (eccentric) muscle actions, compared to shortening (concentric) or isometric muscle actions, because the potential for acute delayed onset of muscle soreness is accentuated and the outcome is similar. The soreness may discourage exercise participation. Muscular strength and endurance can be developed by means of static or dynamic exercises. Although each type of training has advantages and limitations, dynamic resistance exercises are recommended for most adults. Resistance training for the average participant should be rhythmic, performed at a moderate repetition duration (~3 seconds concentric, ~3 seconds eccentric), involve a full range of motion, and not interfere with normal breathing. High-intensity exercise combined with the Valsalva maneuver (forced expiration against a closed glottis) can cause a dramatic, acute increase in both systolic and diastolic blood pressures.[91,92] Currently there is little scientific evidence to indicate that the stimulus for improving muscular strength and muscular endurance in resistance-trained populations is different than for the untrained healthy adult populations.

The following resistance training guidelines are recommended:

- Choose a mode of exercise (free weights, bands, or machines) that is comfortable throughout the full pain free range of motion.
- Perform a minimum of 8 to 10 separate exercises that train the major muscles of the hips, thigh, legs, back, chest, shoulders, arms, and abdomen. A primary goal of the program should be to develop total body strength and endurance in a relatively time-efficient manner. Total exercise training programs lasting longer than 1 hour per session are associated with higher dropout rates.
- Perform one set of each exercise to the point of volitional fatigue for healthy individuals, while maintaining good form.
- While the traditional recommendation of 8 to 12 repetitions is still appropriate, choose a range of repetitions between 3 and 20 (e.g., 3 to 5, 8 to 10, 12 to 15) that can be performed at a moderate repetition duration (~3 sec concentric, ~3 sec eccentric).
- Exercise each muscle group 2 to 3 nonconsecutive days per week and if possible, perform a different exercise for the muscle group every two to three sessions.
- Adhere as closely as possible to the specific techniques for performing a given exercise.
- Allow enough time between exercises to perform the next exercise in proper form.
- For people with high cardiovascular risk or those with chronic disease (hypertension, diabetes), terminate each exercise as the concentric portion of the exercise becomes difficult (RPE 15 to 16) while maintaining good form.
- Perform both the lifting (concentric phase) and lowering (eccentric phase) portion of the resistance exercises in a controlled manner.
- Maintain a normal breathing pattern; breath-holding can induce excessive increases in blood pressure.
- If possible, exercise with a training partner who can provide feedback, assistance, and motivation.

Flexibility Exercise Prescription

Optimal musculoskeletal function requires that an adequate range of motion be maintained in all joints. Therefore, preventive and rehabilitative exercise programs should include activities that promote the maintenance of flexibility. Reductions in flexibility often are evident by the third decade of life and progress with aging. A lack of flexibility combined with a reduced musculoskeletal strength in elderly persons often contributes to a reduced ability to perform activities of daily living. Accordingly, exercise programs for elderly persons, as well as other populations, should emphasize proper stretching for all the major joints, especially for areas affected by a reduction in range of motion. Flexibility is highly individual, specific to each joint, and affected by many factors, including muscular strength and disease (e.g., carpal tunnel syndrome, arthritis).[124]

Stretching can be defined as the systematic elongation of musculotendinous units to create a persistent length of the muscle and a decrease in passive tension. Musculotendinous units are considered the limiting structures preventing greater ranges of motion about the joint.[125] Muscles have viscoelastic properties; that is, elasticity indicates that length changes are directly proportional to the applied force, and viscous properties indicate that the rate of muscle deformation is directly proportional to the applied force. The muscle's viscoelastic property permits a gradual decrease in tension or force within the muscle at a given length. The attenuation of muscular tension over time is termed stress relaxation.[126] The application of stretching can result in a continued deformation (longer length) of the muscle at a lower tension, which is commonly known as improved flexibility.

Although flexibility can improve acutely, there is a lack of scientific evidence as to how long the effect may last. Many experts recommend frequent (daily) stretching because flexibility is believed to be transient. Different types of stretching techniques (e.g., static, dynamic, proprioceptive neuromuscular facilitation [PNF]) can be performed. Static stretching involves slowly stretching a muscle to the end of the range of motion (point of tightness without invoking discomfort) and then holding that position for an extended period of time (usually 15 to 30 seconds). The greatest change in flexibility has been shown in the first 15 seconds of a stretch with no significant improvement after 30 seconds.[127,128] The optimal number of stretches per muscle group is two to four, because no significant additional improvement in muscle elongation is evident in repeated stretching of five to ten repetitions.[126] The risk of injury is low, requires little time and assistance, and is quite effective. For these reasons, static stretching is recommended.

The following two types of stretching techniques are not recommended for the general population; however, certain circumstances (e.g., past history, specific goals, specificity of training) may warrant their use for specific populations. Dynamic stretching uses the momentum created by repetitive bouncing movements to produce muscle stretch. The strain in the muscle has a fast onset and the muscle tension reaches relatively high values. There is a greater risk of strain injury because the muscle is not held at the higher tension to allow the time-dependent stress relaxation response to occur. This type of stretch can result in muscle soreness or injury if the forces generated by the dynamic movements are too great. PNF stretching involves a combination of alternating contraction and relaxation of both agonist and antagonist muscles through a designated series of motions. For example, PNF can be applied to a hamstring stretch by allowing a partner to flex the hip with the knee straight until the participant reports muscle tightness. The participant then actively extends the hip against the partner's resistance. Finally, the participant relaxes the hamstring and allows the partner to passively stretch the hamstring to a greater range of motion by flexing the hip. PNF typically requires a partner trained in the technique, may cause some degree of muscle soreness, and is more time consuming than alternative methods.

Properly performed stretching exercises can aid in improving and maintaining range of motion in a joint or series of joints. Flexibility exercises should be performed in a slow, controlled manner with a gradual progression to greater ranges of motion. A general exercise prescription for achieving and maintaining flexibility should adhere to the following guidelines:[129]

- Precede stretching with a warm-up to elevate muscle temperature
- Do a static stretching routine that exercises the major muscle tendon units that focuses on muscle groups (joints) that have reduced range of motion
- Perform a minimum of 2 to 3 $d \cdot wk^{-1}$, ideally 5 to 7 $d \cdot wk^{-1}$
- Stretch to the end of the range of motion at a point of tightness, without inducing discomfort
- Hold each stretch for 15 to 30 seconds
- Two to four repetitions for each stretch

A series of easy-to-understand stretches are available from various publications that can provide the basis for a prudent flexibility program.[130] Yoga, tai chi, and Pilates movements also may be used to improve flexibility when appropriate. Stretching exercises can be effectively included in the warm-up and/or cool-down periods that precede and follow the aerobic conditioning phase of an exercise session. It is recommended that an active warm-up precede stretching exercises. Some commonly employed stretching exercises may not be appropriate for some participants who may be at greater risk for musculoskeletal injuries because of prior injury, joint insufficiency, or other conditions. Although research concerning the risks of specific exercises is lacking, those activities that require substantial flexibility, skill, or position the joint in a range of motion that stretches ligaments or nerves are not recommended. For example, the following is a list of high-risk stretches (danger to the joint) and safer alternatives.[129]

High-Risk Stretch	Alternative Stretch
Standing toe touch	Seated toe touch or modified hurdler's stretch
Barré stretch	Seated toe touch or modified hurdler's stretch
Hurdler's stretch	Modified hurdler's stretch
Neck circles	Non-twisting directional stretch
Knee hyperflexion	Kneeling hip and thigh stretch
Yoga plow	Seated toe touch

For additional information on the topic, refer to the *ACSM's Resource Manual for Guidelines for Exercise Testing and Prescription* (5th ed.).

Maintenance of the Training Effect

Numerous studies have investigated the physiologic consequences of a reduced exercise dosage or complete cessation of training in physically conditioned people. A significant reduction of 5% to 10% in $\dot{V}O_{2max}$ has been reported within 3 weeks of stopping intense endurance training,[131] with most of the reduction attributed to decreased blood volume. The rapid reduction in maximal oxygen consumption plateaus relatively soon, with a total reduction of only 16% after 12 weeks of detraining.[131] Participants may return to pretraining levels of aerobic fitness in approximately 10 weeks[132] to 8 months of detraining[133] or decrease their gains by half after only 4 to 12 weeks of[134] complete cessation of training. Maintenance of the training effect generally shows a direct relationship to the length of time in training;[131] that is, the longer one remains in a trained state the longer it takes to return to baseline levels, and may be modulated by the level of fitness, age, intervening illness or injury, and specific conditioning practices.

A related series of studies examined the relative effects of decreased exercise frequency,[135] duration,[136] or intensity[137] on the maintenance of $\dot{V}O_{2max}$ during a period of reduced training. All three studies trained young men and women for 40 minutes, 6 d·wk^{-1} for 10 weeks at a moderate to high exercise intensity, followed by 15 weeks of reduced training at one-third and two-third reductions in the frequency, duration, or intensity of training. Only when the intensity of training was reduced was there a significant decrease in $\dot{V}O_{2max}$; moreover, most of the reduction occurred within the first 5 weeks of reduced training.[137] In contrast, decreasing the frequency or duration of training had little influence on the postconditioning $\dot{V}O_{2max}$, provided that the intensity was maintained. Similarly, restricted walk training resulted in rapid deconditioning in cardiac patients who had been jogging, despite an unchanged exercise frequency and duration.[138] Collectively, these findings indicate that exercise intensity is the most important exercise prescription variable to maintain a cardiovascular training response.

The preservation of resistance training effects also has been examined relative to a reduced exercise frequency. In these studies, strength gains were maintained for 12 weeks with one training session per week[139] and only one training session every 2 to 4 weeks,[140] provided that the resistance training loads remained constant. Thus, it appears that a reduced training frequency or duration does not adversely affect $\dot{V}O_{2max}$ or muscular strength if the training intensity is maintained.

Additional evidence, relevant to the maintenance of training effects, suggests that upper body training per se has little influence on the retention of lower body training effects,[141] further reinforcing the principle of training specificity. However, an alternate training modality augments energy expenditure and serves to maintain health benefits.

Program Supervision

Information from health screening, medical evaluation, and exercise testing allow the exercise professional to determine those individuals for whom supervised exercise programs are suggested. Exercise professionals should recognize that most individuals can exercise safely at a moderate intensity without supervision. However, for those who wish to maintain or increase their fitness levels by following the exercise prescription guidelines within this chapter, Table 7-3 provides general guidelines for exercise program supervision.

Table 7-3 represents a hierarchy of supervision. To use this table, determine the health status of the participant through risk stratification, and in conjunction with the participants' functional capacity, determine the level of supervision

TABLE 7-2. Summary of General Exercise Programming

Components of Training Program	Frequency (sessions·wk^{-1})	Intensity	Duration	Activity
Cardiorespiratory	3–5 d·wk^{-1}	40%/50%–85% HRR or VO$_2$R 64/70%–94% HR$_{max}$ 12–16 RPE	20–60 min	Large muscle groups Dynamic activity
Resistance	2–3 d·wk^{-1}	Volitional fatigue (MMF) (e.g., 19–20 RPE) Or Stop 2–3 reps before volitional fatigue (e.g., 16 RPE)	1 set of 3–20 repetitions (e.g., 3–5, 8–10, 12–15)	8–10 exercises Include all major muscle groups
Flexibility	Minimal 2–3 d·wk^{-1} Ideal 5–7 d·wk^{-1}	Stretch to tightness at the end of the range of motion but not to pain	15–30 seconds 2–4 x/stretch	Static stretch all major muscle groups

Abbreviations: HRR, heart rate reserve; VO$_2$R, maximal oxygen uptake reserve; MMF, momentary muscular fatigue.

recommended. For example, if a person's health status is classified as moderate risk, but he or she has a functional capacity of 5 METs, then the clinical professional should supervise the exercise program. If a person is of low risk, but has a functional capacity of <7 METs, then a professional (Table 7-3) should supervise the exercise program. It should be noted that a functional capacity of ≤7 METs is well below the 10th percentile for apparently healthy men, and either at or below the 10th percentile for most apparently healthy women from the Aerobics Center Longitudinal Study (see Table 4-8). *Apparently healthy* individuals within the ACLS cohort would be inclusive of individuals within the ACSM Low and Moderate Risk categories (see Table 2-4).

Supervised exercise programs are recommended for patients with symptoms and cardiorespiratory disease who are considered by their physicians to be clinically stable and who have been medically cleared for participation in such programs. It is recommended that supervised exercise programs for such individuals be under the combined overall guidance of a physician; appropriate nursing staff, and an ACSM-certified Program Director, ACSM Exercise Specialist, or ACSM Registered Clinical Exercise Physiologist (see Appendix F). However, direct supervision of each session by a physician is not necessarily required to ensure safety.[142] These programs can be useful for those who need instruction in proper exercise techniques. For some participants, direct supervision may enhance compliance with an exercise program.

TABLE 7-3. General Guidelines for Exercise Program Supervision

	Level of Supervision		
	Unsupervised	**Professionally Supervised***	**Clinically Supervised†**
Health Status	Low risk (from Table 2-4)	Moderate risk (from Table 2-4) **Or** High risk (from Table 2-4) but with well-controlled, stable CPM disease	High risk (from Table 2-4) with recent onset of CPM that have been cleared by a physician for participation in exercise regimen.
Functional‡ capacity	>7 METs	>7 METs	<7 METs§

*Professionally supervised means supervision by appropriately trained personnel who possess academic training and practical/clinical knowledge, skills, and abilities commensurate with any of the three credentials defined in Appendix F (i.e., ACSM Health/Fitness Instructor, ACSM Exercise Specialist, ACSM RCEP), the ACSM Program Director, or ACSM Health/Fitness Director.

†Clinically supervised means supervision by appropriately trained personnel who possess academic training and practical/clinical knowledge, skills, and abilities commensurate with the ACSM Exercise Specialist or ACSM RCEP credentials defined in Appendix F, or the ACSM Program Director.

‡A functional capacity of ≤7 METs is well below the 10th percentile for apparently healthy men, and either at or below the 10th percentile for most apparently healthy women from the Aerobics Center Longitudinal Study (see Table 4-8). Apparently healthy individuals within the ACLS cohort would be inclusive of individuals within the ACSM Low and Moderate Risk categories (see Table 2-4).

§For functional capacity of <5 METs, a small staff-to-patient ratio (i.e., one clinical staff member for every five to eight patients) also is recommended.

Abbreviation: CPM, cardiovascular, pulmonary, and/or metabolic disease.

Methods for Changing Exercise Behaviors

Despite nearly three decades of the so-called "exercise revolution," structured exercise programs have been only marginally effective in getting people to be more physically active. Fitness and cardiac exercise programs have typically reported dropout rates ranging from 9% to 87% (mean, 45%), highlighting the compliance problem among those who initiate physical conditioning programs.[143,144] Dropout rates are generally high in the first 3 months, increasing to approximately 50% within 1 year. Thus, it appears that exercise is not unlike other health-related behaviors (e.g., medication compliance, smoking cessation, weight reduction) in that typically *half or less* of those who initiate the behavior will continue, irrespective of initial health status or type of program.

To understand why people sometimes lack the motivation for regular physical activity, one must acknowledge a simple yet important fact: Exercise is voluntary and time consuming; therefore, it may extend the day or compete with other valued interests and responsibilities of daily life. According to one recent report, new members of fitness centers typically use these facilities less than twice a month.[145] In another study, patients undergoing gymnasium-based exercise training spent more time in their cars going to and from the programs than patients in a home-training comparison group spent on their cycle ergometers.[146] The traditional approach to the exercise compliance problem has involved attempting to persuade dropouts to become reinvolved. However, an alternative approach involves the

A B C D E	
5 4 3 2 1	1. I get discouraged easily.
5 4 3 2 1	2. I don't work any harder than I have to.
1 2 3 4 5	3. I seldom if ever let myself down.
5 4 3 2 1	4. I'm just not the goal-setting type.
1 2 3 4 5	5. I'm good at keeping promises, especially the ones I make myself.
5 4 3 2 1	6. I don't impose much structure on my activities.
1 2 3 4 5	7. I have a very hard-driving, aggressive personality.

Directions: Circle the number beneath the letter corresponding to the alternative that best describes how characteristic the statement is when applied to you. The alternatives are:

      A. *extremely* uncharacteristic of me.
      B. *somewhat* uncharacteristic of me.
      C. neither characteristic nor uncharacteristic of me.
      D. *somewhat* characteristic of me.
      E. *extremely* characteristic of me.

Scoring: Add together the seven numbers you circled. A score ≤ 24 suggests dropout-prone behavior. The lower the self-motivation score, the greater the likelihood toward exercise noncompliance. If the score suggests dropout proneness, it should be viewed as an incentive to remain active, rather than a self-fulfilling prophecy to quit exercising.

FIGURE 7-6. Self-motivation assessment scale to determine likelihood of exercise compliance. (Copyright 1978, Dishman RK, Ickes W, Morgan WP. Self-motivation and adherence to habitual physical activity. J Appl Social Psychol 1980;10:115–132. From Falls HB, Baylor AM, Dishman RK. Essentials of fitness. Philadelphia: Saunders College, 1980:Appendix A-13. Reproduced by permission of the copyright holders.)

identification and subsequent monitoring of "dropout-prone" individuals, with an aim toward preventing recidivism. A brief questionnaire designed to assess "self-motivation" can be used along with measures of intention and self-efficacy, to predict male and female dropout-prone behavior (Fig. 7-6).[147]

Readiness for change theory has received wide acceptance by health care practitioners in assisting individuals to make permanent lifestyle changes,[148] including regular exercise.[149,150] A preliminary interview/orientation provides an opportunity to identify the client's expectations (realistic or unrealistic), coping techniques/defense mechanisms, belief systems and values, social support systems, and stage of readiness for change (Fig. 7-7). Box 7-2 describes each of these stages. Stage-specific interventions using varied approaches (e.g., structured group programs versus home-based exercise), community resources, and serial monitoring and/or communication should be employed. The latter may include regular telephone contact, mail (e.g., completion of activity logs), fax, video recording, Internet, and transtelephonic ECG monitoring. Unfortunately, some individuals may "exit" from the "preparation phase," and essentially discontinue their sporadic activity patterns. Other persons in the "action" stage also may stop

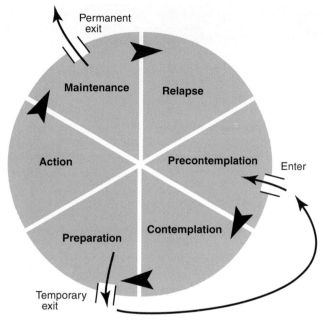

FIGURE 7-7. Progressive stages of readiness for behavior change, with specific reference to temporary and permanent exits and relapse. (Adapted from Prochaska J, DiClemente C. Transtheoretical therapy, toward a more integrative model of change. Psych Theory Res Prac 1982;19:276–288.)

exercising for a variety of reasons (e.g., job change and/or move, intercurrent illness or injury, personal convenience factors, competing priorities [work deadlines]). Such individuals should be taught to deal with inactive lapses or relapses, re-entered at the appropriate stage, and counseled that these behaviors are not necessarily tantamount to failure.

STRATEGIES FOR INCREASING EXERCISE ADHERENCE

Numerous interventions aimed at increasing physical activity levels using behavior change counseling have been described previously with mixed results. Nevertheless, the fervor of the primary physicians' recommendation appears to be one of the most powerful predictors of the patient's participation in exercise,[151] especially if a baseline fitness assessment and an exercise prescription are provided at the point of care.[152] Research and empiric experience suggests that certain program modifications and motivational strategies may enhance participant interest and compliance, as shown in Box 7-3.

ENCOURAGE LIFESTYLE PHYSICAL ACTIVITY

Over the last decade, researchers have re-evaluated the scientific evidence linking physical inactivity with a variety of chronic diseases. These analyses suggest

BOX 7-2	Stages of "Readiness to Change" Model*†

1. *Precontemplation:* Patients express lack of interest in making change. Moving patients through this stage involves use of multiple resources to stress the importance of the desired change. This can be achieved through written materials, educational classes, physician and family persuasion, and other means.
2. *Contemplation:* Patients are "thinking" about making a desired change. This stage can be influenced by helping patients define the risks and benefits of making or not making the desired change (e.g., starting an exercise program).
3. *Preparation:* Patients are doing some physical activity but not meeting the recommended criteria; that is, 30 minutes of moderate intensity physical activity 5 $d \cdot wk^{-1}$ or 3 to 5 $d \cdot wk^{-1}$ of vigorous intensity activity for 20 minutes.
4. *Action:* Patients are meeting the referenced (preparation) criteria on a consistent basis but they have not maintained the behavior for 6 months.
5. *Maintenance:* Patients have been in action for 6 months or more.

*From Dunn AL, Marcus BH, Kampert JB, et al. Reduction in cardiovascular disease risk factors: 6-month results from Project Active. Prev Med 1997;26:883–892; Dunn AL, Marcus BH, Kampert JB, et al. Comparison of lifestyle and structured interventions to increase physical activity and cardiorespiratory fitness: a randomized trial. JAMA 1999;281:327–334.

†Modified for physical activity interventions.

that the intensity of exercise needed to achieve health-related benefits is probably less than that required to improve CR fitness. Thus, frequent bouts of moderate-intensity activity (e.g., brisk walking, household chores, gardening, recreational activities) may serve as an alternative to vigorous exercise, provided that the total energy expenditure is comparable.[153] Recent randomized trials have shown that a lifestyle approach to physical activity among previously sedentary adults is feasible and has similar effects on aerobic fitness, body composition, and coronary risk factors as compared with a traditional structured exercise program.[150,154] Another recent study showed that lifestyle intervention, including at least 150 minutes of physical activity per week, was even more effective than pharmacologic treatment, in reducing the incidence of type 2 diabetes.[155] Collectively, these findings have important implications for public health.[156]

Although lifestyle exercise is not being suggested to replace traditional structured exercise programs, it provides an effective complement to any health and fitness regimen. Accordingly, exercise professionals should consider broadening their client's recommendations beyond the frequency, intensity, duration, and modes of training that are associated with structured programs, by encouraging

BOX 7-3	**Practical Recommendations to Enhance Exercise Adherence**

- Recruit physician support of the exercise program.
- Provide exercise facilities and changing facilities that are appropriately maintained.
- Clarify individual needs to establish the motive to exercise.
- Emphasize short-term, realistic goals.
- Minimize injuries and/or complications with a light to moderate exercise prescription.
- Encourage group participation.
- Emphasize variety and enjoyment in the exercise program.
- Employ periodic fitness testing to assess the client's response to the training program.
- Recruit support of the program among family and friends.
- Include an optional recreational game to the conditioning program format.
- Establish regularity of exercise sessions.
- Use progress charts to record exercise achievements.
- Recognize participant accomplishments through a system of rewards.
- Provide qualified, personable, and enthusiastic exercise professionals.

them to increase physical activity in daily living. To assist with this objective, a five-step counseling plan has been suggested to help clients initiate and maintain a more physically active lifestyle:

1. Ask clients about their current structured exercise and activity habits to determine whether those activities are sufficient to confer health and/or fitness benefits.
2. Provide clients with a traditional exercise prescription.
3. Brainstorm opportunities to increase physical activity in daily living (e.g., increase routine activity by taking the stairs rather than the elevator, increase transportation-related physical activity by walking or cycling versus automobile, and find more convenient forms of leisure physical activity in parks, hiking trails, and bike paths).
4. Emphasize the short- and long-term benefits of these varied approaches.
5. Plan regular follow-up contact to reinforce efforts and devise ways to overcome barriers to regular physical activity.

The Activity Pyramid has been suggested as one way to facilitate these objectives (see Fig. 7-1).[157] In addition, despite a lack of scientific evidence, accelerometers or pedometer use may assist clients in tracking their daily activities[158,159] and facilitate exercise adherence.

REFERENCES

1. Pate RR, Pratt M, Blair SN, et al. Physical activity and public health. A recommendation from the Centers for Disease Control and Prevention and the American College of Sports Medicine. JAMA 1995;273:402–407.
2. United States Department of Health and Human Services. Physical activity and health: a report of the Surgeon General, 1996.
3. Bouchard C. Physical activity and health: introduction to the dose-response symposium. Med Sci Sports Exerc 2001;33:S347–350.
4. Kesaniemi YK, Danforth E Jr, Jensen MD, et al. Dose-response issues concerning physical activity and health: an evidence-based symposium. Med Sci Sports Exerc 2001;33:S351–358.
5. McArdle WD, Margel JR, Delio DJ, et al. Specificity of run training on VO2 max and heart rate changes during running and swimming. Med Sci Sports 1978;10:16–20.
6. Gollnick P. Effects of training on enzyme activity and fiber composition of human skeletal muscle. J Appl Physiol 1973;34:107–111.
7. Thomas TR, Ziogas G, Smith T, et al. Physiological and perceived exertion responses to six modes of submaximal exercise. Res Q Exerc Sport 1995;66:239–246.
8. Bouchard C, Rankinen T. Individual differences in response to regular physical activity. Med Sci Sports Exerc 2001;33:S446–451; discussion S452–453.
9. Southard DR. Modifications of health behavior. In: Roitman JL, ed. ACSM's Resource Manual for Guidelines for Exercise Testing and Prescription. Baltimore: Lippincott Williams & Wilkins, 1998: 523–584.
10. Bishop D. Potential mechanisms and the effects of passive warm-up on exercise performance. Sports Med 2003;33:439–454.
11. Pollock ML, Gaesser GA, Butcher JD. The recommended quantity and quality of exercise for developing and maintaining cardiorespiratory and muscular fitness, and flexibility in healthy adults. Med Sci Sports Exerc 1998;30:975–991.
12. Barnard RJ, Gardner GW, Diaco NV, et al. Cardiovascular responses to sudden strenuous exercise: heart rate, blood pressure, and ECG. J Appl Physiol 1973;34:833–837.
13. Barnard RJ, MacAlpin R, Kattus AA, et al. Ischemic response to sudden strenuous exercise in healthy men. Circulation 1973;48:936–942.
14. Foster C, Anholm JD, Hellman CK, et al. Left ventricular function during sudden strenuous exercise. Circulation 1981;63:592–596.
15. Foster C, Dymond DS, Carpenter J, et al. Effect of warm-up on left ventricular response to sudden strenuous exercise. J Appl Physiol 1982;53:380–383.
16. Chesler RM, Michielli DW, Aron M, et al. Cardiovascular response to sudden strenuous exercise: an exercise echocardiographic study. Med Sci Sports Exerc 1997;29:1299–1303.
17. Stein RA, Berger HJ, Zaret BL. The cardiac response to sudden strenuous exercise in the postmyocardial infarction patient receiving beta blockers. J Cardiopulm Rehabil 1986;6:336–342.
18. Franklin BA, Stoedefalke KG. Games-as-aerobics: activities for cardiac rehabilitation programs. In: Fardy PS, Franklin BA, Porcari JP, Verrill DE, ed. Current Issues in Cardiac Rehabilitation: Training Techniques in Cardiac Rehabilitation. Champaign, IL: Human Kinetics, 1998:106–136.
19. Dimsdale JE, Hartley LH, Guiney T, et al. Postexercise peril. Plasma catecholamines and exercise. JAMA 1984;251:630–432.
20. Wilmore JH, Royce J, Girandola RN, et al. Physiological alterations resulting from a 10-week program of jogging. Med Sci Sports 1970;2:7–14.
21. Tabata I, Nishimura K, Kouzaki M, et al. Effects of moderate-intensity endurance and high-intensity intermittent training on anaerobic capacity and VO2 max. Med Sci Sports Exerc 1996;28:1327–1330.
22. Swain DP, Franklin BA. VO2 reserve and the minimal intensity for improving cardiorespiratory fitness. Med Sci Sports Exerc 2002;34:152–157.
23. Franklin BA, Pamatmat A, Johnson S, et al. Metabolic cost of extremely slow walking in cardiac patients: implications for exercise testing and training. Arch Phys Med Rehabil 1983;64:564–565.
24. Pollock ML, Miller HS Jr, Janeway R, et al. Effects of walking on body composition and cardiovascular function of middle-aged man. J Appl Physiol 1971;30:126–130.
25. Shoenfeld Y, Keren G, Shimoni T, et al. Walking. A method for rapid improvement of physical fitness. JAMA 1980;243:2062–2063.
26. Evans BW, Cureton KJ, Purvis JW. Metabolic and circulatory responses to walking and jogging in water. Res Q 1978;49:442–449.

27. Porcari JP, McCarron R, Kline G. Is fast walking an adequate aerobic training stimulus for 30 to 69 year-old men and women? Phys Sportsmed 1987;15(2):119–129.
28. Spelman CC, Pate RR, Macera CA, et al. Self-selected exercise intensity of habitual walkers. Med Sci Sports Exerc 1993;25:1174–1179.
29. Howley ET. Type of activity: resistance, aerobic and leisure versus occupational physical activity. Med Sci Sports Exerc 2001;33:S364–S369.
30. Swain DP, Leutholtz BC. Heart rate reserve is equivalent to %VO2 reserve, not to %VO2max. Med Sci Sports Exerc 1997;29:410–414.
31. Fox SM 3rd, Naughton JP, Gorman PA. Physical activity and cardiovascular health: III. The exercise prescription: frequency and type of activity. Mod Concepts Cardiovasc Dis 1972;41:25–30.
32. Haskell WL. Design and implementation of cardiac conditioning programs. In: Wenger NK, Hellerstein HK, eds. Rehabilitation of the Coronary Patient. New York: John Wiley & Sons, 1978:203–241.
33. Hellerstein HK, Franklin BA. Exercise testing and prescription. In: Wenger NK, Hellerstein HK, eds. Rehabilitation of the Coronary Patient. New York: John Wiley & Sons, 1978:203–241.
34. Ainsworth BE, Haskell WL, Whitt MC, et al. Compendium of physical activities: an update of activity codes and MET intensities. Med Sci Sports Exerc 2000;32:S498–S516.
35. Robergs RA, Landwehr R. The surprising history of the "HRmax = 220-age" equation. J Exer Physonline 2002;5(2):1–10.
36. Whaley MH, Kaminsky LA, Dwyer GB, et al. Predictions of over- and underachievement of age-predicted maximal heart rate. Med Sci Sports Exerc 1992;24:1173–1179.
37. Miller WC, Wallace JP, Eggert KE. Predicting max HR and the HR-VO2 relationship for exercise prescription in obesity. Med Sci Sports Exerc 1993;25:1077–1081.
38. Londeree BR, Ames SA. Trend analysis of the % VO2 max-HR regression. Med Sci Sports 1976; 8:123–125.
39. Karvonen M, Kentala K, Mustala O. The effects of training on heart rate: a longitudinal study. Ann Med Exp Biol Fenn 1957;35:307–315.
40. Glass SC, Whaley MH, Wegner MS. Ratings of perceived exertion among standard treadmill protocols and steady state running. Int J Sports Med 1991;12:77–82.
41. Brubaker PH, Rejeski WJ, Law HC, et al. Cardiac patients' perception of work intensity during graded exercise testing: Do they generalize to field settings? J Cardiopul Rehab 1994;14: 127–133.
42. Whaley MH, Brubaker PH, Kaminsky LA, et al. Validity of rating of perceived exertion during graded exercise testing in apparently healthy adults and cardiac patients. J Cardiopulm Rehabil 1997;17:261–267.
43. DeBusk RF, Stenestrand U, Sheehan M, et al. Training effects of long versus short bouts of exercise in healthy subjects. Am J Cardiol 1990;65:1010–1013.
44. Murphy MH, Hardman AE. Training effects of short and long bouts of brisk walking in sedentary women. Med Sci Sports Exerc 1998;30:152–157.
45. Jakicic JM, Wing RR, Butler BA, et al. Prescribing exercise in multiple short bouts versus one continuous bout: effects on adherence, cardiorespiratory fitness, and weight loss in overweight women. Int J Obes Relat Metab Disord 1995;19:893–901.
46. Martin JE, Dubbert PM. Adherence to exercise. Exerc Sport Sci Rev 1985;13:137–167.
47. Gettman LR, Pollock ML, Durstine JL, et al. Physiological responses of men to 1, 3, and 5 day per weeek training programs. Res Q 1976;47:638–646.
48. Haskell WL. J.B. Wolffe Memorial Lecture. Health consequences of physical activity: understanding and challenges regarding dose-response. Med Sci Sports Exerc 1994;26:649–660.
49. Lee IM, Skerrett PJ. Physical activity and all-cause mortality: what is the dose-response relation? Med Sci Sports Exerc 2001;33:S459–471; discussion S493–494.
50. American College of Sports Medicine. Position Stand: Appropriate intervention strategies for weight loss and prevention of weight regain for adults. Med Sci Sports Exerc 2001;33:2145–2156.
51. Saris W, Blair SN, van Baak M, et al. How much physical activity is enough to prevent unhealthy weight gain? Outcome of the IASO 1st Stock Conference and consensus statement. Obesity Rev 2003;4:101–114.
52. Food and Nutrition Board, Institute of Medicine. Dietary reference intakes for energy, carbohydrates, fiber, fat, protein and amino acids (macronutrients). Washington, DC: National Academy Press, 2002.
53. Ross R, Janssen I. Physical activity, total and regional obesity: dose-response considerations. Med Sci Sports Exerc 2001;33:S521–527; discussion S528–529.

54. Hendelman D, Miller K, Baggett E, et al. Validity of accelerometry for the assessment of moderate intensity physical activity in the field. Med Sci Sports Exerc 2000;32:S442–S449.
55. Fehling PC, Smith DL, Warner SE, et al. Comparison of accelerometers with oxygen consumption in older adults during exercise. Med Sci Sports Exerc 1999;31:171–175.
56. Ainsworth BE, Haskell WL, Leon AS, et al. Compendium of physical activities: classification of energy costs of human physical activities. Med Sci Sports Exerc 1993;25:71–80.
57. Clausen JP, Trap-Jensen J, Lassen NA. The effects of training on the heart rate during arm and leg exercise. Scand J Clin Lab Invest 1970;26:295–301.
58. Klausen K, Rasmussen B, Clausen JP, et al. Blood lactate from exercising extremities before and after arm or leg training. Am J Physiol 1974;227:67–72.
59. Rasmussen B, Klausen K, Clausen JP, et al. Pulmonary ventilation, blood gases, and blood pH after training of the arms or the legs. J Appl Physiol 1975;38:250–256.
60. Pate RR, Hughes RD, Chandler JV. Effects of arm training on retention of training effects derived from leg training. Med Sci Sports 1978;10:71–74.
61. Henriksson J, Reitman JS. Time course of changes in human skeletal muscle succinate dehydrogenase and cytochrome oxidase activities and maximal oxygen uptake with physical activity and inactivity. Acta Physiol Scand 1977;99:91–97.
62. Clausen JP, Klausen K, Rasmussen B, et al. Central and peripheral circulatory changes after training of the arms or legs. Am J Physiol 1973;225:675–682.
63. McKenzie DC, Fox EL, Cohen K. Specificity of metabolic and circulatory responses to arm or leg interval training. Eur J Appl Physiol Occup Physiol 1978;39:241–248.
64. Thompson PD, Cullinane E, Lazarus B, et al. Effect of exercise training on the untrained limb exercise performance of men with angina pectoris. Am J Cardiol 1981;48:844–850.
65. Detry JM, Rousseau M, Vandenbroucke G, et al. Increased arteriovenous oxygen difference after physical training in coronary heart disease. Circulation 1971;44:109–118.
66. Lewis S, Thompson P, Areskog NH, et al. Transfer effects of endurance training to exercise with untrained limbs. Eur J Appl Physiol Occup Physiol 1980;44:25–34.
67. Winnett RA, Carpinelli RN. Potential health-related benefits of resistance training. Prev Med 2001;33:503–513.
68. Kerr D, Morton A, Dick I, et al. Exercise effects on bone mass in postmenopausal women are site-specific and load-dependent. J Bone Miner Res 1996;11:218–225.
69. Pruitt LA, Taaffe DR, Marcus R. Effects of a one-year high-intensity versus low-intensity resistance training program on bone mineral density in older women. J Bone Miner Res 1995;10:1788–1795.
70. Hurley BF, Hagberg JM, Goldberg AP, et al. Resistance training can reduce coronary risk factors without altering VO2max or percent body fat. Med Sci Sports Exerc 1988;20:150–154.
71. Layne JE, Nelson ME. The effects of progressive resistance training on bone density: a review. Med Sci Sports Exerc 1999;31:25–30.
72. Wilmore JH, Parr RB, Ward P, et al. Energy cost of circuit weight training. Med Sci Sports 1978;10:75–78.
73. Beckham SG, Earnest CP. Metabolic cost of free weight circuit weight training. J Sports Med Phys Fitness 2000;40:118–125.
74. Vincent KR, Vincent HK, Braith RW, et al. Strength training and hemodynamic responses to exercise. Am J Geriatr Cardiol 2003;12:97–196.
75. Phillips WT, Ziuraitis JR. Energy cost of the ACSM single-set resistance training protocol. J Strength Cond Res 2003;17:350–355.
76. Melanson EL, Sharp TA, Seagle HM, et al. Resistance and aerobic exercise have similar effects on 24-h nutrient oxidation. Med Sci Sports Exerc 2002;34:1793–1800.
77. Gore CJ, Withers RT. Effect of exercise intensity and duration on postexercise metabolism. J Appl Physiol 1990;68:2362–2368.
78. Melby C, Scholl C, Edwards G, et al. Effect of acute resistance exercise on postexercise energy expenditure and resting metabolic rate. J Appl Physiol 1993;75:1847–1853.
79. Binzen CA, Swan PD, Manore MM. Postexercise oxygen consumption and substrate use after resistance exercise in women. Med Sci Sports Exerc 2001;33:932–938.
80. Haltom RW, Kraemer RR, Sloan RA, et al. Circuit weight training and its effects on excess postexercise oxygen consumption. Med Sci Sports Exerc 1999;31:1613–1618.
81. Melby CL, Tincknell T, Schmidt WD. Energy expenditure following a bout of non-steady state resistance exercise. J Sports Med Phys Fitness 1992;32:128–135.

82. Bosselaers I, Buemann B, Victor OJ, et al. Twenty-four-hour energy expenditure and substrate utilization in body builders. Am J Clin Nutr 1994;59:10–12.
83. Lemmer JT, Ivey FM, Ryan AS, et al. Effect of strength training on resting metabolic rate and physical activity: age and gender comparisons. Med Sci Sports Exerc 2001;33:532–541.
84. Broeder CE, Burrhus KA, Svanevik LS, et al. The effects of either high-intensity resistance or endurance training on resting metabolic rate. Am J Clin Nutr 1992;55:802–810.
85. Van Etten LM, Westerterp KR, Verstappen FT. Effect of weight-training on energy expenditure and substrate utilization during sleep. Med Sci Sports Exerc 1995;27:188–193.
86. Mazzetti SA, Kraemer WJ, Volek JS, et al. The influence of direct supervision of resistance training on strength performance. Med Sci Sports Exerc 2000;32:1175–1184.
87. Van Etten LM, Verstappen FT, Westerterp KR. Effect of body build on weight-training-induced adaptations in body composition and muscular strength. Med Sci Sports Exerc 1994;26:515–521.
88. Hoeger WW, Barette SL, Hale DR. Relationship between repetition and selected percentages of one repetition maximum. J Appl Sport Sci Res 1987;1(1):11–13.
89. Hoeger WW, Hopkins DR, Bareete SL. Relationship between repetitions and selected percentages of one repetition maximum: a comparison between untrained and trained males and females. J Appl Sport Sci Res 1990;4:47–54.
90. Sale DG. Influence of exercise and training on motor unit activation. Exerc Sport Sci Rev 1987;15:95–151.
91. MacDougall JD, McKelvie RS, Moroz DE, et al. Factors affecting blood pressure during heavy weight lifting and static contractions. J Appl Physiol 1992;73:1590–1597.
92. MacDougall JD, Tuxen D, Sale DG, et al. Arterial blood pressure response to heavy resistance exercise. J Appl Physiol 1985;58:785–790.
93. Sanborn K, Boros R, Hruby J, et al. Short-term performance effects of weight training with multiple sets not to failure vs. a single set to failure in women. J Strength Cond Res 2000;14:328–331.
94. Bemben DA, Fetters NL, Bemben MG, et al. Musculoskeletal responses to high- and low-intensity resistance training in early postmenopausal women. Med Sci Sports Exerc 2000;32:1949–1957.
95. Hass CJ, Garzarella L, de Hoyos D, et al. Single versus multiple sets in long-term recreational weightlifters. Med Sci Sports Exerc 2000;32:235–242.
96. Starkey DB, Pollock ML, Ishida Y, et al. Effect of resistance training volume on strength and muscle thickness. Med Sci Sports Exerc 1996;28:1311–1320.
97. Faigenbaum A, Pollock ML, Ishida Y. Prescription of resistance training for health and disease. Med Sci Sports Exerc 1999;31:38–45.
98. Campos GE, Luecke TJ, Wendeln HK, et al. Muscular adaptations in response to three different resistance-training regimens: specificity of repetition maximum training zones. Eur J Appl Physiol 2002;88:50–60.
99. Anderson T, Kearney JT. Effects of three resistance training programs on muscular strength and absolute and relative endurance. Res Q Exerc Sport 1982;53:1–7.
100. Chestnut JL, Doherty D. The effects of 4 and 10 repetition maximum weight-training protocols on neuromuscular adaptations in untrained men. J Strength Cond Res 1999;13(4):353–359.
101. O'Shea P. Effects of selected weight training programs on the development of strength and muscle hypertrophy. Res Q 1966;37:95–102.
102. Stone WJ, Coulter SP. Strength/endurance effects from three resistance training protocols with women. J Strength Cond Res 1994;8(4):231–234.
103. Weiss LW, Coney HD, Clark FC. Differential functional adaptations to short-term low-, moderate-, high-repetition weight training. J Strength Cond Res 1999;13(3):236–241.
104. Hickson RC, Hidaka K, Foster C. Skeletal muscle fiber type, resistance training, and strength-related performance. Med Sci Sports Exerc 1994;26:593–598.
105. Vincent KR, Braith RW. Resistance exercise and bone turnover in elderly men and women. Med Sci Sports Exerc 2002;34(1):17–23.
106. Taaffe DR, Pruitt L, Pyka G, et al. Comparative effects of high- and low-intensity resistance training on thigh muscle strength, fiber area, and tissue composition in elderly women. Clin Physiol 1996;16:381–392.
107. Borst SE, De Hoyos DV, Garzarella L, et al. Effects of resistance training on insulin-like growth factor-I and IGF binding proteins. Med Sci Sports Exerc 2001;33:648–653.
108. Marx JO, Ratamess NA, Nindl BC, et al. Low-volume circuit versus high-volume periodized resistance training in women. Med Sci Sports Exerc 2001;33:635–643.

109. Rhea MR, Alvar BA, Ball SD, et al. Three sets of weight training superior to 1 set with equal intensity for eliciting strength. J Strength Cond Res 2002;16:525–529.
110. Rhea MR, Alvar BA, Burkett LN. Single versus multiple sets for strength: a meta-analysis to address the controversy. Res Q Exerc Sport 2002;73:485–488.
111. Schlumberger A, Stec J, Schmidtbleicher D. Single- vs. multiple-set strength training in women. J Strength Cond Res 2001;15:284–289.
112. Berger RA. Effect of varied sets of static training on dynamic strength. Am Correct Ther J 1972;26:52–54.
113. Carpinelli RN, Otto RM. Strength training. Single versus multiple sets. Sports Med 1998;26:73–84.
114. Capen EK. Study of four programs of heavy resistance exercise for development of muscular strength. Res Q 1956;27(2):132–142.
115. Coleman AE. Nautilus vs universal gym strength training in adult males. Am Correct Ther J 1977;31:103–107.
116. Graves JE, Holmes BL, Leggett SH. Single versus multiple set dynamic and isometric lumbar extension training. In: Eleventh International Congress of the World Confederation for Physical Therapy. Proceedings Book III. 1991; July 28–August 2:1340–1342.
117. Messier SP, Dill ME. Alterations in strength and maximal oxygen uptake consequent to nautilus circuit weight training. Res Q Exerc Sport 1985;56(4):345–351.
118. Ostrowski KJ, Wilson GJ, Weatherby R. The effect of weight training volume on hormonal output and muscular size and function. J Strength Cond Res 1997;11(3):148–154.
119. Pollock ML, Graves JE, Bamman MM, et al. Frequency and volume of resistance training: effect on cervical extension strength. Arch Phys Med Rehabil 1993;74:1080–1086.
120. Reid CM, Yeater RA, Ullrich IH. Weight training and strength, cardiorespiratory functioning and body composition of men. Br J Sports Med 1987;21:40–44.
121. Silvester LJ, Stiggins C, McGown C. The effect of variable resistance and free-weight training programs on strength and vertical jump. NSCA J 1982;3(6):30–33.
122. Hass CJ, Feigenbaum MS, Franklin BA. Prescription of resistance training for healthy populations. Sports Med 2001;31:953–964.
123. Stowers T, McMillan J, Scala D. The short-term effects of three different strength-power training methods. NSCA J 1983;5:24–27.
124. Marshall JL, Johanson N, Wickiewicz TL, et al. Joint looseness: a function of the person and the joint. Med Sci Sports Exerc 1980;12:189–194.
125. Johns RJ, Wright V. Relative importance of various tissues in joint stiffness. J Appl Physiol 1962;17(5):824–828.
126. Taylor DC, Dalton JD Jr, Seaber AV, et al. Viscoelastic properties of muscle-tendon units. The biomechanical effects of stretching. Am J Sports Med 1990;18:300–309.
127. McHugh MP, Magnusson SP, Gleim GW, et al. Viscoelastic stress relaxation in human skeletal muscle. Med Sci Sports Exerc 1992;24:1375–1382.
128. Bandy WD, Irion JM. The effect of time on static stretch on the flexibility of the hamstring muscles. Phys Ther 1994;74:845–850;discussion 850–852.
129. Knudson D. A review of stretching research. TAHPERD Journal 1995;(Oct):16–18.
130. American College of Sports Medicine. ACSM Fitness Book. 3rd ed. Champaign, IL: Human Kinetics, 2003.
131. Coyle EF, Martin WH 3rd, Sinacore DR, et al. Time course of loss of adaptations after stopping prolonged intense endurance training. J Appl Physiol 1984;57:1857–1864.
132. Fringer MN, Stull GA. Changes in cardiorespiratory parameters during periods of training and detraining in young adult females. Med Sci Sports 1974;6:20–25.
133. Knuttgen HG, Nordesjo LO, Ollander B, et al. Physical conditioning through interval training with young male adults. Med Sci Sports 1973;5:220–226.
134. Kendrick ZV, Pollock ML, Hickman TN, et al. Effects of training and detraining on cardiovascular efficiency. Am Correct Ther J 1971;25:79–83.
135. Hickson RC, Rosenkoetter MA. Reduced training frequencies and maintenance of increased aerobic power. Med Sci Sports Exerc 1981;13:13–16.
136. Hickson RC, Kanakis C Jr, Davis JR, et al. Reduced training duration effects on aerobic power, endurance, and cardiac growth. J Appl Physiol 1982;53:225–229.
137. Hickson RC, Foster C, Pollock ML, et al. Reduced training intensities and loss of aerobic power, endurance, and cardiac growth. J Appl Physiol 1985;58:492–499.

138. Dressendorfer RH, Franklin BA, Smith JL, et al. Rapid cardiac deconditioning in joggers restricted to walking: training heart rate and ischemic threshold. Chest 1997;112:1107–1111.
139. Graves JE, Pollock ML, Leggett SH, et al. Effect of reduced training frequency on muscular strength. Int J Sports Med 1988;9:316–319.
140. Tucci JT, Carpenter DM, Pollock ML, et al. Effect of reduced frequency of training and detraining on lumbar extension strength. Spine 1992;17:1497–1501.
141. Pate RR, Hughes RD, Chandler JV, et al. Effects of arm training on retention of training effects derived from leg training. Med Sci Sports 1978;10:71–74.
142. Franklin BA, Bonzheim K, Gordon S, et al. Safety of medically supervised outpatient cardiac rehabilitation exercise therapy: a 16-year follow-up. Chest 1998;114:902–906.
143. Franklin BA. Program factors that influence exercise adherence: practical adherence skills for clinical staff. In: Dishman R, ed. Exercise Adherence: Its Impact on Public Health. Champaign, IL: Human Kinetics, 1988:237–258.
144. Oldridge, NB. Compliance with exercise rehabilitation. In: Dishman R, ed. Exercise Adherence: Its Impact on Public Health. Champaign, IL: Human Kinetics, 1988:283–304.
145. Franklin BA, Conviser JM, Stewart B. The challenge of enhancing exercise compliance. J Am Coll Cardiol 2001;37:170A.
146. DeBusk RF, Haskell WL, Miller NH, et al. Medically directed at-home rehabilitation soon after clinically uncomplicated acute myocardial infarction: a new model for patient care. Am J Cardiol 1985;55:251–257.
147. Falls HB, Baylor AM, Dishman RK. Essentials for fitness. Philadelphia: Saunders College, 1980: Appendix A-13.
148. Prochaska J, DiClemente C. Transtheoretical therapy, toward a more integrative model of change. Psych Theory Res Prac 1982;19:276–288.
149. Dunn AL, Marcus BH, Kampert JB, et al. Reduction in cardiovascular disease risk factors: 6-month results from Project Active. Prev Med 1997;26:883–892.
150. Dunn AL, Marcus BH, Kampert JB, et al. Comparison of lifestyle and structured interventions to increase physical activity and cardiorespiratory fitness: a randomized trial. JAMA 1999;281: 327–334.
151. Ades PA, Waldmann ML, McCann WJ, et al. Predictors of cardiac rehabilitation participation in older coronary patients. Arch Intern Med 1992;152:1033–1035.
152. Petrella RJ, Koval JJ, Cunningham DA, et al. Can primary care doctors prescribe exercise to improve fitness? The Step Test Exercise Prescription (STEP) project. Am J Prev Med 2003;24: 316–322.
153. Gordon NF, Kohl HI, Blair SN. Life style exercise: a new strategy to promote physical activity for adults. J Cardiopulm Rehabil 1993;13:161–163.
154. Andersen RE, Wadden TA, Bartlett SJ, et al. Effects of lifestyle activity vs structured aerobic exercise in obese women: a randomized trial. JAMA 1999;281:335–340.
155. Knowler WC, Barrett-Connor E, Fowler SE, et al. Reduction in the incidence of type 2 diabetes with lifestyle intervention or metformin. N Engl J Med 2002;346:393–403.
156. Pratt M. Benefits of lifestyle activity vs structured exercise. JAMA 1999;281:375–376.
157. Leon AS, Norstrom J. Evidence of the role of physical activity and cardiorespiratory fitness in the prevention of coronary heart disease. Quest 1995;47:311–319.
158. Bassett DR Jr, Strath SJ. Use of pedometers in assessing physical activity. In: Welk GJ, ed. Physical Activity Assessments for Health-Related Research. Champaign, IL: Human Kinetics, 2002: 163–177.
159. Tudor-Locke C. Taking steps toward increased physical activity: using pedometers to measure and motivate. Research Digest, President's Council on Physical Fitness and Sports 2002;17:1–8.

8

Exercise Prescription Modifications for Cardiac Patients

Contemporary cardiac rehabilitation programs provide several important core components, including baseline patient assessment, nutrition counseling, risk factor management, psychosocial management, and activity counseling. However, appropriately prescribed exercise therapy remains the cornerstone of these programs. Cardiac rehabilitation programs traditionally have been categorized as phase I (inpatient), phase II (up to 12 weeks of electrocardiographic [ECG] monitored exercise and/or education following hospital discharge), phase III (variable length program of intermittent or no ECG monitoring under clinical supervision), and phase IV (no ECG monitoring, professional supervision). New theories of risk stratification, recent data on the safety of exercise, and pressures in the era of managed, capitated health care have contributed to a shortening and acceleration of these phases. There is now movement toward a continuum wherein patients follow a regimen of exercise specific to their vocational and recreational needs, with more individualization of the length of program, degree of ECG monitoring, and level of clinical supervision.[1,2] Outcome analysis is an important part of this evolution and includes not only clinical parameters and quality of life, but also recurrent cardiac events as well as physiologic, functional, and health outcomes.[3]

Inpatient Rehabilitation Programs

Following a documented physician referral, patients hospitalized after a cardiac event or procedure should be provided with a program consisting of early mobilization, identification, and education of cardiovascular disease risk factors; assessment of the patient's level of readiness for physical activity; and comprehensive discharge planning that includes referral to an outpatient cardiac rehabilitation program. The benefits of early mobilization and the other components of the inpatient cardiac rehabilitation program include:

- Offsetting the deleterious psychological and physiologic effects of bed rest during hospitalization
- Providing additional medical surveillance of patients
- Identifying patients with significant cardiovascular, physical, or cognitive impairments that may influence prognosis

- Enabling patients to more safely return to activities of daily living within the limits imposed by their disease
- Preparing the patient and support system at home to optimize recovery following hospital discharge

Before beginning formal physical activity in the inpatient setting, a baseline assessment should be conducted by a health care provider who possesses the skills and competencies necessary to assess and document heart and lung sounds, peripheral pulses, as well as musculoskeletal strength and flexibility.[1] Initiation and progression of physical activity depends on the findings of the initial assessment and varies with level of risk, thus inpatients should be risk-stratified as early as possible following their acute cardiac event. The AACVPR or ACP risk stratification models (see Chapter 2) are useful because they are based on overall prognosis.[1] Furthermore, the clinical indications and contraindications for cardiac rehabilitation (inpatient or outpatient) are listed in Box 8-1; however, exceptions should be considered based on clinical judgment.

Traditional inpatient programs with multiple steps for increasing activity are no longer feasible because of the decreased length of hospital stay for most cardiac patients. In many instances, uncomplicated patients are now seen for only 3 to 4 days before hospital discharge. Activities during the first 48 hours following myocardial infarction (MI) and/or cardiac surgery should be restricted to self-care activities, arm and leg range of motion, and postural change. Simple exposure to orthostatic or gravitational stress, such as intermittent sitting or standing during hospital convalescence, may reduce much of the deterioration in exercise performance that generally follows an acute cardiac event.[4] Structured, formalized, in-hospital exercise programs after acute MI appear to offer little additional physiologic or behavioral (self-efficacy) benefits over routine medical care.[5,6] Patients may progress from self-care activities, to walking short-to-moderate distances (50–500 feet) start with minimal or no assistance, three to four times per day, to independent ambulation on the unit. The optimal dosage of exercise for inpatients depends in part on their medical history, clinical status, and symptoms. The rating of perceived exertion (RPE) provides a useful and complementary guide to heart rate (HR) to gauge exercise intensity. In general, the criteria for terminating an inpatient exercise session are similar to or slightly more conservative than those for terminating a low-level exercise test. Box 8-2 lists potential adverse responses that should result in discontinuation of an inpatient exercise session.

Recommendations for inpatient exercise programming include the following:

Intensity

- RPE <13 (6–20 scale)
- Post-MI: HR <120 beats·min^{-1} or HR$_{rest}$ + 20 beats·min^{-1} (arbitrary upper limit)
- Postsurgery: HR$_{rest}$ + 30 beats·min^{-1} (arbitrary upper limit)
- To tolerance if asymptomatic

Duration

- Begin with intermittent bouts lasting 3 to 5 minutes, as tolerated
- Rest periods can be a slower walk or complete rest at patient's discretion; shorter than exercise bout duration; attempt to achieve 2:1 exercise/rest ratio

BOX 8-1	Clinical Indications and Contraindications for Inpatient and Outpatient Cardiac Rehabilitation

Indications
- Medically stable postmyocardial infarction
- Stable angina
- Coronary artery bypass graft surgery
- Percutaneous transluminal coronary angioplasty (PTCA) or other transcatheter procedure
- Compensated congestive heart failure
- Cardiomyopathy
- Heart or other organ transplantation
- Other cardiac surgery including valvular and pacemaker insertion (including implantable cardioverter defibrillator)
- Peripheral arterial disease
- High-risk cardiovascular disease ineligible for surgical intervention
- Sudden cardiac death syndrome
- End-stage renal disease
- At risk for coronary artery disease, with diagnoses of diabetes mellitus, dyslipidemia, hypertension, etc.
- Other patients who may benefit from structured exercise and/or patient education (based on physician referral and consensus of the rehabilitation team)

Contraindications
- Unstable angina
- Resting systolic blood pressure of >200 mm Hg or resting diastolic blood pressure of >110 mm Hg should be evaluated on a case-by-case basis
- Orthostatic blood pressure drop of >20 mm Hg with symptoms
- Critical aortic stenosis (peak systolic pressure gradient of >50 mm Hg with an aortic valve orifice area of <0.75 cm^2 in an average size adult)
- Acute systemic illness or fever
- Uncontrolled atrial or ventricular dysrhythmias
- Uncontrolled sinus tachycardia (>120 beats·min^{-1})
- Uncompensated congestive heart failure
- 3-degree AV block (without pacemaker)
- Active pericarditis or myocarditis
- Recent embolism
- Thrombophlebitis
- Resting ST segment displacement (>2 mm)
- Uncontrolled diabetes (resting blood glucose of >300 mg·dL^{-1}) or >250 mg·dL^{-1} with ketones present
- Severe orthopedic conditions that would prohibit exercise
- Other metabolic conditions, such as acute thyroiditis, hypokalemia or hyperkalemia, hypovolemia, etc.

BOX 8-2	**Adverse Responses to Inpatient Exercise Leading to Exercise Discontinuation**

- Diastolic BP ≥110 mm Hg
- Decrease in systolic BP >10 mm Hg
- Significant ventricular or atrial dysrhythmias
- Second- or third-degree heart block
- Signs/symptoms of exercise intolerance, including angina, marked dyspnea, and electrocardiogram changes suggestive of ischemia

See reference 1: Reprinted, by permission, from the American Association of Cardiovascular and Pulmonary Rehabilitation, 2004. Guidelines for Cardiac Rehabilitation and Secondary Prevention Programs, 4th ed. (Champaign, IL: Human Kinetics), 36 and 119.

Frequency

- Early mobilization: three to four times per day (days 1–3)
- Later mobilization: two times per day (beginning on day 4) with increased duration of exercise bouts

Progression

- When continuous exercise duration reaches 10 to 15 minutes increase intensity as tolerated

By hospital discharge, the patient should demonstrate an understanding of physical activities that may be inappropriate or excessive. Moreover, a safe, progressive plan of exercise should be formulated before they leave the hospital. Until the patient is evaluated with a submaximal or maximal exercise test, the upper limit of exercise should not exceed levels observed during the inpatient program. The patient also should be apprised of outpatient exercise program options and provided with information regarding the use of home exercise equipment. Selected moderate- to high-risk patients should be encouraged strongly to participate in clinically supervised outpatient rehabilitation programs and, at a minimum, be counseled to identify abnormal signs and symptoms, suggesting exercise intolerance and the need for medical review. Although not all patients may be suitable candidates for inpatient exercise, virtually all benefit from some level of inpatient intervention, including risk factor assessment, activity counseling, and patient and family education.

Outpatient Exercise Programs

Presuming that the goals for inpatient cardiac rehabilitation are met, the goals for outpatient programs are as follows:

- Provide appropriate patient monitoring and supervision to detect deterioration in clinical status and provide ongoing surveillance data to the referring physician to enhance medical management.

- Contingent on patient clinical status, return the patient to premorbid vocational and/or recreational activities, modify these activities as necessary, or find alternate activities.
- Develop and help the patient implement a safe and effective formal exercise and lifestyle activity program.
- Provide patient and family education about comprehensive cardiovascular risk reduction therapies and serial outcome assessments to maximize secondary prevention.

As presented in Chapter 1, exercise training is relatively safe for the vast majority of appropriately assessed cardiac patients. Although not completely preventable, the risk of exercise-induced events can be reduced through appropriate assessment, risk stratification, patient education, and adherence to established recommendations.[1] Prior to starting outpatient exercise rehabilitation, all cardiac patients should be stratified based on their risk for a cardiovascular event during exercise (see Chapter 2). Current risk stratification models for cardiac patients, such as the ones presented in Chapter 2 (see Boxes 2-1 and 2-2),[1,2] allow categorization to a single risk class (e.g., low, moderate, high). Patients who have not undergone exercise testing before entering a program or those with nondiagnostic exercise tests may be inadequately categorized using this approach. Such patients may receive a more cautious approach to risk stratification at program entry and a more conservative exercise prescription. However, risk stratification should be only one factor to consider when making recommendations for outpatient medical supervision and the need for continuous or instantaneous ECG monitoring during exercise. Recommendations for the intensity of supervision and monitoring related to the risk of exercise participation are described in Box 8-3.

The formation of exercise intervention plans for cardiac patients must not only consider safety but also should consider as the patients' vocational and avocational requirements, orthopedic limitations, premorbid and current activities, as well as personal health and fitness goals of the patient. Prescriptive techniques for determining the exercise dosage (i.e., intensity, frequency, and duration) for the general population are detailed in Chapter 7. Generally, the guidelines for appropriate exercise duration and frequency described in Chapter 7 can be applied safely to most low- to moderate-risk cardiac patients. The remainder of this chapter considers specific modifications of the exercise prescription for cardiac patients participating in an outpatient rehabilitation setting, with particular emphasis on intensity because this may be the most critical variable with regard to the safety and effectiveness of exercise training.

EXERCISE INTENSITY FOR THE CARDIAC PATIENT

The prescribed exercise intensity for a cardiac patient should be above a minimal level required to induce a "training effect," yet below the metabolic load that evokes abnormal clinical signs or symptoms.[7–9] Setting the safe upper limit for exercise intensity should be a foremost consideration, regardless of the methods employed, and should be established in order to prevent the signs and symptoms listed in Box 8-4. For most deconditioned cardiac patients, the minimal effective intensity for improving cardiorespiratory fitness approximates 45% of the

BOX 8-3.	Recommendations for Intensity of Supervision and Monitoring Related to Risk of Exercise Participation

Patients at lowest risk for exercise participation
- Direct staff supervision of exercise should occur for a minimum of 6 to 18 exercise sessions or 30 days postevent or postprocedure, beginning with continuous ECG monitoring and decreasing to intermittent ECG monitoring as appropriate (e.g., at 6–12 sessions).
- For a patient to remain at lowest risk, ECG and hemodynamic findings should remain normal, there should be no development of abnormal signs and symptoms either within or away from the exercise program, and progression of the exercise regimen should be appropriate.

Patients at moderate risk for exercise participation
- Direct staff supervision of exercise should occur for a minimum of 12 to 24 exercise sessions or 60 days postevent or postprocedure, beginning with continuous ECG monitoring and decreasing to intermittent ECG monitoring as appropriate (e.g., at 12–18 sessions).
- For a patient to move to the lowest-risk category, ECG and hemodynamic findings should remain normal, there should be no development of abnormal signs and symptoms either within or away from the exercise program, and progression of the exercise regimen should be appropriate.
- Abnormal ECG or hemodynamic findings during exercise, the development of abnormal signs and symptoms either within or away from the exercise program, or the need to severely decrease exercise levels may result in the patient remaining in the moderate-risk category or even moving to the high-risk category.

Patients at highest risk for exercise participation
- Direct staff supervision of exercise should occur for a minimum of 18 to 36 exercise sessions or 90 days postevent or postprocedure, beginning with continuous ECG monitoring and decreasing to intermittent ECG monitoring as appropriate (e.g., at 18, 24, or 30 sessions).
- For a patient to move to the moderate-risk category, ECG and hemodynamic findings should remain normal, there should be no development of abnormal signs and symptoms either within or away from the exercise program, and progression of the exercise regimen should be appropriate.
- Abnormal ECG or hemodynamic findings during exercise, the development of abnormal signs and symptoms either within or away from the exercise program, or significant limitations in the patient's ability to participate in the exercise regimen may result in discontinuation of the exercise program until appropriate evaluation, and intervention where necessary, can take place.

See reference 94: Reprinted from Cardiology Clinics of North America, V19(3) Williams, M.A. Exercise testing in cardiac rehabilitation: Exercise prescription and beyond, 415–431, © 2001, with permission from Elsevier.

BOX 8-4.	Signs and Symptoms Below Which an Upper Limit for Exercise Intensity Should Be Set*

- Onset of angina or other symptoms of cardiovascular insufficiency
- Plateau or decrease in systolic blood pressure, systolic blood pressure of >250 mm Hg or diastolic blood pressure of >115 mm Hg
- ≥1 mm ST-segment depression, horizontal or downsloping
- Radionuclide evidence of left ventricular dysfunction or onset of moderate to severe wall motion abnormalities during exertion
- Increased frequency of ventricular dysrhythmias
- Other significant ECG disturbances (e.g., 2- or 3-degree atrioventricular block, atrial fibrillation, supraventricular tachycardia, complex ventricular ectopy, etc.)
- Other signs/symptoms of intolerance to exercise

*The peak exercise heart rate generally should be at least 10 beats·min^{-1} below the heart rate associated with any of the referenced criteria. Other variables (e.g., the corresponding systolic blood pressure response and perceived exertion); however, also should be considered when establishing exercise intensity.

maximum oxygen uptake reserve ($\dot{V}O_2R$).[10] Improvement in $\dot{V}O_{2max}$ with light-to-moderate training intensities suggests that a decrease in the intensity may be partially or totally compensated for by increases in the exercise duration or frequency, or both.[11] As described in Chapter 7, because heart rate and oxygen consumption are linearly related during dynamic exercise involving large muscle groups, a predetermined training or target heart rate (THR) has become widely used as an index of exercise intensity in a variety of clinical populations, including cardiac patients.[8] The heart rate reserve method appears to closely approximate the same percentage of the oxygen uptake reserve (%$\dot{V}O_2R$) in cardiac patients,[12,13] including those taking β-blockers[13] and diabetics with and without autonomic neuropathy.[14] However, one cannot simply rely on these metabolic or heart rate formulas when prescribing exercise intensity for clinical populations because other variables (e.g., ischemic ST-segment depression, angina symptoms, dysrhythmias, blood pressure responses, perceived exertion) also should be considered.

RPE, when properly explained and practiced, can provide a useful and important adjunct to heart rate as an intensity guide for exercise training.[15] Perceived exertion is particularly valuable when patients enter an exercise-based rehabilitation program without a preliminary exercise test, or when clinical status or medical therapy changes. Although perceived exertion generally correlates well with exercise intensity, even in patients taking β-blockers,[16] ischemic ST-segment depression and serious ventricular dysrhythmias can occur at low heart rates and/or ratings of perceived effort. Generally, exercise rated as 11 to 13 (6–20 scale), between "fairly light" and "somewhat hard," corresponds to the upper limit of prescribed training heart rates during the early stages of outpatient cardiac rehabilitation. For higher-intensity levels of exercise training, rating of perceived exertion of 14 to 16 may be appropriate provided there are no signs or symptoms of ischemia or serious dysrhythmias. However, there is considerable interindividual variation among patients with regard to the relationship between RPE and heart rate or oxygen consumption.[17] One study[18] using cardiac patients in an early outpatient program, observed a wide range in actual physiologic demand (39%–92% of $\dot{V}O_2R$) during an exercise session when patients were instructed to use an RPE of 11 to 13 to regulate exercise training intensity. Consequently, clinicians using RPE exclusively to regulate exercise intensity in cardiac patients should be aware of the intersubject variability of this approach.

It is important to know when myocardial ischemia occurs for cardiac patients with exercise-induced ischemia, so that patients can exercise below the angina or ischemic ECG threshold. Such patients may wish to consider using a heart rate monitor that is highly accurate and offers the advantage of alarms for the upper and lower limits of training, thereby potentially increasing the safety and effectiveness of exercise. A peak exercise training heart rate 10 beats·min^{-1} or more below the threshold has been suggested, because silent myocardial ischemia has been identified as a link between lack of premonitoring symptoms and increased risk of cardiac arrest during physical stress.[19] An alternative is to use heart rate observed at the highest "safe" (i.e., no evidence of ischemia, significant dysrhythmia, hemodynamic abnormalities, or symptoms) workload achieved on an exercise test. It is also important to consider medication effects (see Appendix A), especially β-blockers. For example, at a fixed external work load, patients taking a single morning dose of a β-blocker are more likely to experience tachycardia and ischemic ST-segment depression during late afternoon than during morning exercise bouts.[20] Accordingly, prescribed heart rates for training should be based on an exercise test conducted under conditions as similar as possible, with respect to the timing of medications, to those under which the subject will be exercising.[21]

In two analyses,[10,22] including individuals with and without heart disease, training at higher intensities resulted in greater percentage improvements in aerobic capacity than training at lower intensities, even when the lower-intensity activity was compensated for by an increased exercise duration, frequency, or both, to accomplish the same total amount of work. This finding is clinically relevant in view of epidemiologic data showing lower all-cause mortality for those exercising at vigorous versus moderate intensities, and moderate versus light intensities.[23] Although some studies supporting the *added cardioprotective effect* of vigorous activity were plagued by methodologic limitations (e.g., a one-time assessment of exercise habits and/or failure to control for the total caloric expenditure),[24] several well-designed interventions have come to a similar conclusion.[25–27] Collectively, these data suggest that physicians and allied health professionals should encourage their patients with coronary disease to improve their exercise capacity by initiating a moderate-intensity physical conditioning program and, if possible, strive for the goal of more vigorous exercise, provided there are no contraindications.[28,29]

MODES OF EXERCISE FOR CARDIAC PATIENTS

Whenever possible, patients should be encouraged to engage in multiple activities to promote total physical conditioning (i.e., treadmills, cycle and arm ergometers, stair-climbers, and rowing machines), including range-of-motion exercises and resistance training, if medically appropriate, to maximize the carryover of training benefits to real-life activities.

Physical activity programs initiated early can enhance self-confidence of cardiac patients, without increasing the risk of death, recurrent infarction, or other complications. The inherent neuromuscular limitations to the speed of walking (and, therefore, the rate of energy expenditure) establish it as an appropriate mode of activity for early-unsupervised exercise for coronary patients. Even extremely slow walking (<2 mph) approximates 2 METs and may impose metabolic loads sufficient for exercise training in lower-fit subjects.[30] The CR adaptations to walking are well documented in persons with and without coronary artery disease. Brisk walking programs provide an activity intense enough to increase aerobic capacity and decrease body weight and fat stores in previously sedentary, middle-aged men.[31] Coronary patients undergoing a walking program demonstrated decreases in the rate-pressure product and somatic oxygen requirements at a fixed submaximal work load, suggesting increased mechanical efficiency.[32] Variations of conventional walking training, including walking with a 3- to 6-kg backpack load[33] and swimming pool walking[34] offer additional options for those who wish to reduce body weight and fat stores, improve cardiorespiratory fitness, or both. One study sought to determine if men and women with coronary artery disease could achieve an exercise intensity during a brisk 1-mile walk on a flat track sufficient to induce a training heart rate (THR), arbitrarily defined as ≥70% of measured HR_{max}.[35] These findings suggest that brisk walking is of a sufficient intensity to elicit a THR in all but the most highly fit patients with coronary disease.

PROGRESSION OF EXERCISE FOR THE CARDIAC PATIENT

The recommended rate of progression in a physical conditioning program depends on several variables, including the individual's functional capacity, orthopedic and musculoskeletal status, comorbid conditions (e.g., obesity, diabetes), and their activity goals and preferences. Nevertheless, physical activity progression can be facilitated by gradual increases in the prescribed intensity, frequency, duration, or combinations thereof. Using a prescribed THR provides a built-in regulator for improvements in cardiorespiratory fitness. As the patient becomes more fit, as verified by a conditioning bradycardia, the training work rate must be subtly increased over time to maintain the prescribed heart rate range.

For the low-risk cardiac patient, the endurance component of the exercise prescription generally has three stages of progression: initial, improvement, and maintenance (refer to Table 7-1). The initial phase of structured exercise training should begin with a low total volume of exercise and include only modest increases in frequency, intensity, and duration over the first month. The first week of training might include three sessions at a moderate intensity for only 15 to 20 minutes of continuous or intermittent activity (minimum of 10-minute bouts accumulated throughout the day). For most previously sedentary patients, the initial intensity might range from 2 to 4 METs, corresponding to walking on level ground at a 1.5- to 3.5-mph pace, or stationary cycle ergometry at ~150 to 300 kg·m·min^{-1} (25–50 W), depending on body weight. The improvement stage, which includes months 2 through 6, begins with three to four exercise sessions per week, 25 to 30 minutes per session (excluding warm-up or cool-down periods), at a moderate to hard exercise intensity. Depending on the individual's progress, there are systematic increases in the frequency (up to five sessions per week), intensity (up to 85% heart rate reserve or VO_2R), and duration (up to 40 minutes per session) of training at 6 months. Thereafter, during the maintenance stage, the duration may be lengthened to 60 minutes or longer,[36] especially if weight management is a primary objective, and additional lifestyle activities may be used to complement the conditioning regimen. Clinically stable higher-risk patients, such as those with congestive heart failure, may require an intermittent format of exercise and should be progressed according to symptoms and clinical status. Intensity should be kept low until a continuous duration of 10 to 15 minutes is achieved. An example of a progression from intermittent to continuous exercise is presented in Table 8-1. However, moderate- to high-risk cardiac patients may require more gradual increases in exercise dosage over time.

A scientific statement on preventing heart attack and death in patients with atherosclerotic cardiovascular disease extolled the importance of a minimum of 30 to 60 minutes of moderate-intensity activity three or four times weekly supplemented by an increase in daily lifestyle activities (e.g., walking breaks at work, using stairs, gardening, household chores); 5 to 6 hours a week was suggested for optimal benefits.[37]

RECOMMENDED TOTAL DOSE OR VOLUME OF EXERCISE FOR CARDIAC PATIENTS

As described in Chapter 7, the total dose or volume of exercise can be quantified and subsequently prescribed to target a specific level of energy expenditure. For

TABLE 8-1. Example of Exercise Progression using Intermittent Exercise

| Wk | %FC | Functional Capacity (FC) >4 METs | | | Reps |
		Total Min at %FC	Min Exercise	Min Rest	
1	50–60	15–20	3–5	3–5	3–4
2	50–60	15–20	7–10	2–3	3
3	60–70	20–30	10–15	Optional	2
4	60–70	30–40	15–20	Optional	2

| Wk | %FC | FC ≤4 METs | | | Reps |
		Total Min at %FC	Min Exercise	Min Rest	
1	40–50	10–15	3–5	3–5	3–4
2	40–50	12–20	5–7	3–5	3
3	50–60	15–25	7–10	3–5	3
4	50–60	20–30	10–15	2–3	2
5	60–70	25–40	12–20	2	2
6	Continue with two repetitions of continuous exercise, with one rest period or progress to a single continuous bout				

stable cardiac patients generally it is prudent to progress over a 3- to 6-month period to a total dose or volume of physical activity energy expenditure of more than 1,000 kcal·wk^{-1} because activity below this level was associated with coronary artery progression in one study.[38] Higher levels of physical activity and/or exercise energy expenditure, corresponding to 1,533 ± 122 and 2,204 ± 237 kcal·wk^{-1}, were associated with either no change or a reversal of coronary atherosclerotic lesions, respectively.[38] These goals would require walking approximately 24 and 32 km (15 and 20 miles) per week for most patients. Several investigations have observed that the estimated physical activity energy expenditure of a typical cardiac maintenance program participant is <300 kcal per session.[39,40] Furthermore, physical activity energy expenditure on "nonprogram days" for cardiac rehabilitation participants averaged <200 kcal·d^{-1}.[40] Although weekly amounts of physical activity of these cardiac rehabilitation participants in one study averaged 1,600 kcal·wk^{-1}, there was significant between-subject variability, with a standard deviation of 846 kcal·wk^{-1} and a range of 397 to 4,557 kcal·wk^{-1}.[40] Consequently, only 43% and 19% of participants achieved the target levels of 1,500 and 2,100 kcal·wk^{-1}, respectively. To maximize the potential for coronary artery disease stability and/or regression, patients should focus on achieving a total volume of physical activity of 1,500 to 2,100 kcal·wk^{-1}.[38] Clinicians need to recognize and convey to program participants that three traditional (30–40 minutes of moderate-intensity exercise) sessions per week will fall short of these goals and that physical activity outside of the center-based program is necessary.[40]

Exercise Prescription Without a Preliminary Exercise Test

In patients with known or suspected coronary disease, a pharmacologic stress test may have been recently performed; however, these tests may provide insufficient data to formulate a traditional exercise prescription. Furthermore, symptom-limited exercise testing may be inappropriate for some patients at or soon after hospital discharge, including those with extreme deconditioning, orthopedic limitations, or those with left ventricular dysfunction who are limited by shortness of breath.[41] An initial exercise prescription for patients with no preliminary exercise stress test is shown in Table 8-2. Exercise programs for such patients should be implemented conservatively with close medical surveillance; moreover, a period of continuous ECG-telemetry monitoring is highly recommended. The patient should be observed closely for signs and symptoms of exercise intolerance, and exercise blood pressure measurements should be obtained regularly.

In some instances, dobutamine testing may evoke a considerable rise in heart rate. This is particularly true if atropine is infused at the end of the dobutamine infusion protocol. If the echocardiogram or myocardial perfusion imaging results are negative for ischemia, the highest heart rate obtained may be used as a guide to determine the prescribed THR. However, an abnormal test may signify the need for coronary revascularization, more aggressive medical management (e.g., drug therapy), or both, before initiating an exercise training program. Because these test results may not necessarily define the ischemic ECG threshold, other complementary methods (e.g., symptoms, Holter monitoring, ECG-telemetry, heart rate monitor [watches]) should be used in conjunction with conservative heart rate guidelines to determine the exercise intensity.

TABLE 8-2. Guidelines for Exercise Prescription for Cardiac Patients Without an Entry Exercise Stress Test

Component	Initial Recommendations
Warm-up	
Stretching, low-level calisthenics (ROM)	5–10 minutes
Muscular fitness	
Resistance exercise:* all major muscle groups	10–20 minutes, 2 d·wk^{-1}
Cardiorespiratory fitness	
Frequency	1–2 bouts per day, 5 d·wk^{-1}
Duration†	MI: 30–45 minutes
	CABG: 30–45 minutes
Intensity‡	RHR +20 beats·min^{-1}
	RPE: 11–13
Type of activities§	Treadmill, leg ergometer, arm ergometer, ROM, stairs
Cool-down	
Low-level aerobic exercise, stretching	5–10 minutes

*Resistance training consisting of 10 to 15 repetitions per set, one set of 8 to 10 exercises, 2 d·wk^{-1}.

†For patients who tolerate more than 5 minutes, allow up to 10 minutes on each exercise device for a cumulative exercise duration of 30 to 45 minutes.

‡Use of these techniques may result in significant intersubject variability in exercise intensity as defined by percent of actual HRR or V̇O$_2$R (Joo KC, Brubaker PH, MacDougall AS, et al. Exercise prescription using heart rate plus 20 or perceived exertion in cardiac rehabilitation. J Cardiopulm Rehabil 2004;24:178–186).

§Treadmill, 1 to 2.5 mph, 0% grade; leg ergometer (25–50 W, depending on the patient's body weight); arm ergometer, <25 W.

Abbreviations: ROM, range of motion exercise; MI, myocardial infarction; CABG, coronary artery bypass graft surgery; RHR, resting heart rate; RPE, rating of perceived exertion.

Initial exercise intensities can be determined according to the length of time from the acute cardiac event and associated complications, duration since hospital discharge, and the information obtained during the patient's preliminary outpatient assessment (e.g., activities of daily living, current home walking program, associated signs and symptoms). Patient questionnaires, such as the Duke Activity Status Index (Fig. 8-1)[42] can be used to estimate an individual's activity status and functional capacity in the absence of a preliminary exercise stress test. Nevertheless, initial exercise intensities usually range from 2 to 3 METs, corresponding to 1 to 3 mph, 0% grade on the treadmill, or 100 to 300 kg·m·min^{-1} (or 12.5–50 W) on the cycle ergometer, depending on body weight, with gradual increments of 0.5 to 1.0 METs as tolerated.[1,2] The THR can be set at an arbitrary level of approximately 20 beats·min^{-1} above standing rest, and gradually increased using perceived exertion in the absence of symptoms, abnormal hemodynamics, threatening ventricular dysrhythmias, or ECG changes signifying myocardial ischemia. If ECG-telemetry monitoring suggests new-onset ST-segment depression, this should be confirmed with 12-lead electrocardiography during a simulated exercise session. Use of arbitrarily determined heart rate levels and/or subjective ratings of exertion should be done with caution, because there is significant intersubjective variability

Can you:	Weight
1- Take care of yourself, that is, eat, dress, bathe, or use the toilet?	2.75
2- Walk indoors, such as around your house?	1.75
3- Walk a block or two on level ground?	2.75
4- Climb a flight of stairs or walk up a hill?	5.50
5- Run a short distance?	8.00
6- Do light work around the house like dusting or washing dishes?	2.70
7- Do moderate house work around the house like vacuuming, sweeping floors, or carrying groceries?	3.50
8- Do heavy work around the house like scrubbing floors or lifting or moving heavy furniture?	8.00
9- Do yard work like raking leaves, weeding, or pushing a power mower?	4.50
10- Have sexual relations?	5.25
11- Participate in moderate recreational activities like golf, bowling, dancing, doubles tennis, or throwing a baseball or football?	6.00
12- Participate in strenuous sports like swimming, singles tennis, football, basketball, or skiing?	7.50

FIGURE 8-1. Duke Activity Status Index (DASI). Sum the weights for each "yes" reply and enter into the following equation: VO_2peak (mL·kg^{-1}·min^{-1}) = 0.43 × DASI + 9.

with these approaches.[18] Nonetheless, one study compared the rehabilitation outcomes in 229 post-MI and coronary artery bypass patients who had undergone preliminary symptom-limited exercise testing with 271 matched patients who did not.[43] Program prescription and progression for the former group involved conventional intensities (70%–85% HR$_{max}$, RPE 11–14), whereas the latter group initiated training at approximately 2 to 3 METs and, in the absence of abnormal signs/symptoms, progressed using heart rate and perceived exertion. The program lasted 12 weeks, and all patients underwent continuous ECG telemetry monitoring for the first 3 to 6 weeks. Both groups showed similar physiologic improvements, and there were no cardiovascular events in either group.

Types of Outpatient Exercise Programs

Although traditional supervised group programs are associated with increased cost and extended travel time,[3] considerable data are available regarding the safety, efficacy, and cost effectiveness of this model.[44] Such programs also are more appropriate for the growing medical complexity of candidates who may be at increased risk for future cardiac events, as well as those unable to self-regulate, or those whose adherence depends heavily on group support. Ideally, most cardiac patients should participate in a supervised rehabilitation program for some period of time to facilitate both exercise and lifestyle management changes. Advantages to exercising in a structured program include group support, professional feedback and monitoring, increased access to varied training modalities, recreational opportunities, and the availability of direct medical surveillance and emergency support. Outpatient cardiac rehabilitation programs traditionally have been divided into phases II and III, often separated arbitrarily based on length of participation or number of exercise sessions attended. In the current era, the outpatient rehabilitation process is viewed more on a continuum from early outpatient to long-term (lifelong) maintenance.[1] Movement along this continuum should be individualized to the patients' medical and psychosocial needs and not simply based on length of participation. Guidelines for the intensity of supervision and degree of monitoring are described in Box 8-3. The decision to progress a patient from a clinically and/or professionally supervised program to a nonsupervised environment is best made by the physician with input from the rehabilitation team. General criteria for such decisions are presented in Box 8-5.

Not all patients are able to, or wish to, participate in a supervised rehabilitation program. Accordingly, home exercise rehabilitation should be promulgated as an alternative, because of its lower cost, convenience, and potential to promote independence and self-responsibility.[45] For low-risk patients, medically directed, home-based rehabilitation and supervised group programs have shown comparable safety and efficacy. Smoking cessation programs and dyslipidemia management also can be successfully achieved in a home-based rehabilitation setting.[46] A variety of techniques may be used to facilitate monitoring and/or communication between patients managed at home and rehabilitation staff,

---

BOX 8-5 — **Guidelines for Progression from Clinical or Professional Supervision to Independent Exercise**

- Estimated functional capacity of ≥7 METs (or measured ≥5 METs) or twice the level of occupational demand
- Appropriate hemodynamic response to exercise (increase in systolic blood pressure with increasing work load) and recovery
- Appropriate ECG response at peak exercise with normal or unchanged conduction, stable or benign dysrhythmias, and nondiagnostic ischemic response (i.e., <1 mm ST-segment depression)
- Cardiac symptoms stable or absent
- Stable and/or controlled baseline heart rate and blood pressure
- Adequate management of risk factor intervention strategy and safe exercise participation such that the patient demonstrates independent and effective management of risk factors with favorable changes in those risk factors
- Demonstrated knowledge of the disease process, abnormal signs and symptoms, medication use, and side effects

including regular telephone contact, mail (e.g., completion of activity logs), fax, video recording, Internet, and transtelephonic ECG monitoring.

Benefits of Endurance Exercise Training in Cardiac Patients

There are multiple physiologic and psychosocial mechanisms by which moderate to vigorous physical activity may decrease morbidity and mortality rates associated with the secondary prevention of cardiovascular disease (Fig. 8-2). Aerobic exercise training programs can reduce stress and depression and promote decreases in body weight and fat stores, blood pressure (particularly among hypertensive individuals), total blood cholesterol, serum triglycerides, and low-density lipoprotein cholesterol, and increases in the "antiatherogenic" high density lipoprotein subfraction.[47] The beneficial effect of exercise on a variety of lipid and lipoprotein variables, independent of changes in body weight, is seen most clearly with higher amount, higher intensity regimens.[48] Considerable data now strongly support the role of aerobic fitness and regular physical activity in improving both glucose and insulin homeostasis.[49,50] Moreover, recent cross-sectional studies have reported an inverse relationship between C-reactive protein, a marker of inflammation, and CR fitness in men[51] and women.[52] The effects of chronic exercise training on the autonomic nervous system act to reduce heart rate at rest, during exercise and in recovery.[53] Vagal tone appears to be increased at rest, whereas sympathetic drive (circulating catecholamines, particularly norepinephrine) is decreased during exercise. The result is a reduction in the heart rate–blood pressure product and myocardial

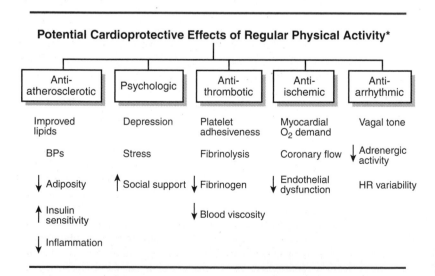

FIGURE 8-2. A structured endurance exercise program sufficient to maintain and enhance cardiorespiratory fitness may provide multiple mechanisms to reduce nonfatal and fatal cardiovascular events.
*Moderate to vigorous exercise intensities (i.e., ≥55% HR max, ≥12–13 rating of perceived exertion (6–20 scale). Abbreviations: BP, blood pressure; HR, heart rate.

aerobic requirements at any given oxygen uptake or submaximal workload, even when low to moderate exercise training intensities are used.[54] The beneficial effects of exercise training on myocardial perfusion and/or indices of myocardial ischemia include less ST-segment depression during exercise testing, reduced anginal symptoms, and resolution of reversible myocardial perfusion abnormalities.[55,56] Additionally, short-term aerobic exercise training has now been shown to improve endothelium-dependent vasodilation both in epicardial coronary vessels and in resistance vessels in patients with asymptomatic coronary atherosclerosis.[57] Finally, it has been suggested that exercise training improves hemostatic/fibrinolytic parameters in patients with and without coronary artery disease, reducing the potential for thrombosis and plaque expansion, and simultaneously elevating red blood cell transport efficiency.[58] Ischemic preconditioning; that is, brief periods of myocardial ischemia before coronary occlusion,[59] also may help to reduce infarct size and/or the potential for threatening ventricular dysrhythmias.[60] Although endurance exercise training has been shown to increase baroreflex sensitivity and heart rate variability in patients with coronary artery disease,[61] reports that described changes in ventricular dysrhythmias related to exercise-based cardiac rehabilitation have yielded inconsistent results.[44]

Resistance Training for Cardiac Patients

Many cardiac patients lack the physical strength and/or self-confidence to perform common activities of daily living. Resistance training provides an effective method for improving muscular strength and endurance, preventing and managing a variety of chronic medical conditions, modifying coronary risk factors, and enhancing functional independence.[62] Resistance training also appears to decrease cardiac demands (i.e., reduced rate pressure product) during daily activities like carrying groceries or lifting moderate to heavy objects, while simultaneously increasing endurance capacity.[63]

ELIGIBILITY AND EXCLUSION CRITERIA FOR RESISTANCE TRAINING

Many low- to moderate-risk patients should be encouraged to incorporate resistance training into their physical conditioning program, especially those who rely on their upper extremities for work or recreational pursuits. Box 8-6 lists criteria and time course recommendations for resistance training in low to moderate risk cardiac patients. The safety and effectiveness of resistance training in higher risk cardiac patients (i.e., those with severe left ventricular dysfunction, severe valvular disease, uncontrolled dysrhythmias, uncontrolled hypertension, or unstable symptoms) have not been well studied.[44] Accordingly, these patient subsets may require more careful evaluation, initial monitoring, and progression. General absolute and relative contraindications to resistance training are similar to those used for the aerobic component of cardiac exercise programs (see Box 8-1) and should be evaluated in each patient. Participation in resistance training ultimately should be contingent on approval of the medical director and/or the patients' personal physician. Box 8-6 lists the general guidelines of resistance training for cardiac patients.

BOX 8-6.	Patient Criteria for a Resistance Exercise Program*,†

- Minimum of 5 weeks after date of MI or cardiac surgery, *including* 4 weeks of consistent participation in a supervised CR endurance training program‡
- Minimum of 3 weeks following transcatheter procedure (PTCA, other), *including* 2 weeks of consistent participation in a supervised CR endurance training program‡
- No evidence of the following conditions:
  - Congestive heart failure
  - Uncontrolled dysrhythmias
  - Severe valvular disease
  - Uncontrolled hypertension. Patients with moderate hypertension (systolic BP >160 mm Hg or diastolic BP >100) should be referred for appropriate management, although these values are not absolute contraindications for participation in a resistance training program
  - Unstable symptoms

*Reprinted, with permission, from the American Association of Cardiovascular and Pulmonary Rehabilitation, 2004. Guidelines for Cardiac Rehabilitatoin and Secondary Prevention Programs, 4th ed. (Champaign, IL: Human Kinetics). 36 and 119.

†In this box, a resistance exercise program is defined as one in which patients lift weights 50% or greater of 1 RM. The use of elastic bands, 1- to 3-lb hand weights, and light free weights may be initiated in a progressive fashion at phase II program entry, provided no other contraindications exist.

‡Entry should be a staff decision with approval of the medical director and surgeon as appropriate.

TIME COURSE FOR RESISTANCE TRAINING

Many patients can safely perform static-dynamic activity equivalent to carrying up to 30 pounds by 3 weeks after acute MI.[64] Thus, it is possible that resistance exercise could be initiated sooner if a continuum of modalities is employed. A traditional resistance training program has been defined as one in which patients lift weights corresponding to 50% or more of the maximum weight that could be used to complete one repetition (i.e., 1 repetition maximum, 1 RM).[1] However, the use of elastic bands, light (1- to 5-lb) cuff and hand weights, light free weights, and wall pulleys may be initiated in a progressive fashion at immediate outpatient program entry (i.e., phase II) in the absence of contraindications.

RESISTANCE TRAINING PRESCRIPTION FOR CARDIAC PATIENTS

The cardiac patient should start at a low weight and perform one set of 10 to 15 repetitions to moderate fatigue using 8 to 10 different exercises. Weight is increased slowly as the patient adapts to the program (approximately 2 to 5 lbs·wk^{-1} for arms and 5 to 10 lbs·wk^{-1} for legs). The rate-pressure product should not exceed that during prescribed endurance exercise, and perceived exertion should range from 11 to 13 ("light" to "somewhat hard") on the Borg category scale.[15] Additionally, patients should be counseled to raise weights with slow, controlled movements to full extension, exhale during the exertion phase of the lift, avoid straining and the Valsalva maneuver, and stop exercise in the event of warning signs and symptoms.[1] Tight gripping of the weight handles or bar should be avoided to prevent an excessive blood pressure response to lifting.

Exercise Training for Return to Work

Failure to return to work after a cardiac event can stem from a variety of factors, including low functional capacity, poor prognosis, reduced self-efficacy, or inappropriate perceptions of actual job demands.[65] Exercise training may enhance the return to work decision and long-term employment by helping selected patients to improve their work capacity and self-efficacy for physical work. Nevertheless, it appears that exercise-based cardiac rehabilitation exerts less of an influence on the rates of return to work than many nonexercise variables, including employer attitudes, prior employment status, and economic incentives.[44]

In addition to enhancing work capacity, exercise training may help patients gain a better appreciation of their ability to perform physical work within reasonable levels of safety. Monitoring the physiologic responses to a simulated work environment also may be helpful in this regard. Enhanced self-efficacy, in turn, may lead to a greater willingness on the part of patients to resume work and/or more willingness to remain employed long-term following a cardiac event. Patients who plan to resume work combined with environmental heat stress should consider a gradual exposure to an outdoor exercise program during convalescence rather than restricting all exercise to an air-conditioned environment.[65] A few days of relatively short periods of mild to moderate exercise in a warm environment can enhance thermoregulation that, in turn, can lower the cardiovascular demand of work combined with heat stress.[66] Refer to Appendix E for further discussion of the impact of environmental factors on vocational requirements.

Special Cardiac Patient Populations

Cardiac patients who have specific needs to consider when formulating the exercise prescription include those with history of myocardial ischemia, congestive heart failure, pacemakers, and/or implanted cardioverter defibrillators (ICDs), cardiac transplantation, as well as revascularization or valve surgery. A more comprehensive description of exercise testing and training protocols for these patient subsets is available elsewhere.[67] A brief description of each population and specific modifications to the exercise prescription is provided.

MYOCARDIAL ISCHEMIA

Ischemia generally occurs when clinically significant lesions (i.e., 70% or more of the vessel's cross-sectional area) result in blood flow inadequate to meet myocardial oxygen demands, causing significant ST-segment depression, angina pectoris, transient myocardial perfusion abnormalities, or combinations thereof. When ischemic ECG changes occur in the absence of symptoms it is referred to as silent ischemia. For a given patient, stable angina predictably occurs with progressive exercise at approximately the same rate-pressure product. In contrast, unstable angina may be characterized by an abrupt increase in the frequency of angina, angina at rest, or both. This acceleration of symptoms may herald an impending cardiovascular event, serves as a contraindication to exercise, and requires immediate medical attention.

Exercise training can decrease the severity of angina at submaximal levels of exertion by reducing heart rate, systolic blood pressure and subsequent myocardial oxygen consumption ($M\dot{V}O_2$). In addition to the reduction in myocardial demand, exercise training may improve myocardial blood supply through changes in endothelial function and vascular smooth muscle.[57]

Exercise Prescription and Training Considerations for the Angina Patient

- Exercise may be inappropriate for those who experience exertional angina at aerobic requirements of <3 METs.
- The primary goal for persons with angina is to increase the anginal and ischemic ECG threshold by decreasing the rate-pressure product at any given level of submaximal exertion.
- Patients should be taught to recognize the symptoms that may represent classic angina pectoris, such as substernal pressure radiating across the chest and/or down the left arm, back, jaw, or stomach, or lower neck pain or discomfort.
- The exercise session should be discontinued, or at least decreased in intensity, when the discomfort reaches a moderate level (i.e., >2 on 1–4 scale) level.
- The exercise session should include a prolonged warm-up and cool down (≥10 minutes), both of which may have an antianginal effect, and consist of range of motion, stretching, and low-level aerobic activities.[68] The goal of the warm-up is to gradually raise the heart rate response within 10 to 20 beats·min^{-1} of the lower limit prescribed for endurance training.
- Because symptomatic or silent ischemia may be arrhythmogenic,[19] the THR for endurance exercise should be set safely below (≥10 beats·min^{-1}) the ischemic ECG or anginal threshold. Alternatively, the upper heart level can be set as the highest "nonischemic" workload from the GXT.
- Patients with stable angina should be counseled regarding the potential exacerbation of symptoms while exercising in the cold.
- Upper body exercises may precipitate angina more readily than lower body exercises because of a higher pressor response.
- Patients with stable angina may, in selected cases, also benefit from prophylactic (preexercise) nitroglycerin. However, the use of prophylactic nitroglycerin should be cleared with the supervising physician and/or referring physician.
- Blood pressure should be checked routinely before and after the administration of nitroglycerin to reduce the potential for hypotensive sequelae.

- Intermittent, shorter duration-type exercise on a more frequent basis (e.g., 4–6 d·wk^{-1} with 5 to 10 minutes per session and two or three sessions per day)[68] may be useful.
- Any increase or change in anginal symptoms should be recorded and receive immediate medical attention as it may reflect a change in coronary status.
- If anginal symptoms are not relieved by termination of exercise or by the use of three sublingual nitroglycerin tablets (one taken every 5 minutes), the patient should be transported to the nearest hospital emergency center.

CONGESTIVE HEART FAILURE

Congestive heart failure (CHF) is characterized by the inability of the heart to adequately deliver oxygenated blood to metabolizing tissue, secondary to impairment in cardiac output. Impaired left ventricular systolic function and/or diastolic dysfunction can result in abnormalities in skeletal muscle metabolism and morphology, vascular function, neurohormonal responses, or pulmonary function.[69] Although treatment with bed rest and restricted physical activity is still appropriate for acute or unstable conditions, exercise can be safe and beneficial for those with chronic heart failure.[70] Previous concerns[71] regarding the potential deleterious effects of early exercise training in patients recovering from large anterior wall MI, causing abnormal ventricular remodeling and infarct expansion, now have been resolved. Two randomized controlled trials in patients with anterior Q-wave MI and decreased ejection fraction showed no significant difference in left ventricular dysfunction between exercise training and control patients.[72,73]

Physical conditioning in patients with heart failure and moderate to severe left ventricular dysfunction results in improved functional capacity and quality of life, and reduced symptoms.[74,75] Peripheral adaptations (increased skeletal muscle oxidative enzymes and improved mitochondrial size and density) are largely responsible for the increase in exercise tolerance.[70] Whether these physiological adaptations will ultimately decrease fatal and nonfatal cardiovascular events is yet to be determined by a large prospective trial, although there is at least one small trial that showed a reduction in hospital admissions and improved 1-year survival.[74] A large prospective randomized trial, **H**eart **F**ailure and **A C**ontrolled **T**rial **I**nvestigating **O**utcomes of **E**xercise Trai**N**ing (HF-ACTION), funded by the National Institutes of Health, is underway currently. This trial proposes to randomize patients with CHF to a formal exercise training program (12 weeks), followed by home-based exercise (~3 years), or usual care, with the primary endpoints of all-cause mortality or all-cause hospitalizations.

Exercise Prescription and Training Considerations for Heart Failure Patients

- CHF patients who are selected for exercise training should be stable on medical therapy without absolute contraindications (particularly obstruction to left ventricular outflow, decompensated CHF, or threatening dysrhythmias) and have an exercise capacity of more than 3 METs.

- If possible, peak oxygen consumption should be determined by direct gas exchange measurements because aerobic capacity may be markedly overestimated from treadmill exercise time in this patient subset.[69]
- Many of these patients also may be taking multiple medications, including digoxin, diuretics, vasodilators, ACE inhibitors, β-blockers, and antiarrhythmics, which have the potential to influence the ECG and hemodynamic response to exercise. Moreover, hypokalemia commonly results from chronic diuretic therapy.
- Because malignant ventricular dysrhythmias are the most common cause of sudden cardiac death in CHF patients, supervisory staff should be especially vigilant of worsening signs and/or symptoms (e.g., increasing fatigue, worse-than-usual dyspnea or shortness of breath or angina on exertion, edema, sudden weight gain, or malignant ventricular dysrhythmias) that may suggest deterioration in clinical status. Serial ECG and blood pressure monitoring may be helpful in this regard.
- Exercise intensity should be based on a symptom-limited treadmill or cycle ergometer evaluation, using a THR range corresponding to approximately 40% to 75% $\dot{V}O_{2max}$, 3 to 7 d·wk^{-1}, 20 to 40 minutes per session.[69]
- If possible, ancillary study data (e.g., exercise echocardiogram, radionuclide studies, gas analysis) may be helpful when formulating the exercise intensity to avoid work rates that produce ischemic wall motion abnormalities,[19] a drop in ejection fraction, a pulmonary wedge pressure greater than 20 mm Hg, or a response exceeding the ventilatory threshold.[69]
- Warm-up and cool-down periods should be lengthened to a minimum of 10 to 15 minutes each, and patients should be advised to avoid isometric exertion.
- Training sessions initially should be brief (e.g., 10–20 minutes), including exercise for intervals of 2 to 6 minutes separated by 1 to 2 minutes of rest, and progressively lengthened as the patient's tolerance improves. Interval exercise training has been used in patients with chronic CHF, applying short bouts of intense muscular loading, with good clinical results and accelerated rehabilitation outcomes.[76]
- Walking, stationary cycling, and other aerobic activities, including arm exercise training, generally are recommended. These moderate-intensity activities may be safely and effectively complemented by a resistance training program in patients with stable CHF to improve symptoms of fatigue, dyspnea, and quality of life.[77]
- Because the chronotropic response may be impaired, perceived exertion and dyspnea may be used preferentially over heart rate or workload targets. Perceived exertion ratings of 11 to 14 (on the 6–20 scale) are useful guides.

PACEMAKERS AND IMPLANTABLE CARDIOVERTER DEFIBRILLATORS

Patients with a history of resuscitated sudden cardiac death, threatening ventricular dysrhythmias, or disease of the sinus node or conduction system with permanent pacemakers or an ICD, are being increasingly referred to exercise-based cardiac rehabilitation programs.[78] Although these patients traditionally were cautioned to avoid vigorous physical activity because of the pacemaker's fixed rate, advances in technology now enable dual chamber pacing with atrioventricular (AV) synchrony as well as dynamic adjustment of the heart rate to match increasing levels of metabolic demand.[79] Moreover, the safety and effectiveness of exercise training in this patient subset now has been demonstrated.[80]

Because some upper body movements may dislodge implanted leads, there is a brief period (~2–3 weeks) following pacemaker implantation during which the patient should avoid raising the arm on the affected side above the shoulder. Thereafter, patients may participate in physical activities that are compatible with their functional capacity. Although vigorous upper body activities and contact sports are not advised for patients with pacemakers, most physicians permit routine activities involving the upper extremities. Initial ECG telemetry monitoring may be useful to ensure proper functioning of the pacemaker during progressive physical activity. Particularly important is maintenance of the proper emergency and resuscitation equipment, including a cardioverter/defibrillator with R-wave synchronizing capability.[79] The North American Society of Pacing and Electrophysiology (NASPE)/British Pacing and Electrophysiology Group (BPEG) have developed a standard international five-letter code to provide a universal description of pacemaker characteristics (Table 8-3). Pacemakers are categorized by these codes (e.g., AAI, VVI, DDD, VVIR, and AATOP). The first letter position represents the chamber(s) paced, the second letter position describes the chamber(s) sensed, and the third letter position signifies the response of the pacemaker to a sensed event. The fourth letter represents rate-responsive properties, and the fifth position denotes any antitachyarrhythmia function of the pacemaker.

Considerations for Patients with Fixed Rate Pacemakers

For many patients, the pacemaker is programmed in VVI to manage ventricular bradycardias effectively.[81] However, limitations of VVI pacing include the lack of AV synchronization, absence of an atrial contribution to end-diastolic volume, and intermittent valvular regurgitation. Consequently, the patient demonstrates an attenuated rise in cardiac output during physical activity, and functional capacity may be severely compromised. Other individuals with VVI pacemakers may have little or no chronotropic reserve. Although previously it was believed that exercise training programs were ineffective for patients with a fixed heart rate response, it appears that these patients adapt to physical conditioning in a manner similar to patients with coronary artery disease who are heart rate-responsive.[82] Exercise prescription and training considerations for patients with fixed rate pacemakers include the following:

- Because of the nonlinear relationship between oxygen consumption and heart rate, in patients without rate-adaptive pacemakers, adjunctive target MET levels and perceived exertion limits should be provided
- Exercise intensity can be determined by modifying the Karvonen[83] equation from heart rate to systolic blood pressure (SBP), as follows (modified Karvonen formula):

$$TSBP = (SBP_{max} - SBP_{rest}) (50\% \text{ to } 80\%) + SBP_{rest}$$

where TSBP equals training systolic blood pressure.

TABLE 8-3. NASPE/BPEG Generic Pacemaker Code

Position	I	II	III
Category	Chamber(s) Paced	Chambers Sensed	Response to Sensing
	0 = None	0 = None	0 = None
	A = Atrium	A = Atrium	T = Triggered
	V = Ventricular	V = Ventrcular-	I = Inhibited
	D = Dual (A and V)	D = Dual (A and V)	D = Dual (T and I)

- Systolic blood pressure should be monitored throughout exercise to ensure safe and effective exercise intensity.
- Extended warm-up and cool-down periods are recommended.
- Such patients also should work at a markedly reduced intensity for the first few minutes of exercise to avoid dyspnea or premature fatigue.[81]
- Finally, it should be emphasized that without rate adaptive pacing, the functional capacity of VVI-paced patients may be greatly reduced when compared with those with rate modulation and AV synchrony.

Considerations for Patients with Rate Responsive Pacemakers

Rate responsiveness to exercise can be achieved in patients with chronotropic incompetence with VVIR or DDD pacing. The pacing rate for these modalities is determined by physiologic variables or atrial tracking. Various rate-responsive sensors have relative advantages and disadvantages. Exercise recommendations for patients with nonphysiologic sensors, such as a motion sensitive piezoelectric crystal device or accelerometer, should be designed carefully with respect to the type and intensity of activity. For example, treadmill exercise should use speed increments more than gradient changes because these units may respond at an inappropriately slower rate during uphill walking, despite comparable aerobic requirements. Similarly, stationary cycle ergometry may not produce sufficient motion of the thorax to yield an adequate rise in heart rate. A combined arm-leg ergometer that uses the levers and pedals simultaneously may elicit a more appropriate chronotropic response.[81]

For patients with adequate sinus node function but high-grade AV block, the DDD pacemaker offers the advantage of AV synchrony as well as rate responsiveness during activity via atrial tracking. Pacing in the VVIR mode provides rate responsiveness to activity, but without AV synchrony. Nevertheless, it should augment cardiac output during activity in appropriately selected patients. Finally, the DDDR pacemaker most closely resembles the normal heart's conduction system because it provides AV synchrony and uses sinus rhythm for the sensor-driven heart rate. The R in the pacemaker coding system indicates that physiologic or nonphysiologic sensors are used for rate modulation.

Exercise intensity for pacemaker patients should approximate 50% to 85% of HRR, 4 to 7 d·wk^{-1}, 20 to 60 minutes per session.[78] Exercise intensity for patients with rate-modulating pacemakers can be prescribed using the following methods, alone or in combination:[81]

IV	V
Programmability and Modulation	**Antitachyarrhythmia Functioning**
0 = None	0 = None
P = Simple programmable	P = Pacing (antitachyarrhythmia)
M = Multiprogram	S = Shock
C = Communicating	D = Dual (P and S)
R = Rate modulation	

- Maximal heart rate reserve method of Karvonen[83]
- A fixed percentage of the maximal heart rate[9]
- Rating of perceived exertion[15]
- METs

If either of the heart rate methods is used, consideration should be given to the upper- and lower-rate limits of the pacemaker device. If signs or symptoms of myocardial ischemia occur during exercise, the upper limit for prescribed heart rate in DDD and VVIR pacemakers should be set at 10 beats·min^{-1} or more below the person's ischemic threshold. Reprogramming of maximum heart rate below the ischemic threshold also should be considered.

Considerations for Patients with Antitachycardia Pacemakers and Implanted Cardioverter Defibrillators

Antitachycardia pacemakers and ICDs are commonly used to manage tachydys-rhythmias (usually with burst pacing or shock). An ICD consists of a cardioverter device and a lead system. The unit is designed to recognize rapid rhythms and respond in a tiered fashion. Because the device is programmed to detect dysrhythmias using heart rate and intervals as the main criteria, it is critical to know the cutoff rate. Persons with ICDs are at risk of receiving inappropriate shocks during exercise if the sinus heart rate exceeds the programmed threshold or the patient develops an exercise-induced supraventricular tachycardia.[78] For this reason, patients with ICDs should be closely monitored using continuous or instantaneous ECG telemetry monitoring, pulse palpation, or both, to titrate a safe and effective exercise dose. A magnet should be readily available to override or inactivate the device should it malfunction.

CARDIAC TRANSPLANT RECIPIENT

Cardiac transplantation represents a therapeutic alternative for nearly 3,000 patients each year with end-stage heart failure. Moreover, 1- and 3-year survival rates for transplant recipients now approximate 86% and 80%, respectively.[84] Despite surgery, cardiac transplant patients continue to experience exercise intolerance because of extended inactivity and convalescence, associated skeletal muscle derangements, loss of muscle mass and strength, and the absence (complete or partial) of autonomic cardiac innervation. Because of the adverse side effects of immunosuppressive drug therapy (cyclosporine and prednisone), such as dyslipidemia, hypertension, obesity, and diabetes, these individuals are at increased risk of developing coronary atherosclerosis of the donor heart. As a result, increasing numbers of patients are being referred to exercise rehabilitation early after cardiac transplantation to improve functional capacity, coronary risk factors, and quality of life.[85]

Because of the surgical procedure, the transplanted heart essentially is denervated, although some evidence for partial reinnervation exists.[86] As a result of the denervation, there are numerous differences in the cardiorespiratory, ECG (e.g., two separate P waves may be apparent), hemodynamic, and neuroendocrine responses at rest and during exercise when comparing transplant recipients with age- and gender-matched healthy individuals. Resting sinus tachycardia (90–110 beats·min^{-1}) is common, and systolic and diastolic hypertension may result from elevated catecholamine levels, the effects of immunosuppressive medications, altered baroreceptor sensitivity, or combinations thereof. In the normally innervated heart, the increase in cardiac output during exercise is elicited by a significant increase in heart rate, and, to a lesser extent, in stroke volume. In the denervated heart, the cardioacceleratory response to exercise is delayed, yet cardiac output increases to support the metabolic demand. Studies in cardiac transplant recipients have shown that the initial increase in cardiac output with submaximal exercise is achieved by an increase in stroke volume via the Frank-Starling mechanism because immediate cardioacceleratory stimulation is lacking. However, at higher work rates the myocardium responds with tachycardia to humoral adrenergic stimulation, largely to rising plasma norepinephrine levels.[87] Postexercise heart rates often rise or remain elevated longer than normal because of the continued presence of norepinephrine and/or the lack of parasympathetic innervation. Peak oxygen consumption in untrained cardiac transplant recipients generally is 50% of normal and ranges from 10 to 22 mL·kg^{-1}·min^{-1}.[84] Collectively, these data indicate an earlier onset of anaerobiosis in transplant recipients than in healthy individuals.

Exercise Prescription and Training Considerations for Cardiac Transplant Patients

- The exercise prescription for the cardiac transplant recipient should be based on data derived from exercise testing to volitional fatigue, using "graded" protocols with 1 to 2 MET increments per 3-minute stage.[84]
- Although isolated cases of chest pain have been reported in cardiac transplant recipients, generally there is an absence of anginal symptoms because of partial or complete denervation.
- The sensitivity of the exercise ECG in this patient subset is extremely low relative to the detection of myocardial ischemia. Consequently, radionuclide testing or exercise echocardiography may be more appropriate in assessing atherosclerotic heart disease.
- Exercise intensity in cardiac transplant recipients can be established using the following methods:
  - 50% to 75% $\dot{V}O_{2peak}$
  - Rating of perceived exertion (11–15 on the 6–20 scale)
  - Ventilatory threshold
  - Dyspnea

Because the initial heart rate response is attenuated and may not correspond with exercise intensity, predetermined work rates or MET loads may be preferred, using perceived exertion and dyspnea ratings as adjunctive guides for training. However, large interindividual variations in RPE at a given oxygen uptake have been reported in this patient population.[88] With continued exercise it is not uncommon for cardiac transplant patients to approach or exceed the maximal heart rate achieved on a previous exercise test.[84] Longer periods of warm-up and cool-down are indicated because the physiologic responses to exercise and recovery take longer. Cardiac transplant recipients should perform aerobic exercises 4 to 6 d·wk^{-1} while progressively increasing the duration of training from 15 to 60 minutes per session.[84] Low- to moderate-intensity resistance training and range-of-motion activities performed 2 to 3 d·wk^{-1} may be used to complement this regimen. Moreover, 6 months of resistance training prevents glucocorticoid-induced myopathy in heart transplant recipients and restores fat-free mass to levels greater than before transplantation surgery.[89]

Surveillance of the transplant patient during exercise training should focus on resting and exercise blood pressures, possible adverse effects of immunosuppressive drug therapy, and evidence of rejection. Blood pressure should be monitored carefully because hypertension is a common side effect of cyclosporin. Moreover, prednisone therapy may result in numerous side effects, including sodium and fluid retention; loss of muscle mass; glucose intolerance and/or diabetes mellitus; osteoporosis; fat redistribution from the extremities to the torso; gastric irritation; increased appetite; increased susceptibility to infection; predisposition to peptic ulcers; and increased potassium excretion. Finally, knowledge of the most recent cardiac biopsy score is important because rejection exacerbates exercise intolerance. If evidence of rejection is present, the prescribed exercise regimen should be discontinued until this is reversed.

CARDIAC SURGERY AND PERCUTANEOUS TRANSLUMINAL CORONARY INTERVENTION

The two most common approaches to revascularize occluded coronary arteries are coronary artery bypass graft surgery (CABGS) and percutaneous transluminal coronary interventions (PTCIs) which include angioplasty (PTCA) and/or intracoronary stenting. In the United States alone, more than 519,000 CABGS and 561,000 PTCIs were performed in 2000.[90] Valve replacements/repairs are also commonly performed, particularly for aortic and mitral valve disease.[91] Generally, the uncomplicated PTCI patient is discharged in 24 hours, whereas cardiac surgery patients (CABGs or valvular) are hospitalized for 4 to 6 days. To counteract the deleterious effects of bed rest and complications associated with the cardiac surgery, range-of-motion activities and very light (i.e., 1- to 3-pounds) hand weights, as well as mobilization are initiated while in the hospital or in the early outpatient setting. Stretching or flexibility activities can begin as early as 24 and 48 hours after bypass surgery or uncomplicated MI, respectively. Patients may be seen once daily and perform 10 to 15 repetitions of each exercise. However, as outlined in Box 8-7, postsurgery patients should avoid traditional resistance training exercises (with moderate to heavy weights), until the sternum has healed sufficiently, generally by 3 months.[62] Surgery patients who experience sternal movement or wound complications should perform lower extremity exercises only. Nevertheless, significant soft-tissue and bone damage of the chest wall can occur during surgery. If this area does not receive range-of-motion exercise, adhesions may develop and the musculature can become weaker and shorten, accentuating postural problems and hindering strength gains. Aerobic exercise training for the postsurgical inpatient can be guided initially using resting HR + 30 beats·min^{-1} (or other techniques described in the inpatient section of this chapter) until more objective data from a symptom-limited exercise test is generated. Valve surgery patients generally can follow the same exercise prescription guidelines as the CABGs patient, although these patients may have had greater activity restrictions and/or longer periods of symptoms prior to surgery. The resulting low functional capacity, as well as advanced age, may require valve surgery patients to start and progress at a slower rate.[92]

For PTCI patients, aerobic and resistance training can begin almost immediately as long as the catheter access site has healed properly. The exercise

---

BOX 8-7 | Resistance Training Guidelines*

- To prevent soreness and minimize the risk of injury, the initial load should allow 12 to 15 repetitions comfortably. If a 1 RM pretest is used, this load would be approximately 30% to 40% 1RM for the upper body and 50% to 60% for hips and legs. Low-risk-stratified, well-trained patients may progress to higher relative loads depending on program goals.
- Perform one set of 8 to 10 exercises (major muscle groups) 2 to 3 days/week. An additional set may be added, but additional gains are not proportionate.
- Some specific considerations are as follows:
  - Exercise large muscle groups before small muscle groups.
  - Increase loads by 5% when the patient can comfortably lift 12 to 15 repetitions.
  - Raise weights with slow, controlled movements; emphasize complete extension of the limbs when lifting.
  - Avoid straining.
  - Exhale (blow out) during the exertion phase of the lift (e.g., exhale when pushing a weight stack overhead and inhale when lowering it).
  - Avoid sustained, tight gripping, which may evoke an excessive BP response to lifting.
  - An RPE of 11 to 13 may be used as a subjective guide to effort.
  - Stop exercise if warning signs or symptoms occur, especially dizziness, dysrhythmias, unusual shortness of breath, or anginal discomfort.

Reprinted, by permission, from the American Association of Cardiovascular and Pulmonary Rehabilitation, 2004. Guidelines for Cardiac Rehabilitation and Secondary Prevention Programs, 4th ed. (Champaign, IL: Human Kinetics), 182.

prescription for PTCIs is similar to other cardiac patients although these patients may be able to progress more rapidly if there was no myocardial damage and less inactivity preprocedure and postprocedure. In the current era of stenting and aggressive pharmacotherapy, the risk for restenosis in PTCI patient is reduced considerably from early experiences with PTCA alone. However, the PTCI patient should still be observed closely in the exercise program for potential recurrence of ischemic signs and symptoms.[93]

REFERENCES

1. American Association of Cardiovascular and Pulmonary Rehabilitation. Guidelines for Cardiac Rehabilitation and Secondary Prevention Programs, 4th ed. Champaign, IL: Human Kinetics, 2003.
2. Fletcher GF, Balady GJ, Amsterdam EA, et al. Exercise Standards for testing and training: a statement for healthcare professionals from the American Heart Association. Circulation 2001;104:1694–1740.
3. Franklin BA, Hall L, Timmis GC. Contemporary cardiac rehabilitation services. Am J Cardiol 1997;79:1075–1077.
4. Convertino VA. Effect of orthostatic stress on exercise performance after bed rest: relation to in-hospital rehabilitation. J Cardiac Rehab 1983;3:660–663.
5. Sivarajan ES, Bruce RA, Almes MJ, et al. In-hospital exercise after myocardial infarction does not improve treadmill performance. N Engl J Med 1981;305:357–362.
6. Oldridge NB, Rogowski BL. Self-efficacy and in-patient cardiac rehabilitation. Am J Cardiol 1990;66:362–365.
7. Franklin BA, Gordon S, Timmis GC. Amount of exercise necessary for the patient with coronary artery disease. Am J Cardiol 1992;69:1426–1432.
8. Wilmore JH. Exercise prescription: role of the physiatrist and allied health professional. Arch Phys Med Rehabil 1976;57:315–319.
9. American Heart Association. Exercise testing and training of individuals with heart disease or at high risk for its development: a handbook for physicians. Dallas, 1975.
10. Swain DR, Franklin BA. Is there a threshold intensity for aerobic training in cardiac patients? Med Sci Sports Exerc 2002;34:1071–1075.
11. Pollock ML, Gaesser GA, Butcher JD. The recommended quantity and quality of exercise for developing and maintaining cardiorespiratory and muscular fitness, and flexibility in healthy adults. Med Sci Sports Exerc 1998;30:975–991.
12. Franklin BA, Swain DP. New insights on the threshold intensity for improving cardiorespiratory fitness. Prev Cardiol 2003;6:118–121.
13. Brawner CA, Keteyian SJ, Ehrman JK. The relationship of heart rate reserve to VO2 reserve in patients with heart disease. Med Sci Sports Exerc 2002;34:418–422.
14. Colberg SR, Swain DP, Vinik AI. Use of heart rate reserve and rating of perceived exertion to prescribe exercise intensity in diabetic autonomic neuropathy. Diabetes Care 2003;26:986–990.
15. Borg GAV. Borg's Perceived Exertion and Pain Scales. Champaign, IL: Human Kinetics, 1998.
16. Pollock ML, Lowenthal DT, Foster C. Acute and chronic responses to exercise in patients treated with beta-blockers. J Cardiopulm Rehabil 1991;11:132–144.
17. Whaley MH, Brubaker PH, Kaminsky LA, et al. Validity of rating of perceived exertion during graded exercise testing in apparently healthy adults and cardiac patients. J Cardiopulm Rehabil 1997;17:261–267.
18. Joo KC, Brubaker PH, MacDougall AS, et al. Exercise prescription using heart rate plus 20 or perceived exertion in cardiac rehabilitation. J Cardiopulm Rehabil 2004;24:178–186.
19. Hoberg E, Schuler G, Kunze B, et al. Silent myocardial ischemia as a potential link between lack of premonitoring symptoms and increased risk of cardiac arrest during physical stress. Am J Cardiol 1990;65:583–589.
20. Franklin BA, Gordon S, Timmis GC. Diurnal variation of ischemic response to exercise in patients receiving a once-daily dose of beta-blockers. Implications for exercise testing and prescription of exercise and training heart rates. Chest 1996;109:253–257.
21. Wilmore JH, Freund BJ, Joyner MJ, et al. Acute response to submaximal and maximal exercise consequent to beta-adrenergic blockade: implications for the prescription of exercise. Am J Cardiol 1985;55:135D(141D.

22. Swain DP, Franklin BA. VO2 reserve and the minimal intensity for improving cardiorespiratory fitness. Med Sci Sports Exerc 2002;34:152–157.

23. Lee IM, Paffenbarger RS Jr. Associations of light, moderate, and vigorous intensity physical activity with longevity. The Harvard Alumni Health Study. Am J Epidemiol 2000;151:293–299.

24. Yu S, Yarnell JW, Sweetnam PM, et al. What level of physical activity protects against premature cardiovascular death? The Caerphilly study. Heart 2003;89:502–506.

25. Lee IM, Hsieh CC, Paffenbarger RS Jr. Exercise intensity and longevity in men. The Harvard Alumni Health Study. JAMA 1995;273:1179–1184.

26. Tanasescu M, Leitzmann MF, Rimm EB, et al. Exercise type and intensity in relation to coronary heart disease in men. JAMA 2002;288:1994–2000.

27. Lee IM, Sesso HD, Oguma Y, et al. Relative intensity of physical activity and risk of coronary heart disease. Circulation 2003;107:1110–1116.

28. Lee IM, Paffenbarger RS Jr. The role of physical activity in the prevention of coronary artery disease. In: Thompson PD, ed. Exercise and Sports Cardiology. New York: McGraw-Hill, 2001.

29. Franklin BA. Survival of the fittest: evidence for high-risk and cardioprotective fitness levels. Curr Sports Med Rep 2002;1:257–259.

30. Franklin BA, Pamatmat A, Johnson S, et al. Metabolic cost of extremely slow walking in cardiac patients: implications for exercise testing and training. Arch Phys Med Rehabil 1983;64:564–565.

31. Pollock ML, Miller HS Jr, Janeway R, et al. Effects of walking on body composition and cardiovascular function of middle-aged man. J Appl Physiol 1971;30:126–130.

32. Dressendorfer RH, Smith JL, Amsterdam EA, et al. Reduction of submaximal exercise myocardial oxygen demand post-walk training program in coronary patients due to improved physical work efficiency. Am Heart J 1982;103:358–362.

33. Shoenfeld Y, Keren G, Shimoni T, et al. Walking. A method for rapid improvement of physical fitness. JAMA 1980;243:2062–2063.

34. Evans BW, Cureton KJ, Purvis JW. Metabolic and circulatory responses to walking and jogging in water. Res Q 1978;49:442–449.

35. Quell KJ, Porcari JP, Franklin BA, et al. Is brisk walking an adequate aerobic training stimulus for cardiac patients? Chest 2002;122:1852–1856.

36. US Department of Agriculture/US Department of Health and Human Services. Nutrition and Your Health: Dietary Guidelines for Americans, 6th ed. Home and Garden Bulletin No. 232. Washington, DC: US Department of Agriculture/US Department of Health and Human Services, 2002.

37. Smith SC Jr, Blair SN, Bonow RO, et al. AHA/ACC Scientific Statement: AHA/ACC guidelines for preventing heart attack and death in patients with atherosclerotic cardiovascular disease: 2001 update. A statement for healthcare professionals from the American Heart Association and the American College of Cardiology. Circulation 2001;104:1577–1579.

38. Hambrecht R, Niebauer J, Marburger C. Various intensities of leisure time physical activity in patients with coronary artery disease: effects on cardiorespiratory fitness and progression of coronary atherosclerotic lesions. J Am Coll Cardiol 1993;22:468–477.

39. Schairer JR, Kostelnik T, Proffitt SM, et al. Caloric expenditure during cardiac rehabilitation. J Cardiopulm Rehabil 1998;18:290–294.

40. Ayabe M, Brubaker PH, Doborosielski D, et al. The physical activity patterns of cardiac rehabilitation program participants. J Cardiopulm Rehab, 2004;24(2):80–86.

41. McConnell TR. Exercise prescription when the guidelines do not work. J Cardiopulm Rehabil 1996;16:34–37.

42. Hlatky MA, Boineau RE, Higginbotham MB, et al. A brief self-administered questionnaire to determine functional capacity (the Duke Activity Status Index). Am J Cardiol 1989;64:651–654.

43. McConnell TR, Klinger TA, Gardner JK, et al. Cardiac rehabilitation without exercise tests for post-myocardial infarction and post-bypass surgery patients. J Cardiopulm Rehabil 1998;18:458–463.

44. Wenger NK, Froelicher ES, Smith LK, et al. Cardiac rehabilitation. Clinical Practice Guideline No. 17. Rockville, MD: US Department of Health and Human Services, Public Health, Agency for Health Care Policy and Research and National Heart, Lung, and Blood Institute. AHCPR Publication No. 96-0672. 1995:1–23.

45. DeBusk RF, Haskell WL, Miller NH, et al. Medically directed at-home rehabilitation soon after clinically uncomplicated acute myocardial infarction: a new model for patient care. Am J Cardiol 1985;55:251–257.

46. DeBusk RF, Miller NH, Superko HR, et al. A case-management system for coronary risk factor modification after acute myocardial infarction. Ann Intern Med 1994;120:721–729.

47. Tran ZV, Brammell HL. Effects of exercise training on serum lipid and lipoprotein levels in post-MI patients: a meta-analysis. J Cardiopulm Rehabil 1989;9:250–255.
48. Kraus WE, Houmard JA, Duscha BD, et al. Effects of the amount and intensity of exercise on plasma lipoproteins. N Engl J Med 2002;347:1483–1492.
49. Wei M, Gibbons LW, Mitchell TL, et al. The association between cardiorespiratory fitness and impaired fasting glucose and type 2 diabetes mellitus in men. Ann Intern Med 1999;130:89–96.
50. Knowler WC, Barrett-Connor E, Fowler SE, et al. Reduction in the incidence of type 2 diabetes with lifestyle intervention or metformin. N Engl J Med 2002;346:393–403.
51. Church TS, Barlow CE, Earnest CP, et al. Associations between cardiorespiratory fitness and C-reactive protein in men. Arterioscler Thromb Vasc Biol 2002;22:1869–1876.
52. LaMonte MJ, Durstine JL, Yanowitz FG, et al. Cardiorespiratory fitness and C-reactive protein among a tri-ethnic sample of women. Circulation 2002;106:403–406.
53. Tiukinhoy S, Beohar N, Hsie M. Improvement in heart rate recovery after cardiac rehabilitation. J Cardiopulm Rehabil 2003;23:84–87.
54. Franklin BA, Besseghini I, Golden LH. Low intensity physical conditioning: effects on patients with coronary heart disease. Arch Phys Med Rehabil 1978;59:276–280.
55. Shephard RJ, Balady GJ. Exercise as cardiovascular therapy. Circulation 1999;99:963–972.
56. Sdringola S, Nakagawa K, Nakagawa Y, et al. Combined intense lifestyle and pharmacologic lipid treatment further reduce coronary events and myocardial perfusion abnormalities compared with usual-care cholesterol-lowering drugs in coronary artery disease. J Am Coll Cardiol 2003;41:263–272.
57. Hambrecht R, Wolf A, Gielen S, et al. Effect of exercise on coronary endothelial function in patients with coronary artery disease. N Engl J Med 2000;342:454–460.
58. Church TS, Lavie CJ, Milani RV, et al. Improvements in blood rheology after cardiac rehabilitation and exercise training in patients with coronary heart disease. Am Heart J 2002;143:349–355.
59. Kloner RA, Bolli R, Marban E, et al. Medical and cellular implications of stunning, hibernation, and preconditioning: an NHLBI workshop. Circulation 1998;97:1848–1867.
60. Hull SS Jr, Vanoli E, Adamson PB, et al. Exercise training confers anticipatory protection from sudden death during acute myocardial ischemia. Circulation 1994;89:548–552.
61. Iellamo F, Legramante JM, Massaro M, et al. Effects of a residential exercise training on baroreflex sensitivity and heart rate variability in patients with coronary artery disease: a randomized, controlled study. Circulation 2000;102:2588–2592.
62. Pollock ML, Franklin BA, Balady GJ. Resistance exercise in individuals with and without cardiovascular disease: benefits, rationale, safety, and prescription. Circulation 2000;101:828–833.
63. Hickson RC, Rosenkoetter MA, Brown MM. Strength training effects on aerobic power and short-term endurance. Med Sci Sports Exerc 1980;12:336–339.
64. Wilke NA, Sheldahl LM, Tristani FE, et al. The safety of static-dynamic effort soon after myocardial infarction. Am Heart J 1985;110:542–545.
65. Sheldahl LM, Wilke NA, Tristani FE. Evaluation and training for resumption of occupational and leisure-time physical activities in patients after a major cardiac event. Med Exerc Nutr Health 1995;4:273–289.
66. Folinsbee LJ. Heat and air pollution. In: Pollock ML, Schmidt DH, eds. Heart Disease and Rehabilitation, 3rd ed. Champaign, IL: Human Kinetics, 1995:327–342.
67. Durstine JL, Moore GE, eds. American College of Sports Medicine's Exercise Management for Persons with Chronic Diseases and Disabilities, 2nd ed. Champaign, IL: Human Kinetics, 2003.
68. Gitkin A, Canulette M, Friedman D. Angina and silent ischemia. In: Durstine JL, Moore GE, eds. American College of Sports Medicine's Exercise Management for Persons with Chronic Diseases and Disabilities, 2nd ed. Champaign, IL: Human Kinetics, 2003:40–46.
69. Myers JN, Brubaker PH. Chronic heart failure. In: Durstine JL, Moore GE, eds. American College of Sports Medicine's Exercise Management for Persons with Chronic Diseases and Disabilities, 2nd ed. Champaign, IL: Human Kinetics, 2003:64–69.
70. Pina IL, Apstein CS, Balady G. Exercise and heart failure. A statement from the American Heart Association Committee on Exercise, Rehabilitation, and Prevention. Circulation 2003;107:1210–1225.
71. Jugdutt BI, Michorowski BL, Kappagoda CT. Exercise training after anterior Q wave myocardial infarction: importance of regional left ventricular function and topography. J Am Coll Cardiol 1988;12:362–372.
72. Giannuzzi P, Tavazzi L, Temporelli PL, et al. Long-term physical training and left ventricular remodeling after anterior myocardial infarction: results of the Exercise in Anterior Myocardial Infarction (EAMI) trial. EAMI Study Group. J Am Coll Cardiol 1993;22:1821–1829.

73. Giannuzzi P, Temporelli PL, Tavazzi L, et al. EAMI—exercise training in anterior myocardial infarction: an ongoing multicenter randomized study. Preliminary results on left ventricular function and remodeling. The EAMI Study Group. Chest 1992;101:315S(321S.

74. Belardinelli R, Georgiou D, Cianci G, et al. Randomized, controlled trial of long-term moderate exercise training in chronic heart failure: effects on functional capacity, quality of life, and clinical outcome. Circulation 1999;99:1173–1182.

75. McKelvie RS, Teo KK, Roberts R, et al. Effects of exercise training in patients with heart failure: the Exercise Rehabilitation Trial (EXERT). Am Heart J 2002;144:23–30.

76. Meyer K. Exercise training in heart failure: recommendations based on current research. Med Sci Sports Exerc 2001;33:525–531.

77. Oka RK, De Marco T, Haskell WL, et al. Impact of a home-based walking and resistance training program on quality of life in patients with heart failure. Am J Cardiol 2000;85:365–369.

78. West M, Roberts SO. Pacemakers and implantable cardioverter defibrillators. In: Durstine JL, Moore GE, eds. American College of Sports Medicine's Exercise Management for Persons with Chronic Diseases and Disabilities, 2nd ed. Champaign, IL: Human Kinetics, 2003:52–57.

79. Schweikert RA, Pashkow FJ, Wilkoff BL. Rehabilitation of patients with arrhythmias, pacemakers, and defibrillators. In: Pashkow FJ, Dafoe WA, eds. Clinical Cardiac Rehabilitation: A Cardiologist's Guide, 2nd ed. Baltimore: Williams & Wilkins, 1999:192–203.

80. Vanhees L, Schepers D, Heidbuchel H, et al. Exercise performance and training in patients with implantable cardioverter-defibrillators and coronary heart disease. Am J Cardiol 2001;87:712–715.

81. Sharp CT, Busse EF, Burgess JJ, et al. Exercise prescription for patients with pacemakers. J Cardiopulm Rehabil 1998;18:421–431.

82. Superko HR. Effects of cardiac rehabilitation in permanently paced patients with third-degree heart block. J Cardiac Rehab 1983;3:561–568.

83. Karvonen M, Kentala K, Mustala O. The effects of training on heart rate: a longitudinal study. Annales Medicinae Experimentalis et Biological Fennial 1957;35(3):307–315.

84. Keteyian SJ, Brawner C. Cardiac transplant. In: Durstine JL, Moore GE, eds. American College of Sports Medicine's Exercise Management for Persons with Chronic Diseases and Disabilities. Champaign, IL: Human Kinetics, 1997:70–75.

85. Kobashigawa JA, Leaf DA, Lee N, et al. A controlled trial of exercise rehabilitation after heart transplantation. N Engl J Med 1999;340:272–277.

86. Kaye DM, Esler M, Kingwell B, et al. Functional and neuralchemical evidence for partial cardiac sympathetic reinnervation after cardiac transplantation in humans. Circulation 1993;88:1110–1118.

87. Shepard RJ. Responses of the cardiac transplant patient to exercise and training. Exerc Sport Sci Rev 1992;7:297–320.

88. Shephard RJ, Kavanagh T, Mertens DJ, et al. The place of perceived exertion ratings in exercise prescription for cardiac transplant patients before and after training. Br J Sports Med 1996;30:116–121.

89. Braith RW, Welsch MA, Mills RM Jr, et al. Resistance exercise prevents glucocorticoid-induced myopathy in heart transplant recipients. Med Sci Sports Exerc 1998;30:483–489.

90. American Heart Association. Heart Disease and Stroke Statistics, 2003 Update. 2002.

91. Canulette M, Gitkin A, Friedman D. Valvular heart disease. In: Durstine JL, Moore GE, eds. American College of Sports Medicine's Exercise Management for Persons with Chronic Diseases and Disabilities. Champaign, IL: Human Kinetics, 2003:58–63.

92. Stewart KJ, Badenhop D, Brubaker PH, et al. Cardiac rehabilitation following percutaneous revascularization, heart transplant, heart valve surgery, and for chronic heart failure. Chest 2003;123:2104–2111.

93. Franklin B. Coronary artery bypass surgery and percutaneous transluminal coronary angioplasty. In: Durstine JL, Moore GE, eds. American College of Sports Medicine's Exercise Management for Persons with Chronic Diseases and Disabilities. Champaign, IL: Human Kinetics, 2003:32–39.

94. Williams MA. Exercise testing in cardiac rehabiliatation: exercise prescription and beyond. Cardiol Clin 2001;19:415–431.

Other Clinical Conditions Influencing Exercise Prescription

Although the general principles of exercise prescription apply to persons with and without chronic disease, certain clinical conditions may require differences in programming to maximize effectiveness and avoid complications. This chapter extends the general exercise prescription guidelines presented in Chapter 7 for persons with one or more of the following conditions: arthritis, diabetes, dyslipidemia, hypertension, obesity, metabolic syndrome, immunologic disorders, osteoporosis, peripheral arterial disease, pulmonary disease, and pregnancy. Each condition is highlighted with a brief overview of pathophysiology, divergence for exercise testing and exercise prescription relative to the general exercise prescription (Table 9-1), and special considerations to ensure safety. If modifications of exercise testing and exercise prescriptions are not noted, the guidelines from the preceding chapters apply. Refer to the ACSM Resource Manual (Section 4) for a comprehensive and detailed analysis of each condition.

Arthritis

Arthritis and rheumatoid disease typically affect almost 14% of Americans and cause muscle weakness, fatigue, and pain, stiffness, and swelling in joints and other supporting structures of the body such as muscles, tendons, ligaments, and bones. The two most common conditions of arthritis and rheumatic diseases are osteoarthritis and rheumatoid arthritis. Osteoarthritis is a degenerative joint disease that typically impacts the knees, hips, feet, spine, and hands. Rheumatoid arthritis is a chronic, systemic inflammatory disease affecting the synovial membrane of joints. The complications of arthritis may lead to a less active lifestyle. However, individuals with either inflammatory or degenerative joint disease generally are able to engage in regular exercise to improve their health status. The goals for many arthritis patients are to engage in normal everyday activities without undue fatigue and pain, improve cardiovascular, muscular, and flexibility fitness, enhance functional status, and decrease joint swelling and pain.

The ACSM makes the following recommendations regarding exercise testing and training for patients with arthritis.

TABLE 9-1. Summary of Exercise Programming

Components of Training Program	Frequency (sessions·wk^{-1})	Intensity	Duration	Activity
Cardiorespiratory	3–5 d·wk^{-1}	40%/50%–85% HRR or VO$_2$R 64/70%–94% HR$_{max}$ 12–16 RPE	20–60 min	Large muscle groups Dynamic activity
Resistance	2–3 d·wk^{-1}	Volitional fatigue (MMF) (e.g., 19–20 RPE) Or Stop 2–3 reps before volitional fatigue (e.g., 16 RPE)	1 set of 3–20 repetitions (e.g., 3–5, 8–10, 12–15)	8–10 exercises Include all major muscle groups
Flexibility	Minimal 2–3 d·wk^{-1} Ideal 5–7 d·wk^{-1}	Stretch to tightness at the end of the range of motion but not to pain	15–30 seconds 2–4 x/stretch	Static stretch all major muscle groups

Abbreviations: HRR, heart rate reserve; VO$_2$R, maximal oxygen uptake reserve; MMF, momentary muscular fatigue.

EXERCISE TESTING

- Assessment of physiologic function should include cardiopulmonary capacity, neuromuscular status, and flexibility.
- Modifications of traditional protocols may be warranted depending on functional limitations and an early onset of fatigue.
- Choose a mode of exercise based on the most pain-free method for exercise. Although treadmill and cycle ergometer protocols can be tolerated, cycle testing or combined arm and leg ergometry may provide a more accurate measurement of cardiopulmonary function if the patient is less limited by pain.
- Most patients are able to perform a symptom-limited graded exercise test.

EXERCISE PRESCRIPTION

- The recommended mode, intensity, frequency, duration, and overload generally are consistent with those in Chapter 7 for cardiorespiratory, resistance, and flexibility exercise stimuli (see summary in Table 9-1).
- Focus on improvement of both functional status as well as physical fitness.
- In a single exercise session, progress from flexibility exercises (affected joints), to neuromuscular muscle function exercises (strength and endurance), to aerobic activities (weight-bearing and/or non–weight bearing).

- Perform flexibility exercise one to two times daily, using the pain-free range of motion as an index of intensity.[1]
- Perform cardiovascular exercise initially in short bouts (~10 minutes). Add 5 minutes per session up to 30 minutes and progress with duration versus intensity. Aquatic, walking, and cycling activities are preferred.[1]
- Perform resistance training (free weights, machines, elastic bands, isometrics) of two to three repetitions progressing to 10 to 12 repetitions, 2 to 3 $d \cdot wk^{-1}$ using pain threshold as an index of intensity.[1]
- Functional activities (e.g., climbing stairs, sit to stand) should be performed daily.
- Use low-intensity and low-duration during the initial phase of programming. Discontinuous exercise bouts of 5 to 10 minutes may be necessary with deconditioned patients.
- Alternate exercise modes or cross-training should be incorporated in the program.
- Avoid exercise during arthritic flare-up.
- Conditions for exercise termination include unusual or persistent fatigue, increased weakness, decreased range of motion, increased joint swelling, and continuing pain that lasts more than 1 hour after exercise.

SPECIAL CONSIDERATIONS

- Hydrotherapy may attenuate pain and stiffness and reduce reliance on nonsteroidal antiinflammatory drugs (NSAIDs).
- Regular use of NSAIDs may cause anemia because of gastrointestinal bleeding and mask the musculoskeletal pain.
- Contraindications to exercise include vigorous, highly repetitive exercise with unstable joints, overstretching and hypermobility, and morning exercise with rheumatoid arthritis because of significant morning stiffness.
- Morning exercise often is avoided for rheumatoid arthritis patients, who have significant morning stiffness. However, some patients may benefit from the enhanced circulation.

Diabetes Mellitus

Diabetes mellitus is a group of metabolic diseases resulting from defects in insulin secretion, insulin action, or both. Since 1997, the types of diabetes have been classified by the etiologic origins. Type 1 diabetes is caused by the autoimmune destruction of the insulin producing β cells of the pancreas. Absolute insulin deficiency and a high propensity for ketoacidosis are the common characteristics of type 1 diabetic patients. Type 2 diabetes (NIDDM) is caused by insulin resistance with an insulin secretory defect. Approximately 90% to 95% of all diabetics are type 2.[2] Although type 2 diabetes is associated with excess body fat, the primary feature is an upper body fat distribution regardless of the amount of total body fat. In contrast to type 1 diabetes, type 2 diabetes often is associated with elevated insulin concentrations.

The treatment goal for diabetes is glucose control, which includes diet, medications, and exercise. Intensive treatment to control blood glucose has been documented to reduce the risk of progression of diabetic complications 50% to 75% in type 1 diabetic adults[3] and has been considered to be of similar efficacy in type 2 diabetic adults.[4] The 2003 report from the ADA Expert Panel on Diagnosis of Diabetes Mellitus includes the following:[5]

- Normal fasting plasma glucose <100 mg·dL^{-1} (5.6 mmol·L^{-1})
- Cutpoint between non-diabetic and diabetic is fasting plasma glucose ≥126 mg·dL^{-1} (7.0 mmol·L^{-1})
- Fasting plasma glucose values between 100 and 125 mg·dL^{-1} indicate impaired fasting glucose (IFG)
- 2-Hour plasma glucose level in an oral glucose tolerance test (OGTT) >200 mg·dL^{-1} (11.1 mmol·L^{-1}) is diagnostic criteria for diabetes
- The use of HbA$_{1c}$ as a diagnostic test for diabetes is not recommended because of a lack of standardized methodologies

ACSM makes the following recommendations regarding exercise testing and training for patients with diabetes.

EXERCISE TESTING

- Prior to beginning an exercise program, diabetic patients should undergo an extensive medical evaluation particularly for the cardiovascular, nervous, renal, and visual systems because they are related to diabetic complications.[6]
- Some patients, who exhibit nonspecific electrocardiographic (ECG) changes in response to exercise or who have nonspecific ST and T wave changes on resting ECG, may require additional radionuclide stress testing to rule out atherosclerotic heart disease.[7]
- Simple cardiovascular tests of resting heart rate (tachycardia) as well as heart rate and blood pressure response to orthostatic challenge, deep breathing, and Valsalva can provide information on the extent of autonomic neuropathy.[8]

EXERCISE PRESCRIPTION

- Exercise is effective in glucose control because exercise has an insulin-like effect that enhances the uptake of glucose even in the presence of insulin deficiency.
- Outcomes of exercise treatment in diabetes include improved glucose tolerance, increased insulin sensitivity, decreased glycosylated hemoglobin, and decreased insulin requirements.[9] Additional benefits of exercise for diabetic patients include improved lipid profiles, blood pressure reduction, weight management, increased physical work capacity, and improved well-being.[10–12]
- The basic elements of a cardiorespiratory exercise prescription[7]

  - Frequency: 3–4 d·wk^{-1}
  - Duration: 20–60 minutes
  - Intensity: 50%–80% $\dot{V}O_2R$ or heart rate reserve (HRR)

Within this recommended prescription, patients with type 2 diabetes should strive to accumulate a minimum of 1,000 kcal·wk^{-1} of physical activity.[9] Greater amounts of caloric expenditure ($\geq$2000 kcal·wk^{-1}), including daily exercise, may be required if weight loss is a goal.

- For resistance training, lower resistance (40%–60% of one repetition maximum [RM]), and lower intensity (avoiding MMF) is recommended.

  - One set of exercises for the major muscle groups with 10 to 15 repetitions; progress to 15 to 20.
  - The minimum frequency is two per week, with at least 48 hours between sessions.
  - Proper technique, including minimizing sustained gripping, static work and Valsalva are essential to prevent a hypertensive response.[13]

- Hypoglycemia is the most common problem for diabetics who exercise. See Table 9-2 for common symptoms associated with hypoglycemia.
- Hyperglycemia during exercise is a risk, particularly for type 1 diabetics, who are not in glycemic control. See Table 9-2 for common symptoms associated with hyperglycemia.
- Because of the increase of glucose uptake during exercise, the risk of hypoglycemia exists during and after exercise. Hypoglycemia, usually considered <80 mg·dL^{-1} is relative. Rapid drops in blood glucose also can cause the signs and symptoms of hypoglycemia in elevated glycemic states.
- Hypoglycemia, associated with exercise, may last as long as 48 hours after exercise.[14] To prevent postexercise hypoglycemia, monitor plasma glucose levels and ingest carbohydrates as needed.
- For diabetic patients with retinopathy, exercise that produces high arterial pressures may increase the risk of retinal detachment and vitreous hemorrhage.[15] Diabetic patients with overt nephropathy often have a reduced capacity for exercise.[6]
- Peripheral neuropathy may result in balance and gait abnormalities during exercise[16] as well as foot ulceration and fracture.[6]

TABLE 9-2. Signs and Symptoms of Hyperglycemia and Hypoglycemia

Hyperglycemia (>300 mg·dL^{-1})	Hypoglycemia (<80 mg·dL^{-1} or a rapid drop in glucose)	
Weakness	Crying	Apathy
Increased thirst	Drowsy	Blurred vision
Dry mouth	Fainting or feeling faint	Confusion
Soft eyeballs	Hand tremors	Delusion
Frequent, scant urination	Sweat	Double vision
Decreased appetite	Dizziness	Loss of Consciousness
Nausea	Excessive hunger	Convulsions
Vomiting	Fatigue	Headache
Abdominal tenderness	Irritability	Inability to concentrate
Acetone breath	Unsteady gait	Nervousness
Kussmaul respirations		Slurred speech
		Somnolence
		Poor coordination

- Autonomic neuropathy may cause chronotropic incompetence, blunted systolic blood pressure response, blunted oxygen uptake kinetics, and anhydrosis.[6,17,18] Consequently, RPE may be needed to regulate exercise intensity.
- Dehydration resulting from polyuria contributes to compromised thermoregulation.[19]
- Sudden death and silent ischemia during exercise also are associated with autonomic neuropathy.[6] The incidence of silent myocardial infarction is six to seven times greater in the diabetic population.[19] Cardiac patients reported angina during exercise approximately 50% more often than diabetic cardiac patients with similar thallium scintigraphy.[20] Sudden death during exercise may be attributed to sympathetic imbalance and prolonged QT interval.[21]

SPECIAL CONSIDERATIONS

- Glycosylated hemoglobin (HbA_{1C}) should be an additional blood chemistry test, because this measure provides information on long-term glycemic control.[9] As mentioned, HbA_{1C} is not recommended as a screening tool for diabetes.
- Hyperglycemia, common to diabetes may cause polyuria, polydipsia, weight loss (sometimes with polyphagia), and blurred vision.
- Brittle diabetic patients must be in glycemic control before starting an exercise program to prevent hypoglycemic and hyperglycemic events.[7]
- Exercise with a partner or under supervision to reduce the risk of problems associated with hypoglycemic events.
- Monitor blood glucose to prevent hypoglycemia or hyperglycemia associated with exercise, especially if taking insulin or oral hypoglycemic agents that increase insulin production.
  - Monitor blood glucose prior to exercise and following exercise, especially when beginning or modifying the exercise program.
  - A late-onset hypoglycemia can occur up to 48 hours following exercise, especially when beginning or modifying the exercise program.
  - See Table 9-2 for signs and symptoms of hyperglycemia and hypoglycemia.
  - Avoid physical activity if fasting glucose >250 mg·dL^{-1} and ketosis are present, and use caution if glucose >300 mg·dL^{-1} and no ketosis is present.[7]
  - Adjust carbohydrate intake or insulin injections prior to exercise based on blood glucose and exercise intensity to prevent hypoglycemia associated with exercise. Twenty to thirty grams of additional carbohydrates should be ingested if preexercise blood glucose is <100 mg·dL^{-1}.
  - To lower the risk of hypoglycemia associated with exercise,[19,22] avoid injecting insulin into exercising limbs; an abdominal injection site is preferred.
  - When exercising late in the evening, an increased consumption of carbohydrates may be required to minimize the risk of nocturnal hypoglycemia.
  - *Intense* resistance exercise often produces an acute hyperglycemic effect, whereas postexercise hypoglycemia in the hours following *basic* resistance training is an increased risk for patients on insulin or oral hypoglycemic agents.[13]

- For diabetic patients with retinopathy, prevent retinal detachment and vitreous hemorrhage associated with exercise:[15]
  - For moderate nonproliferative diabetic retinopathy, avoid activities that dramatically elevate blood pressure.
  - For severe nonproliferative diabetic retinopathy, avoid exercise that increases systolic blood pressure >170 mm Hg.
  - For proliferative diabetic retinopathy avoid strenuous activities, Valsalva maneuvers, or activities of pounding or jarring
- For diabetic patients with autonomic neuropathy:[6,19]
  - Monitor for signs and symptoms of hypoglycemia because of the inability of the patient to recognize them.
  - Monitor for signs and symptoms of silent ischemia because of the inability to perceive angina.
  - Monitor blood pressure following exercise to manage hypotension and hypertension associated with vigorous exercise.[19]
  - Understand that the heart rate and blood pressure response to exercise may be blunted and that the use of perceived exertion may help guide exercise intensity.[19]
  - Use precautions for poor thermoregulation in both hot and cold environments.
- For the patient with peripheral neuropathy:[6]
  - Take proper care of the feet to prevent foot ulcers.[23]
  - Limit weight-bearing exercise for patients with significant peripheral neuropathy.
- For the patient with nephropathy:[6]
  - Limit exercise to low to moderate intensities and discourage strenuous intensities when physical work capacity is low.

Dyslipidemia

Dyslipidemia, or abnormalities in blood lipid and lipoprotein concentrations, is a major modifiable cause of coronary heart disease (CHD) and a widespread problem. For example, 49% of adult men and 43% of adult women in the United States have elevated low-density lipoprotein cholesterol (LDL-C) concentrations (e.g., $\geq$130 mg·dL^{-1}).[24] Elevated blood LDL-C and triglyceride (TG) concentrations and low high-density lipoprotein cholesterol (HDL-C) concentrations are all independent risk factors for CHD.[25] The National Cholesterol Education Program's classifications for cholesterol and TG measurements are presented in Table 3-2. Current detection, evaluation, and treatment guidelines for dyslipidemia are available within the NCEP ATP III report.[25] The ATP III report recognizes the importance of lifestyle modification in the treatment of dyslipidemia.[25] These recommendations include increased physical activity and weight reduction, if needed.

A recent review of 28 randomized clinical trials involving over 4,700 participants[26] revealed that aerobic exercise training has varying influences on blood lipids and lipoproteins. The most common lipoprotein adaptation, observed in 40% of the studies, was a 4.6% increase in HDL-C, which occurred in both men and women and across all age groups. Changes in HDL-C were inversely related to the baseline concentrations, and were associated, in part, with changes in body and fat mass. Changes in LDL-C (-5.0%), triglycerides (-3.7%), and total cholesterol (-1.0%, nonsignificant) occurred less consistently than the changes in HDL-C. The available studies that evaluated a dose-response relationship between training intensity and lipid changes provide conflicting results.

Based on the known therapeutic effects of habitual physical activity, ACSM makes the following recommendations regarding exercise testing and training of persons with dyslipidemia.[26,27]

EXERCISE TESTING

- Individuals with dyslipidemia should be screened and stratified prior to exercise testing (see Table 2-4).
- Standard exercise testing methods and protocols are appropriate for use with dyslipidemic patients cleared for exercise testing. Special consideration should be given to the presence of other conditions (e.g., obesity, hypertension) that may require modifications to standard exercise testing protocols and modalities.
- Alternative testing modes may be required if the individual has xanthomas that cause biomechanical problems.

EXERCISE PRESCRIPTION

- The recommended mode, intensity, frequency, duration, and overload generally are consistent with those in Chapter 7 for cardiorespiratory, resistance, and flexibility exercise stimuli (see summary in Table 9-1).
- Primary mode should be large muscle group aerobic activities.
- Exercise intensity between 40% to 70% of $\dot{V}O_2R$ or HRR
- Frequency of training: 5 or more days per week to maximize caloric expenditure
- Duration of training session: 40 to 60 minutes (or two sessions per day of 20 to 30 minutes)
- This prescription is consistent with recommendations for long-term weight control (e.g., 200 to 300 min·wk^{-1}, $\geq$2,000 kcal·wk^{-1}).[28]

SPECIAL CONSIDERATIONS

- Consideration should be given to the presence of other conditions, such as obesity and hypertension, which may necessitate modification in the exercise prescription (see relevant sections in this chapter).
- Consideration should be given if the individual takes lipid-lowering medications (e.g., HMG CoA reductase inhibitors, fibric acid) that have the potential to cause muscle damage.
- Improvement in blood lipids/lipoproteins with aerobic exercise training may take several weeks or months, depending on the blood lipid/lipoprotein of interest and the weekly caloric expenditure.[27]

HYPERTENSION

Hypertension is defined clinically as an elevation in arterial blood pressure equal to or exceeding a systolic blood pressure of 140 mm Hg and/or a diastolic blood pressure of 90 mm Hg. The Seventh Report of the Joint National Committee on Prevention, Detection, Evaluation, and Treatment of Hypertension (JNC7) classification system for hypertension is presented in Table 3-1.[29] Hypertension is one of the most prevalent forms of cardiovascular disease affecting approximately 50 million Americans and approximately 1 billion individuals worldwide.[29] The prevalence of hypertension increases with advancing age and is higher in men than women and in blacks than in whites.[30] Hypertension is the major contributor to the more than 700,000 strokes and 280,000 stroke deaths annually in the United States and is a major factor contributing to the more than 1 million heart attacks and 500,000 heart attack deaths annually.[24] Hypertension is also an important risk factor for congestive heart failure, peripheral vascular disease, and kidney failure.[24] Furthermore, the risk of many of these diseases increases at levels of blood pressure well below the diagnostic threshold of 140/90 mm Hg.[31] Therefore, lowering blood pressure may benefit individuals with any elevation above optimal levels. In addition, the association between obesity and hypertension is well established. Risk estimates from the Framingham Heart Study suggest that approximately 75% and 65% of the cases of hypertension in men and women, respectively, are directly attributable to overweight and obesity.[32]

Although advances in the detection, treatment, and control of hypertension have taken place over the past few decades, control rates (SBP <140 mm Hg and DBP <90 mm Hg) are still well below the Healthy People 2010 goal of 50%; and approximately 30% of hypertensive individuals remain undiagnosed.[29] The goal of hypertension prevention and management is to reduce morbidity and mortality by the least intrusive means possible. This may be accomplished by achieving and maintaining blood pressure <140/90 mm Hg or lower if tolerated, while controlling other cardiovascular disease risk factors.[29] Persons with systolic blood pressure 120 to 139 mm Hg and/or diastolic blood pressure of 80 to 89 mm Hg are classified prehypertensive and should also engage in lifestyle modifications to prevent cardiovascular disease.[29] Table 9-3 presents lifestyle modifications recommended alone, or in combination with pharmacologic treatment by JNC 7.[29] Regular physical activity and weight control are at the core of current recommendations for both the primary prevention and treatment of high blood pressure.[29,33]

Recent meta-analyses[34,35] from over 54 randomized clinical trials, involving more than 2,600 subjects indicate that aerobic exercise training will elicit average reductions of 3 to 4 mm Hg and 2 to 3 mm Hg for systolic and diastolic pressure, respectively. However, the reductions subsequent to aerobic training appear to be more pronounced in hypertensive subjects (i.e., −7.4 and −5.8 mm Hg for systolic and diastolic pressure).[35] With respect to training protocols, changes in blood pressure following aerobic training appear to be similar with training intensities between 40% and 70% of $\dot{V}O_{2max}$, for training frequencies 3 to 5 d·wk^{-1}, and for training durations of 30 to 60 minutes.[35] Reductions in blood pressure following aerobic exercise training appear to be independent of both baseline obesity status and weight loss during training.[34]

ACSM makes the following recommendations regarding exercise testing and training of persons with hypertension.[36,37]

TABLE 9-3. Lifestyle Modifications to Manage Hypertension*

Modification	Recommendation	Approximate SBP Reduction (range)
Weight reduction	Maintain normal body weight (BMI 18.5–24.9 kg·m^{-2})	5–20 mm Hg per 10 kg weight loss [104,105]
Adopt DASH eating plan	Consume a diet risk in fruits, vegetables, and low-fat dairy products with a reduced content of saturated fat	8–14 mm Hg [106,107]
Dietary sodium restriction	Reduce dietary sodium intake to no more than 100 mmol per day (2.4 g sodium or 6 g sodium chloride)	2–8 mm Hg [106–108]
Physical activity	Engage in regular aerobic physical activity such as brisk walking (at least 30 min per day, most days of the week)	4–9 mm Hg [34,109]
Moderation of alcohol consumption	Limit consumption to no more than 2 drinks (1 oz or 30 mL ethanol; e.g., 24 oz beer, 10 oz wine, or 3 oz 80-proof whiskey) per day in most men and to no more than one drink per day in women and lighter-weight persons	2–4 mm Hg [110]

*See reference 29: Reprinted with permission from National High Blood Pressure Education Program. The Seventh Report of the Joint National Committee on Prevention, Detection, Evaluation, and Treatment of High Blood Pressure (JNC7), 2003, 03-5233. National Heart, Lung, and Blood Institute U.S. Department of Health and Human Services.

Abbreviations: DASH, Dietary Approaches to Stop Hypertension; BMI, body mass index; SBP, systolic blood pressure; g, gram; oz, ounce.

EXERCISE TESTING

- Medical clearance of hypertensive persons is advised before maximal exercise testing or prior to their participation in vigorous exercise (see Table 2-1).
- Standard exercise testing methods and protocols are appropriate for use with hypertensive patients cleared for exercise testing. Other comorbidities (e.g., obesity) or concerns (e.g., advanced age) may dictate modifications to the testing procedures.
- Medications should be taken at the usual time relative to the exercise bout.
- Carefully monitor blood pressure for exaggerated response (systolic >250 mm Hg or diastolic >115 mm Hg are indications for test termination).
- Mass exercise testing is not advocated to determine those individuals at high risk for developing hypertension in the future as a result of an exaggerated exercise blood pressure response. However, if exercise test results are available and an individual has a hypertensive response to exercise, this information does provide some indication of risk stratification for that patient and the

necessity for appropriate lifestyle counseling to ameliorate this increase. Medication changes may be appropriate in certain instances.

EXERCISE PRESCRIPTION

- The recommended mode, duration, and overload are consistent with those in Chapter 7 for cardiovascular, resistance, and flexibility exercise stimuli (see summary in Table 9-1).
- Primary mode should be large muscle group aerobic activities.
- Exercise intensity 40% to 70% $\dot{V}O_2R$ or HRR appears to reduce blood pressure as much as, if not more than, exercise at higher intensities.[35] This may be especially important for specific hypertensive populations, such as the elderly and obese.
- Frequency of aerobic training: 3 to 7 $d\cdot wk^{-1}$ are effective in reducing BP. However, because of the acute reduction in BP that may last many hours after a single bout of aerobic exercise, *daily exercise* may provide more optimal control of BP.[37,38]
- Duration of aerobic training session: 30 to 60 minutes
- Resistance training is not recommended as the primary form of exercise training for hypertensive individuals, but should be combined with aerobic training. Resistance training regimens should incorporate lower resistance with higher repetitions.

SPECIAL CONSIDERATIONS

- Do not exercise if resting systolic BP >200 mm Hg or diastolic BP >110 mm Hg (see Box 3-5).
- β-Blockers attenuate heart rate response during submaximal and maximal exercise and may decrease exercise capacity, particularly in patients without myocardial ischemia (see Appendix A).
- β-Blockers and diuretics may impair thermoregulation during exercise in hot and/or humid environments. Hypertensive patients taking these medications should be well informed about signs and symptoms of heat intolerance, along with prudent modifications in the exercise routine to prevent heat illness (see Appendix E).
- α_1-Blockers, α_2-blockers, calcium channel blockers, and vasodilators may provoke postexertion hypotension so emphasize a gradual cool-down period following the exercise session.
- Diuretics may cause a decrease in $[K^+]$, potentially leading to cardiac dysrhythmias and a false positive exercise ECG (see Appendix A).
- Although BP termination criteria for exercise testing are established at >250/115 mm Hg, lower BP thresholds for termination of an exercise training session may be prudent (i.e., >220/105 mm Hg).[37]
- Avoid Valsalva maneuvers during resistance training.
- Individuals with more marked elevations in BP (i.e., ≥160/100) should add endurance exercise training to their treatment regimen only after initiating pharmacologic therapy.[37] Exercise may reduce their BP further and, thus, allow them to decrease their antihypertensive medications and attenuate their risk for premature mortality.

Obesity

Obesity is a serious and common public health problem in the United States and other industrialized countries. During the past decade the number of overweight (BMI $\geq$25 to <30 kg·m^{-2}) and obese (BMI $\geq$30 kg·m^{-2}) individuals has increased dramatically. According to the most recent National Health and Nutrition Examination Survey (NHANES III), ~65% of Americans are overweight and 31% are obese.[39] An excess accumulation of fat, particularly in the intraabdominal region, is associated with an increased risk of a number of chronic diseases including hypertension, coronary heart disease, and type 2 diabetes and reduced life expectancy and early mortality.[40,41] In turn, obesity places a significant burden on the economy by increasing rates of health care usage and associated costs.

Obesity is caused by a complex interplay between genetic and environmental factors.[41] Ultimately, a cumulative positive energy balance causes obesity. Energy balance is determined by the difference between energy intake (calories consumed) and energy expenditure (calories expended through resting energy metabolism, the thermic effect of food, and physical activity). Therefore, weight gain occurs when energy intake exceeds energy expenditure (i.e., positive energy balance) and body weight is lost when the opposite occurs (i.e., negative energy balance). One pound of fat is equivalent to approximately 3,500 kcal of energy (1 kg is approximately equal to 7,700 kcal). The modern environment is driving the current obesity epidemic by favoring sedentary behavior and overconsumption;[42] therefore, physical activity and sound nutrition form the basis of obesity prevention and treatment.

A failure to fully appreciate the expected weight loss following exercise training has led to disappointment on the part of many participants and, in some cases, health care providers. This could serve to discourage health care providers from making physical activity recommendations to their obese patients. Results from recent meta-analysis[43] of short-term exercise intervention studies (i.e., $\leq$16 weeks) in which subjects consumed an isocaloric diet revealed that physical activity was associated with reductions in total body fat in a dose-response manner, with an average weight loss of 0.26 kg·wk^{-1} and fat loss of 0.25 kg·wk^{-1}. Longer duration studies reported a smaller effect (i.e., 0.06 kg·wk^{-1} reduction in body weight and total fat). However, the above results were derived from studies that: 1) incorporated isocaloric diets to isolate the "exercise effect," and 2) reported an average energy expenditure typically less than 1500 kcal·wk^{-1}. Intervention programs that incorporate dietary modification and greater energy expenditure would likely produce greater weight and fat losses.[28] Overall, reductions in body weight and fat resulting from increased exercise appear to be proportional to the amount of aerobic exercise performed.[28,43]

However, it is important to emphasize that there is considerable interindividual variability in the magnitude of weight loss produced by exercise. Some individuals actually may gain small amounts of weight, whereas others experience dramatic weight loss. The degree to which an individual compensates with changes in energy intake and/or physical activity during the remaining nonexercise portions of the day is an important determinant of the degree of weight loss experienced with exercise. For example, if two individuals expend 300 kcal·d^{-1} with exercise and one of these individuals reduces their activity during the remainder of the day by 150 kilocalories (or consumes an additional 150 kcal) then the difference in weight loss between these individuals over time could be considerable (i.e., approximately 30 lbs versus 15 lbs in 1 year). Therefore, it is important to emphasize the concept of energy balance in both causing and treating obesity.

Obesity often carries a negative social stigma and obese individuals are almost invariably sedentary, have low physical work capacities, and many have had negative experiences with exercise in the past. The exercise professional should interview the obese participant to determine goals, past exercise history, perceived barriers to exercise participation, and the locations where exercise might be performed (e.g., sports club, home, street, school gym, or track). This may increase adherence to an agreed-on exercise program. In addition, because reduction in adiposity is often a goal and need of many obese exercise program participants, exercise prescriptions should be designed to aid in accomplishing this objective. However, normalization of body weight and composition is not a realistic goal for most obese clients. In this regard, it is important to emphasize that it is not necessary to achieve an optimal body weight to experience health benefits. Even modest levels of weight loss (5% to 10% reduction in body weight) are associated with clinically significant reductions in blood pressure, increases in insulin sensitivity, and improvements in lipid and lipoproteins concentrations.[28] The prevention of further weight gain should be the first priority for obese individuals. Subsequently, the obese patient should be encouraged to focus on gradual but permanent weight loss, improving cardiorespiratory fitness and reducing overall cardiovascular disease risk.

ACSM makes the following recommendations regarding exercise testing and training of overweight and obese persons.[28,44]

EXERCISE TESTING

- Although standard exercise testing methods and protocols are generally appropriate with obese patients cleared for exercise testing, the level of deconditioning typically observed within this population will necessitate a low initial workload (2 to 3 metabolic equivalents [METs]) and small workload increments per test stage (0.5 to 1.0 METs).
- Other comorbidities (e.g., hypertension other chronic diseases) or concerns (e.g., orthopedic limitations or elderly) may dictate modifications to the testing procedures.
- Use of leg or arm ergometry may enhance testing performance.
- Medications should be taken at usual time relative to the exercise bout.
- For those who have difficulty adjusting to the exercise equipment, the initial stage may need to be extended, the test restarted, or the test repeated.
- Special attention to proper cuff size is necessary for accurate blood pressure measurements.

EXERCISE PRESCRIPTION

- The recommended mode, intensity, duration, and overload are consistent with those in Chapter 7 for cardiovascular, resistance, and flexibility exercise stimuli (see summary in Table 9-1). However, modifications should be made to encourage greater overall energy expenditure within the program for the obese individual.

- The needs and goals of the obese subject must be individually matched with the proper exercise program to achieve long-term weight management.
- Primary mode should be large muscle group aerobic activities.
- The *initial* exercise training intensity should be moderate (e.g., 40% to 60% $\dot{V}O_2R$ or HRR) with more emphasis placed on increased duration and frequency. Eventual progression to higher exercise intensities (50% to 75% $\dot{V}O_2R$ or HRR) allows for further increases in $\dot{V}O_{2max}$, which in turn allows for a more efficient exercise session (i.e., attainment of goal energy expenditure in reasonable amount of time).[44] However, for some (especially older) obese subjects, a walking or other moderate-intensity exercise program may be all they desire, and movement toward a more intense program may not be warranted.
- Frequency of training: 5 to 7 $d \cdot wk^{-1}$
- Duration of training session: 45 to 60 minutes[28,44]
- Volume of training: Initial training volume should follow the progressions outlined in Table 7-1, focusing on attainment of 150 minutes of moderate intensity exercise weekly. However, the optimal maintenance dose of physical activity is $\geq 2,000$ $kcal \cdot wk^{-1}$ (200–300 minutes per week for most).[28,44]
- Obese individuals benefit from additional resistance exercise training in a manner similar to otherwise healthy adults. However, the addition of resistance exercise to endurance exercise and diet modification does not appear to minimize the loss of fat-free mass or resting energy expenditure compared to that observed with diet modification alone, or the combination of diet modification and endurance exercise training.[28]

SPECIAL CONSIDERATIONS

- When the exercise component of a weight loss program is designed, the balance between intensity and duration of exercise should be manipulated to promote a high total caloric expenditure.
- Obese individuals are at an increased risk for orthopedic injury, and this may require that the intensity of exercise be maintained at or below the intensity recommended for improvement of CR fitness.
- Non–weight-bearing activities (and/or rotation of exercise modalities) may be necessary, and frequent modifications in frequency and duration also may be required.
- Obese individuals have an increased risk of hyperthermia during exercise.
- Equipment modifications may be necessary (i.e., wide seats on cycle ergometers and rowers).[45]
- It should be emphasized that increases in physical activity, even in the absence of weight loss, can reduce the risk of cardiovascular disease in obese subjects.
- Physical activity is the best predictor of long-term weight maintenance.[40]

RECOMMENDED WEIGHT LOSS PROGRAMS

Unfortunately, there is little evidence that exercise alone or in combination with dietary energy restriction produces magnitudes of weight loss achieved with dietary energy restriction alone.[40] However, the optimal approach to weight loss is one that combines a mild caloric restriction with regular endurance exercise. ACSM makes the following recommendations for weight loss programs:[28]

- Targets a long-term reduction in body weight of at least 5% to 10%
- Includes the exercise recommendations outlined in the preceding section
- Includes a reduction in dietary fat intake to <30% of total energy intake and emphasizes fruits, vegetables, whole grains, and lean sources of protein
- Includes foods that are acceptable in terms of sociocultural background, preferences, costs, and ease in acquisition and preparation
- Provides in a negative energy balance of 500 to 1,000 kcal·d^{-1}, resulting in gradual weight loss of 0.5 to 1 kg·wk^{-1} (1 kg approximately equal to 7,700 kcal)
- Includes the use of behavior modification techniques including relapse prevention
- Provides physical activity and dietary habits that can be continued for life to maintain the achieved lower body weight

Metabolic Syndrome

The metabolic syndrome, also referred to as syndrome X or the insulin resistance syndrome, describes a condition in which several coronary heart disease (CHD) risk factors (e.g., dyslipidemia, insulin resistance, elevated blood pressure, impaired fibrinolysis, and chronic low-grade inflammation) are clustered together.[46] Visceral obesity (e.g., increased intra-abdominal adipose tissue) appears to be a central feature of this syndrome.[47] The prevalence of the metabolic syndrome has been estimated to be approximately 22% in the United States, which corresponds to about 47 million adults.[48] The risk factors associated with this syndrome act synergistically to increase cardiovascular disease morbidity and mortality.[49]

Several mechanisms have been proposed to explain how visceral obesity might lead to insulin resistance and the other abnormalities associated with the syndrome. Visceral adipose tissue secretes factors including PAI-1, cytokines (e.g., IL-6, TNF-α), and angiotensinogen that are associated with one or more features of this syndrome.[50] In addition, visceral adipose tissue, which is drained by the portal vein, is highly lipolytically active, thereby increasing non–esterified fatty acid (NEFA) flux to the liver.[50] Increased hepatic NEFA uptake may lead to hyperglycemia, hyperinsulinemia, and hypertriglyceridemia.[50]

Diagnosis of the metabolic syndrome is made when three or more of the risk determinants shown in Table 9-4 are present.[25] However, abdominal obesity, as assessed by waist circumference, is more highly correlated with metabolic risk factors than is an elevated body mass index (BMI).[25] Therefore, waist circumference should be used as the primary anthropometric marker of the metabolic syndrome. Some male patients exhibit metabolic risk factors with lower levels of abdominal obesity (e.g., waist circumference of 94–102 cm [37–40 in.]).[25] These patients are thought to have strong genetic contribution to insulin resistance.[25]

There are two major objectives for the clinical management of the metabolic syndrome: 1) reduce underlying causes of the disorder (e.g., obesity and physical inactivity), and 2) treat the associated risk factors.[25] Thus, the initial treatment

TABLE 9-4. Clinical Identification of the Metabolic Syndrome*,†

Risk Factor	Defining Level
Abdominal obesity	Waist circumference‡
Men	>102 cm (>40 in.)
Women	>88 cm (>35 in.)
Triglycerides	≥150 mg·dL^{-1}
High-density lipoprotein cholesterol	
Men	<40 mg·dL^{-1}
Women	<50 mg·dL^{-1}
Blood pressure	≥130/≥85 mm Hg
Fasting glucose	≥110 mg·dL^{-1}

*See reference 25: From the National Cholesterol Education Program. Third Report of the National Cholesterol Education Program (NCEP) Expert Panel on Detection, Evaluation, and Treatment of High Blood Cholesterol in Adults (Adult Treatment Panel III). 2002. NIH Publication No. 02-5215.

†The ATP III panel did not find adequate evidence to recommend routine measurement of insulin resistance (e.g., plasma insulin), proinflammatory state (e.g., high-sensitivity C-reactive protein), or prothrombotic state (e.g., fibrinogen or PAI-1) in the diagnosis of the metabolic syndrome.

‡Some males can develop multiple metabolic risk factors when the waist circumference is only marginally increased (e.g., 94–102 cm [37–39 in.]). Such persons may have a strong genetic contribution to insulin resistance. They should benefit from changes in life habits, similar to men with categorical increases in waist circumference.

approach is weight reduction and increased physical activity. Even a modest 5% to 10% reduction in body weight results in significant improvements in metabolic risk factors.[47] Treatment of risk factors also may involve treatment of hypertension, aspirin use in patients with CHD, and the treatment of elevated TG and low HDL-C concentrations.[25]

EXERCISE TESTING AND PRESCRIPTION

Standard exercise testing methods and protocols are recommended for individuals with the metabolic syndrome. However, consideration should be given to specific elements of the syndrome (e.g., hypertension, diabetes, and obesity), which may necessitate alterations in standardized testing methods (see appropriate sections of this chapter for testing considerations).

Because obesity is at the core of the metabolic syndrome, exercise prescription guidelines should be based on those for obese patients (see preceding section on obesity). However, as the syndrome represents a clustering of metabolic disorders, the exercise guidelines related to the other components of the syndrome (i.e., dyslipidemia, hypertension, and if necessary, diabetes) also should be taken into consideration. Furthermore, as the metabolic syndrome has been associated with both sedentary lifestyle[25] and low CR fitness,[51] the eventual exercise progression should incorporate an increased training intensity (50% to 75% VO$_2$R or maximal HR reserve) to provide the stimulus to improve cardiorespiratory fitness and allow for more efficient exercise sessions (i.e., attainment of goal energy expenditure in reasonable amount of time).[44]

Immunology

The majority of human research in exercise immunology has focused on the influence of exercise on susceptibility to upper respiratory tract infections (URTIs; e.g., common cold or influenza [flu]). Thus, this section focuses on the relationship between exercise and URTI symptomatology and on basic immune responses to exercise, from which recommendations for exercise testing and prescription are derived. For more detailed information on exercise immunology, particularly as it relates to cancer patients/survivors and people infected with a human immunodeficiency virus (HIV), consult ACSM's Resource Manual, 5th ed., Chapter 28.[52–55]

EXERCISE AND UPPER RESPIRATORY TRACT INFECTIONS

The generally accepted "J" curve model proposes a relationship between the amount and intensity of exercise and susceptibility to URTI (Fig. 9-1).[56] This model proposes that moderate exercise training reduces the risk of developing URTI below that of a sedentary person, whereas the risk rises to above-average levels after intense exercise. Epidemiologic studies have demonstrated a higher incidence of self-reported symptoms of URTI in endurance athletes after both competition (e.g., marathon) and intensified training relative to the general public.[56–58] Moderate exercise training (e.g., brisk walking) in untrained healthy individuals on the other hand, may reduce the incidence and/or the duration of URTI

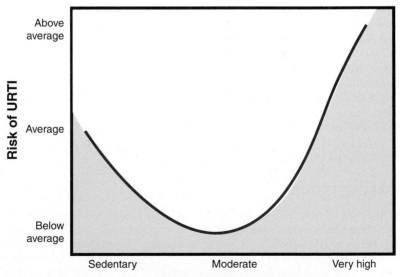

FIGURE 9-1. Proposed relationship between the amount and intensity of exercise and susceptibility to upper respiratory tract infections. (Reprinted with permission from Nieman DC. Exercise, upper respiratory tract infection, and the immune system. Med Sci Sports Exerc 1994;26:128–139.)

symptomatology.[56,58,59] Short-term (10 days) moderate exercise training (55% of HRR) does not appear to increase the severity of mild symptoms associated with a rhinovirus-induced URTI (~50% of URTI are caused by rhinoviruses) nor negatively affect resting pulmonary function, submaximal exercise responses, or maximal exercise performance.[60,61]

IMMUNE RESPONSES TO EXERCISE

Reductions in selected measures of immune function during recovery from endurance exercise may provide an "open window" for viruses and bacteria to gain a foothold.[53,56] Vigorous (e.g., >80% HRR), but not moderate, intensity exercise may increase the probability of developing a subclinical (i.e., without symptoms) or a clinical (i.e., with symptoms) infection 1 to 4 days after the exercise.

Changes in immune function after a single bout of intense endurance exercise or after intense training does not appear to chronically enhance nor suppress immunity in the resting state.[53,54] In addition, no studies have demonstrated that endurance athletes during intensified training are clinically immune deficient. Similarly, moderate endurance training and resistance training in healthy individuals does not appear to chronically influence immune function in the resting state.[53,54,62] Larger long-term prospective studies are needed to confirm the "J" curve model and the "open window" hypothesis. In addition to exercise, the immune system is influenced by many factors, including psychological stress, underlying disease, nutrition, medications, smoking, alcohol consumption, obesity, weight loss, aging, allergies, socioeconomic factors, and environmental conditions.[53,54,63,64] Thus, clinicians should not confuse the apparent association between acute and chronic exercise and altered susceptibility to URTI with causation. Changes in URTI symptomatology may occur in the absence of exercise. Because clinical populations (e.g., cardiovascular diseased, cancer patients/survivors, HIV-infected individuals, and elderly people) exhibit many of the aforementioned factors, the immune response to exercise may be different from the responses observed in healthy or younger individuals.[55,65,66] Thus, the overall health status of the client must be taken into account when assessing the impact of exercise on immunity.

ACSM makes the following recommendations regarding exercise testing and training for patients with URTI.

EXERCISE TESTING

- It is probably safe to test clients at a submaximal intensity, whose symptoms are mild and limited to the upper respiratory tract (e.g., common cold symptoms of a runny or congested nose, sneezing, and/or sore throat). Maximal testing of subjects exhibiting URTI symptoms does not elicit diminished performance, and thus it is not necessary to postpone testing.[60,61] However, for the comfort of the patient and because of a lack of information regarding long-term effects, it is prudent to delay maximal testing until the symptoms have resolved.
- Exercise testing should be postponed in clients who demonstrate symptoms of systemic involvement (e.g., fever, tiredness, diarrhea, and myalgia) until the symptoms have resolved (generally 1 to 2 weeks). Exercising with a systemic

infection could increase the virulence of some viruses, lead to severe dehydration, exacerbate existing conditions (e.g., pulmonary or cardiovascular disease), and increase the risk of developing secondary complications (e.g., bronchitis, chronic fatigue syndrome, and exacerbations of cardiopulmonary conditions). Persons aged 65 years and older, pregnant women, HIV-infected individuals, and people of any age with chronic medical conditions are more likely to experience secondary complications (e.g., pneumonia, myocarditis) from the flu.[52]

- Prescribed or over-the-counter medications should be taken into account, because they may affect cardiovascular responses to testing and exercise performance.

EXERCISE PRESCRIPTION

- Healthy individuals with symptoms of a URTI could follow the *above the neck rule*.[53] That is, if the symptoms of a URTI are mild and limited to the mouth, nose, and throat (above the neck) exercise could be performed, albeit at a lower intensity and volume. Exercise should be discontinued if symptoms worsen. If the symptoms are moderate to severe and/or indicate a systemic involvement (e.g., fever, tiredness, diarrhea, and myalgia), then exercise should be postponed until the symptoms have resolved.
- Resumption of training after URTI should begin at a modest level and the progression should be gradual.
- Clients with a mild URTI should be encouraged not to exercise in a group exercise setting to prevent the spread of their infection to other clients.
- Closely monitor exercise tolerance to avoid overtraining and chronic fatigue.

SPECIAL CONSIDERATIONS

- Encourage clients to get adequate rest, maintain a well-balanced diet, ingest ample fluids, and minimize psychological stress, particularly during periods of intense training.
- To reduce viral self-inoculation, encourage clients to wash hands with warm soapy water and minimize hand-to-eye and hand-to-nose contact, particularly during the cold and flu season.
- Clients should minimize their exposure to individuals with a URTI because URTI is spread from person to person primarily through coughing and sneezing of infected persons.
- Clients should be encouraged to consult with their physician on the appropriateness and timing of receiving a flu vaccine, particularly those at high risk for developing secondary complications from the flu (persons aged 65 years and older, pregnant women, and people of any age with chronic medical conditions).[52] Clinicians who have frequent contact with these high-risk populations should obtain a flu vaccine.[52]

Osteoporosis

Osteoporosis is defined as a systemic skeletal disease characterized by low bone mass and microarchitectural deterioration of bone tissue with a consequent increase in generalized skeletal fragility, such that fractures occur with minimal trauma.[67] Osteoporosis involves reductions in both bone mineral density (BMD) and bone quality. Osteopenia is defined as a bone density between 1 and 2.5 standard deviation units below average and places the individual at greater risk for osteoporosis.[68] The risk of fracture increases with age for the osteopenia patient. An estimated 44 million Americans are at risk of osteoporosis, with 10 million displaying the disease and 34 million having low bone mass.[*]

Osteoporosis has a debilitating effect on independence and quality of life. Risk factors for osteoporosis are family history, female gender, estrogen deficiency, low weight, dietary factors, prolonged use of corticosteroids, smoking, and physical inactivity.[69] Exercise therapy, particularly resistance-based and weight-bearing activity may increase bone material and modify several risk factors for osteoporotic fracture, including muscle strength, bone-mineral density, and dynamic balance.[68,70] Bone mass attained early in life is perhaps the most important determinant of lifelong skeletal health.[71] Nutrition, exercise, and body composition all play a key role in bone density. Exercise can positively affect peak bone mass in children and adolescents, maintain or even modestly increase bone density in adulthood, and assist in minimizing age-related bone loss in older adults. Therefore, exercise programming should be presented to optimize bone health and to safely prescribe exercise for individuals with existing low BMD.

ACSM makes the following recommendations regarding exercise testing and training for patients with osteoporosis.

EXERCISE TESTING

- Physician approval is warranted prior to graded exercise testing to determine the risk/ benefit ratio of testing.
- The patient should maintain an upright posture at all times, as any sort of spinal flexion is contraindicated. A cycle ergometer protocol is preferred.
- Premature termination may occur from osteoporotic pain.
- Severe kyphosis, which can exist as a functional limitation imposed by multiple vertebral fractures, may result in compromised ventilatory capacity and a forward shift in center of gravity.
- Care must be taken to ensure the patient does not trip or fall if a traditional treadmill exercise test is performed. Additional testing may include balance, muscular strength, and gait biomechanics.

EXERCISE PRESCRIPTION

- Consider pain status of patient. If the patient is relatively pain-free, aerobic weight bearing activity (4 d·wk^{-1}) and resistance training (2–3 d·wk^{-1}) is recommended.
- Specific exercises focusing on improving balance and modifying activities of daily living are recommended.[70]
- Improving muscle strength helps to conserve bone mass and enhance dynamic balance.[70] When prescribing exercise for patients who are severely limited

---

[*]National Institutes of Health, Osteoporosis and Related Bone Diseases National Resource Center (www.osteo.org).

by pain, the physician should be consulted prior to exercise participation.
- Perform cardiovascular exercise (aquatic, walking, cycling) at 40% to 70% of $\dot{V}O_2R$ or HRR.[69]
- Perform resistance exercise (free weights, machines, calisthenics, elastic bands) with the load directed over the long axis of the bone, 2 d·wk^{-1} for 8 to 10 repetitions at a submaximal intensity (RPE 13–15) for one to two sets.[69] Avoid exercises with spinal flexion and perform all exercises in an upright posture.
- Perform flexibility exercise 5 to 7 d·wk^{-1}.[69]
- Perform functional exercise activities (chair exercise, chair sit and stand, vigorous walking) 2 to 5 d·wk^{-1}. [69]

SPECIAL CONSIDERATIONS

- Contraindicated exercises include explosive movement and high-impact loading activities to the skeleton, such as jumping, running, or jogging.[68]
- Dynamic abdominal exercises (e.g., sit-ups), excessive trunk flexion, and twisting movements can be dangerous. Exercises that require bending forward at the waist or excessive twisting at the waist (golf swing) produce high compressive forces in the spinal area and increase the vulnerability to fracture. Daily activities such as sitting and bending to pick up objects can cause vertebral fracture.

Peripheral Arterial Disease

Peripheral arterial disease (PAD) is a manifestation of systemic atherosclerosis that affects approximately 8 to 10 million people in the United States.[72,73] PAD diminishes blood flow to the lower extremities, which leads to a mismatch of oxygen delivery and metabolic demand during physical activity. Claudication is the primary symptom of PAD and is characterized as walking-induced pain in one or both legs that does not go away with continued walking and is relieved by rest. Claudication primarily affects the calves but may begin in the buttock region and radiate down the leg. The symptoms commonly are described as burning, searing, aching, tightness, or cramping. Claudication is present in 15% to 40% of persons with PAD.[74] To avoid leg discomfort, patients with claudication alter their gait by decreasing their ambulatory pace and distance. Daily physical activity and maximal oxygen uptake are reduced by 50% in those with claudication compared to healthy subjects of similar age. Many affected patients are so deconditioned that they become housebound or dependent on others.[75] In more advanced cases, ischemic limb symptoms can occur at rest ("critical limb ischemia") and often requires surgery or amputation.

The goals of treatment for patients with claudication are to relieve their exertional symptoms, improve their walking capacity and quality of life, and reduce their atherosclerosis risk burden.[76] Patients are treated initially with cardiovascular disease risk factor modification, exercise training, and medications. The goals for risk factor modification in patients with peripheral arterial disease are similar to those in patients with coronary artery disease.

ACSM makes the following recommendations regarding exercise testing and training for patients with PAD.

EXERCISE TESTING

- Patients with PAD generally are classified as high risk; thus, exercise testing should be conducted in the presence of a physician.
- Because of the high risk of cardiovascular disease in this population, exercise testing with ECG monitoring should be performed so that ischemic symptoms, ST-T wave changes, or dysrhythmias may be identified.
- Graded treadmill protocol at 2 mph with modest increases in grade of 3.5% every 3 minutes or 2% every 2 minutes or a gradual ramp protocols may be used.[77] Record time or distance to the onset of claudication pain (see Chapter 5 for claudication scale) and the maximal walking time or distance.
- Arm ergometry or pharmacologic stress testing can be used in patients who cannot perform leg exercise to assess cardiovascular status.
- Questionnaires are a useful adjunct to exercise testing to assess community-based activity levels.[75,78,79]

EXERCISE PRESCRIPTION[77,80,81]

- The recommended mode, frequency, duration, and overload generally are consistent with those in Chapter 7 for cardiorespiratory, resistance, and flexibility exercise stimuli (see summary in Table 9-1).
- Initial enrollment in a medically supervised program with ECG, heart rate, and blood pressure monitoring is encouraged (see Table 7-3).
- Warm-up and cool down period of 5 to 10 minutes each.
- Treadmill and track walking are the most effective approaches to reduce claudication and should be performed 3 to 5 d·wk^{-1}.[82]
- Initial treadmill workload is set to elicit claudication symptoms within 3 to 5 minutes. Patients walk at this workload until they reach claudication of moderate severity (level 3). This is followed by a brief period of standing or sitting to allow symptoms to resolve.
- The exercise-rest-exercise pattern is repeated throughout the exercise session. The initial duration is a total of 35 minutes of intermittent walking, and increased by 5 minutes each session until 50 minutes of intermittent walking can be completed. Ultimately, 35 to 50 minutes of continuous walking is desired.
- Cardiac signs and symptoms may appear as patients increase their exercise capacity and reach higher heart rates and blood pressure.
- Resistance training and/or upper body ergometry is complementary to but not a substitute for walking.

SPECIAL CONSIDERATIONS

- The most common procedure for assessing the peripheral circulation is the ratio of ankle to arm systolic blood pressure (ankle-brachial index [ABI])
  - Normal: 0.91 to 1.30
  - Mild to moderate PAD: 0.41 to 0.90
  - Severe PAD: 0.00 to 0.40
  - Noncompressible, calcified vessel: >1.30

- Ankle systolic BP and ABI are further reduced after exercise because blood flow is shunted into the proximal leg musculature at the expense of the periphery and distal circulation in the leg.
- Although serial measurements of ABI are used for assessing progression in disease severity, an increase in leg blood flow is not a common response to exercise training. Hence, ABI is not useful for assessing the efficacy of intervention.
- Time to onset of intermittent claudication on exercise test is valuable outcome measure.

Pulmonary Diseases

Pulmonary diseases typically result in dyspnea or shortness of breath with exertion. As a result of this dyspnea, pulmonary patients limit their physical activity, and deconditioning results. Consequentially, pulmonary patients experience even greater dyspnea with even lower levels of physical exertion. Unless this vicious cycle can be broken, the pulmonary patient eventually becomes disabled and functionally impaired. Exercise has been shown to be an effective intervention that can break this cycle and prevent disability and functional impairment.[83,84]

Pulmonary function abnormalities often are divided into restrictive and obstructive dysfunction. Restrictive lung dysfunction is an abnormal reduction in pulmonary ventilation that may be the result of many different diseases, trauma, radiation, or certain drugs. In contrast, chronic obstructive pulmonary disease (COPD) is defined as a permanent diminution of airflow, usually associated with chronic bronchitis, emphysema, and asthma. Current evidence suggests that standard principles of exercise prescription (mode, frequency, intensity, and duration) generally can be applied to patients with pulmonary diseases. However, the majority of published data on exercise testing and prescription in this population have been obtained from those with COPD.[85,86] Individuals with well-controlled asthma can exercise following the general guidelines presented in Chapter 7. However, patients with asthma, particularly those with exercise-induced asthma (EIA), should pay special attention to avoiding environmental "triggers" such as cold, dry, dusty air and/or inhaled pollutants, chemicals. Individuals suffering from acute asthma should not exercise until symptoms have subsided.

ACSM makes the following recommendations regarding exercise testing and training for patients with pulmonary disease.

EXERCISE TESTING

- Assessment of physiologic function should include cardiopulmonary capacity, pulmonary function and determination of arterial blood gases and/or arterial oxygen saturation (S_aO_2).
- Modifications of traditional protocols (extended stages, smaller increments, slower progression) may be warranted depending on functional limitations and the early onset of dyspnea.
- Exercise testing may be terminated because of arterial oxygen desaturation.

- The exercise testing mode is typically walking or stationary cycling. If arm ergometry is to be used, it is important to remember that upper extremity aerobic–type exercise can result in increased dyspnea that can limit the duration of the activity.[87]

EXERCISE PRESCRIPTION

- The recommended mode, frequency, duration, and overload generally are consistent with those in Chapter 7 for cardiorespiratory, resistance, and flexibility exercise stimuli (see summary in Table 9-1).
- Walking is recommended strongly as the mode of exercise because it is involved in most activities of daily living. Stationary cycling may be used as an alternate mode of training. As with testing, upper extremity aerobic exercise training can result in increased levels of dyspnea.
- The recommended minimal goal for exercise frequency is 3 to 5 d·wk^{-1}. Individuals with a reduced functional capacity may require more frequent (i.e., daily) exercise training for optimal improvement.
- At present, there is no consensus as to the "optimal" intensity of exercise training for pulmonary patients. Two major approaches that have been evaluated are to exercise at 50% of peak $\dot{V}O_2$ or at maximal limits as tolerated by symptoms.[84,88,89]
- No matter what the prescribed intensity, the exercise professional should closely monitor initial exercise sessions and be ready to adjust intensity and/or duration according to patient responses. In many cases, the presence of symptoms, particularly dyspnea/breathlessness supersedes objective methods of exercise prescription.
- The traditional method for monitoring the training intensity has been heart rate. An alternative approach is to use a dyspnea rating obtained from a GXT as a "target" for exercise training. Most patients with COPD can accurately and reliably produce a desired exercise intensity using a dyspnea target of 2 to 3 (on 4-point scale) or between 3 and 5 ("moderate to severe") on the 0 to 10 category-ratio scale during submaximal exercise of 10 to 30 minutes' duration.[90,91] It is probably unrealistic for most patients with a chronic respiratory disease to perform 20 to 30 minutes of continuous exercise at the start of a physical training program. Therefore, some patients may be able to exercise only at a specified intensity for a few minutes. Intermittent exercise, that is, repetitive exercise-rest periods, may be necessary for the initial training sessions until the patient can achieve sustained higher intensities.
- It is now recognized that respiratory diseases, COPD in particular, not only affect the lungs but skeletal muscle as well. As such, resistance training of skeletal muscle should be an integral part of pulmonary rehabilitation programs.[92–94] The exercise prescription for resistance training with pulmonary patients should follow the same principles as those with older healthy adults.[94–96]
- Because respiratory disease patients can experience greater dyspnea while performing activities of daily living involving the upper extremities,[87] it may be beneficial for these patients to focus on the muscles of the shoulder girdle when performing resistance exercises.

- Inspiratory muscle weakness has been identified as a contributor to exercise intolerance and dyspnea.[97,98] As such, training of these muscles has the potential to reduce dyspnea and improve exercise capacity. Respiratory muscle strength and/or endurance can be specifically increased with inspiratory muscle training. Although positive benefits from inspiratory muscle training have not been demonstrated conclusively, there is emerging evidence to suggest that inspiratory muscle training does have positive effects in those patients presenting with inspiratory muscle weakness.[85,99]
- Guidelines for inspiratory muscle training for individual patients include: a minimum frequency of 4 to 5 $d \cdot wk^{-1}$, an intensity of 30% of maximal inspiratory pressure measured at functional residual capacity, and a duration of 30 minutes a day or two 15-minute sessions per day.

SPECIAL CONSIDERATIONS

- Unlike healthy individuals and heart disease patients, pulmonary disease patients may exhibit arterial oxygen desaturation with exercise. Therefore, some measure of the blood oxygenation, either the partial pressure of arterial oxygen (P_aO_2) or percent saturation of arterial oxygen (S_aO_2), should be made during the initial GXT. In addition, oximetry is recommended for the initial exercise training sessions to evaluate possible exercise-induced O_2 desaturation.
- Based on the recommendations of the Nocturnal Oxygen Therapy Trial,[100] supplemental O_2 is indicated for patients with a P_aO_2 of 55 mm Hg or less, or an S_aO_2 of 88% or less while breathing room air. These same guidelines apply when considering supplemental oxygen during exercise training.

Pregnancy

The physiologic changes associated with pregnancy warrant evaluation of obstetric and medical risks prior to engaging in regular physical exercise. Concerns regarding the possible adverse effects of exercise participation have focused on: 1) inadequate availability of oxygen or substrate for mother and fetus, 2) hyperthermia-induced fetal distress or birth abnormalities, and/or 3) increased uterine contractions. However, current studies indicate that healthy women with uncomplicated pregnancy do not need to limit their exercise for fear of adverse effects.[101] Generally, participation in a wide range of recreational activities appears safe during and after pregnancy. Women should be encouraged to engage in a consistent, moderate-intensity physical activity to reap the health-related benefits associated with exercise. Overly vigorous activity in the third trimester, activities that have a high potential for contact, or activities with a high risk of falling should be avoided. In addition, during pregnancy refrain from activities with a risk of abdominal trauma, exertion at altitude greater than 6,000 feet, and scuba diving.[101] Interestingly, the benefits of chronic exercise reside with the mother, whereas the risks of overexercise predominantly affect the fetus.

The American College of Obstetricians and Gynecologists (ACOG)[101] have established relative and absolute contraindications (Box 9-1) for exercise during pregnancy. If the aforementioned contraindications do not preclude

| BOX 9-1 | Contraindications for Exercising During Pregnancy* |

Relative
- Severe anemia
- Unevaluated maternal cardiac dysrhythmia
- Chronic bronchitis
- Poorly controlled type I diabetes
- Extreme morbid obesity
- Extreme underweight (BMI <12)
- History of extremely sedentary lifestyle
- Intrauterine growth restriction in current pregnancy
- Poorly controlled hypertension
- Orthopedic limitations
- Poorly controlled seizure disorder
- Poorly controlled hyperthyroidism
- Heavy smoker

Absolute
- Hemodynamically significant heart disease
- Restrictive lung disease
- Incompetent cervix/cerclage
- Multiple gestation at risk for premature labor
- Persistent second- or third-trimester bleeding
- Placenta previa after 26 weeks of gestation
- Premature labor during the current pregnancy
- Ruptured membranes
- Preeclampsia/pregnancy-induced hypertension

*See reference 101: From American College of Obstetricians and Gynecologists. Exercise during pregnancy and the postpartum period. ACOG Committee Opinion No. 267. Obstet Gynecol 2002;99:171–173.

participation, guidelines for safe exercise participation for women with no risk factors for adverse maternal or perinatal outcomes are suggested. Women who currently participate in exercise can continue their exercise program without major modifications. However, many active women modify their program based on symptoms, discomfort, and risk associated with joint laxity and body mass gain. Precautions may include using a treadmill or track for walking or running instead of exercising along the sidewalks or roadways. Exercising indoors may provide more environmental control to avoid excess heat, cold, or air pollution.

Lactation is an energy-demanding physiologic process; however, exercise has no detrimental effects on lactation for milk composition, milk volume, or maternal health. Many of the physiologic changes associated with pregnancy persist 4 to 6 weeks postpartum. Prepregnancy exercise programs should be resumed gradually depending on birth complications (i.e., Caesarean section) and physical symptoms. Although there is no evidence that a rapid return to training is associated with maternal complications, the rate of return to prepregnancy levels differs among individuals.[102] Moderate weight reduction while nursing is safe and does not compromise neonatal weight gain.

ACSM makes the following recommendations regarding exercise testing and training during and following pregnancy.

EXERCISE TESTING

- Unless a clinical condition dictates maximal exercise testing, it is not recommended for pregnant women, and only under the supervision of a physician.
- Submaximal testing can be performed with an endpoint of <75% heart rate reserve.
- Women who were less active or sedentary prior to pregnancy should seek the approval of a physician prior to engaging in physical activity.

EXERCISE PRESCRIPTION

- The recommended mode, frequency, duration, and overload generally are consistent with those in Chapter 7 for cardiorespiratory, resistance, and flexibility exercise stimuli (see summary in Table 9-1).
- In the absence of either medical or obstetric complications, 30 to 40 minutes or more of moderate physical activity on most, if not all, days of the week is recommended.
- Regular exercise (e.g., at least 3 $d \cdot wk^{-1}$) is preferable to intermittent activity.
- Monitor exercise intensity by use of ratings of perceived exertion (RPE 11–13) (light to somewhat hard), rather than heart rate.
- Women who were sedentary or relatively inactive prior to pregnancy should begin with light-intensity (20%–39% HRR), low- (or non-) impact activities, such as walking and swimming.
- Avoid exercise in the supine position after the first trimester because mild obstruction of venous return attenuates cardiac output and may facilitate orthostatic hypotension.

SPECIAL CONSIDERATIONS

- Pregnancy requires an additional 300 $kcal \cdot d^{-1}$ to maintain metabolic homeostasis.[103] Therefore, ingest additional calories to meet the needs of exercise and pregnancy.
- Motionless standing results in venous blood pooling, so it should be avoided.
- Heat dissipation is important throughout pregnancy. Appropriate clothing, environmental considerations, and adequate hydration should be priorities during the exercise program to prevent the possibility of hyperthermia and the corresponding risk to the fetus. Drink ample water to prevent dehydration. Avoid brisk exercise in hot, humid weather or when you have a fever.
- Maternal hypoglycemia may be associated with strenuous exercise during the last trimester of pregnancy. The reduction in blood glucose may result from increased glucose uptake by the fetus and mother, decreased maternal liver glycogen stores, or reduced maternal liver glycogenolysis.[103] Attenuate the

---

BOX 9-2 | **Conditions for Exercise Termination During Pregnancy***

- Vaginal bleeding
- Dyspnea prior to exertion
- Dizziness
- Headache
- Chest pain
- Muscle weakness
- Calf pain or swelling (need to rule out thrombophlebitis)
- Preterm labor
- Decreased fetal movement
- Amniotic fluid leakage

*See reference 101: From American College of Obstetricians and Gynecologists. Exercise during pregnancy and the postpartum period. ACOG Committee Opinion No. 267. Obstet Gynecol 2002;99:171–173.

---

opportunity for hypoglycemia with increased carbohydrate intake (e.g., 30 to 50 g) with food and/or a sports drink prior to exercise.
- Avoid exercise that involves the risk of abdominal trauma, falls, and excessive joint stress. Sport activities such as softball, basketball, and racquet sports are not recommended because of the increased risk of abdominal injury. When exercising, pregnant women should be aware of signs and symptoms for discontinuing exercise and seeking medical advice (Box 9-2).

REFERENCES

1. Minor MA, Kay DR. Arthritis. In: Durstine JL, Moore GE, eds. ACSM's Exercise Management for Persons with Chronic Diseases and Disabilities, 2nd ed. Champaign, IL: Human Kinetics, 2003:210–216.
2. Centers for Disease Control and Prevention. National Diabetes Fact Sheet: National Estimates and General Information on Diabetes in the United States, 1999.
3. American Diabetes Association. Standards of medical care for patients with diabetes mellitus. Diabetes Care 2003;26:S33–S50.
4. American Diabetes Association. Implications of the Diabetes Control and Complications Trial. Diabetes Care 1997;21:S88–S90.
5. Expert Committee on the Diagnosis and Classification of Diabetes Mellitus. Follow-up report on the diagnosis of diabetes mellitus. Diabetes Care 2003;26:3160–3167.
6. Anonymous. Diabetes mellitus and exercise. Diabetes Care 1997;20:1908–1912.
7. American Diabetes Association. Physical Activity/Exercise and Diabetes. Diabetes Care 2003; 26:S73–S77.
8. Ewing DJ, Martyn CN, Young RJ, et al. The value of cardiovascular autonomic function tests: 10 years experience in diabetes. Diabetes Care 1985;8:491–498.
9. American College of Sports Medicine. Position Stand: Exercise and type 2 diabetes. Med Sci Sports Exerc 2000;32:1345–1360.
10. Ruderman N, Ganda O, Johansen K. The effects of physical training on glucose tolerance and plasma lipids in maturity-onset diabetes. Diabetes 1979:89–92.
11. Pasternostro-Bayles M, Wing RR, Robertson RI. Effect of life-style activity of varying duration on glycemic control in type II diabetic women. Diabetes Care 1989;12:34–37.
12. Kaplan R, Hartwell SL, Wilson KJ, et al. Effects of diet and exercise interventions upon control and the quality of life in non-insulin dependent diabetes mellitus (NIDDM). J Gen Int Med 1987;2: 220–228.

13. Hornsby WG. Resistance training. In: Ruderman NB, Devlin JT, eds. The Health Professional's Guide to Diabetes and Exercise. Alexandria, VA: American Diabetes Association, 1995:85–87.

14. McDonald MS. Postexercise late-onset hypoglycemia in insulin-dependent diabetic patients. Diabetes Care 1987;10:584–588.

15. Aiello LM, Cavakkerano J, Aiello LP, et al. Retinopathy. In: Ruderman NB, Devlin JT, eds. The Health Professional's Guide to Diabetes and Exercise. Alexandria, VA: American Diabetes Association, 1995:143–152.

16. Cavanagh PR, Derr JA, Ulbrecht JS, et al. Problems with gait and posture in neuropathic patients with insulin-dependent diabetes mellitus. Diabetes Medicine 1992;9:469–474.

17. Goodman JI. Diabetic anhidrosis. Am J Med 1966;41:831–835.

18. Kremser CB, Levitt NS, Borow KM, et al. Oxygen uptake kinetics during exercise in diabetic neuropathy. J Appl Physiol 1988;65:2665–2671.

19. Vinik AI. Neuropathy. In: Ruderman NB, Devlin JT, eds. The Health Professional's Guide to Diabetes and Exercise. Alexandria, VA: American Diabetes Association, 1995:183–197.

20. Nesto RW, Phillips RT, Kett KG, et al. Angina and exertional myocardial ischemia in diabetic and nondiabetic patients: assessment by exercise thallium scintigraphy. Ann Intern Med 1988;108:107–175.

21. Kahn JK, Sisson JC, Vinik AI. QT interval prolongation and sudden cardiac death in diabetic autonomic neuropathy. J Clin Endocrinol Metab 1987;64:751–754.

22. Gordon NF. The exercise prescription. In: Ruderman NB, Devlin JT, eds. The Health Professional's Guide to Diabetes and Exercise. Alexandria, VA: American Diabetes Association, 1995:67–82.

23. Levin ME. The diabetic foot. In: Ruderman NB, Devlin JT, eds. The Health Professional's Guide to Diabetes and Exercise. Alexandria, VA: American Diabetes Association, 1995:137–142.

24. American Heart Association. Heart Disease and Stroke Statistics, 2003 Update. 2002.

25. National Cholesterol Education Program. Third Report of the National Cholesterol Education Program (NCEP) Expert Panel on Detection, Evaluation, and Treatment of High Blood Cholesterol in Adults (Adult Treatment Panel III). 2002. NIH Publication No. 02-5215.

26. Leon AS, Sanchez O. Response of blood lipids to exercise training alone or in combined with dietary intervention. Med Sci Sports Exerc 2001;33:S502–515.

27. Durstine J, Moore G, Thompson P. Hyperlipidemia. In: Durstine JL, Moore GE, eds. ACSM's Exercise Management for Persons with Chronic Diseases and Disabilities, 2nd ed. Champaign, IL: Human Kinetics, 2003:142–148.

28. American College of Sports Medicine. Position Stand: Appropriate intervention strategies for weight loss and prevention of weight regain for adults. Med Sci Sports Exerc 2001;33:2145–2156.

29. National High Blood Pressure Education Program. The Seventh Report of the Joint National Committee on Prevention, Detection, Evaluation, and Treatment of High Blood Pressure (JNC7), 2003, 03-5233.

30. Burt VL, Cutler JA, Higgins M, et al. Trends in the prevalence, awareness, treatment, and control of hypertension in the adult US population. Data from the health examination surveys, 1960 to 1991. Hypertension 1995;26:60–69.

31. Nesbitt SD, Julius S. Prehypertension: a possible target for antihypertensive medication. Curr Hypertension Repts 2000;2:356–361.

32. Garrison RJ, Kannel WB, Stokes J 3rd, et al. Incidence and precursors of hypertension in young adults: the Framingham Offspring Study. Prev Med 1987;16:235–251.

33. Whelton PK, He J, Appel LJ, et al. Primary prevention of hypertension: clinical and public health advisory from The National High Blood Pressure Education Program. JAMA 2002;288:1882–1888.

34. Whelton SP, Chin A, Xin X, et al. Effect of aerobic exercise on blood pressure: a meta-analysis of randomized, controlled trials. Ann Intern Med 2002;136:493–503.

35. Fagard R. Exercise characteristics and the blood pressure response to dynamic physical training. Med Sci Sports Exerc 2001;33:S484–S492.

36. American College of Sports Medicine. In: Durstine JL, Moore GE, eds. ACSM's Exercise Management for Persons with Chronic Diseases and Disabilities, 2nd ed. Champaign, IL: Human Kinetics, 2003.

37. American College of Sports Medicine. Position Stand: Exercise and Hypertension. Med Sci Sports Exerc 2004;36:533–553.

38. Thompson PD, Crouse SF, Goodpaster B, et al. The acute versus the chronic response to exercise. Med Sci Sports Exerc 2001;33:S438–S445.

39. Flegal KM, Carroll MD, Ogden CL, et al. Prevalence and trends in obesity among US adults, 1999–2000. JAMA 2002;288:1723–1727.

40. National Institutes of Health. Clinical Guidelines on the Identification, Evaluation, and Treatment of Overweight and Obesity in Adults: The Evidence Report. National Institutes of Health. Obes Res 1998;6(suppl 2):51S–209S.

41. Pi-Sunyer FX. The obesity epidemic: pathophysiology and consequences of obesity. Obes Res 2002;10(suppl 2):97S–104S.

42. Hill JO, Wyatt HR, Reed GW, et al. Obesity and the environment: where do we go from here? Science 2003;299:853–855.

43. Ross R, Janssen I. Physical activity, total and regional obesity: dose-response considerations. Med Sci Sports Exerc 2001;33:S521–527;discussion S528–529.

44. Saris W, Blair SN, van Baak M, et al. How much physical activity is enough to prevent unhealthy weight gain? Outcome of the IASO 1st Stock Conference and consensus statement. Obes Rev 2003;4:101–114.

45. Wallace JP. Obesity. In: Durstine JL, Moore GE, eds. ACSM's Exercise Management for Persons with Chronic Diseases and Disabilities, 2nd ed. Champaign, IL: Human Kinetics, 2003: 149–156.

46. Reaven GM. Diet and syndrome X. Curr Atheroscler Rep 2000;2:503–507.

47. Despres JP, Lemieux I, Prud'homme D. Treatment of obesity: need to focus on high risk abdominally obese patients. BMJ 2001;322:716–720.

48. Ford ES, Giles WH, Dietz WH. Prevalence of the metabolic syndrome among US adults: findings from the third National Health and Nutrition Examination Survey. JAMA 2002;287:356–359.

49. Isomaa B, Almgren P, Tuomi T, et al. Cardiovascular morbidity and mortality associated with the metabolic syndrome. Diabetes Care 2001;24:683–689.

50. Frayn KN. Visceral fat and insulin resistance(causative or correlative? Br J Nutr 2000;83(suppl 1):S71–77.

51. Whaley MH, Kampert JB, Kohl HW, et al. Physical fitness and clustering of risk factors associated with the metabolic syndrome. Med Sci Sports Exerc 1999;31:287–293.

52. Bridges CB, Fukuda K, Cox NJ, et al. Prevention and control of influenza. Recommendations of the Advisory Committee on Immunization Practices (ACIP). MMWR Recomm Rep 2001;50:1–44.

53. Mackinnon LT. Physical activity, diet, and the immune system. In: Myers JN, Herbert WG, Humphrey R, eds. ACSM's Resources for Clinical Exercise Physiology: Musculoskeletal, Neuromuscular, Neoplastic, Immunologic, and Hematologic Conditions. Baltimore: Lippincott Williams & Wilkins, 2002:192–205.

54. Pedersen BK, Hoffman-Goetz L. Exercise and the immune system: regulation, integration, and adaptation. Physiol Rev 2000;80:1055–1081.

55. Schmitz HR, Layne JE, Roubenoff R. Exercise and HIV infection. In: Myers JN, Herbert WG, Humphrey R, eds. ACSM's Resources for Clinical Exercise Physiology: Musculoskeletal, Neuromuscular, Neoplastic, Immunologic, and Hematologic Conditions. Baltimore: Lippincott Williams & Wilkins, 2002.

56. Nieman DC. Exercise, upper respiratory tract infection, and the immune system. Med Sci Sports Exerc 1994;26:128–139.

57. Peters EM. Exercise, immunology and upper respiratory tract infections. Int J Sports Med 1997;18(suppl 1):S69–77.

58. Shephard RJ. Special feature for the Olympics: effects of exercise on the immune system: overview of the epidemiology of exercise immunology. Immunol Cell Biol 2000;78:485–495.

59. Matthews CE, Ockene IS, Freedson PS, et al. Moderate to vigorous physical activity and risk of upper-respiratory tract infection. Med Sci Sports Exerc 2002;34:1242–1248.

60. Weidner TG, Anderson BN, Kaminsky LA, et al. Effect of a rhinovirus-caused upper respiratory tract illness on pulmonary function test and exercise responses. Med Sci Sports Exerc 1997;29(5):604–610.

61. Weidner TG, Cranston T, Schurr T, et al. The effect of exercise training on the severity and duration of a viral upper respiratory illness. Med Sci Sports Exerc 1998;30:1578–1583.

62. Flynn MG, Fahlman M, Braun WA, et al. Effect of resistance training on selected indexes of immune function in elderly women. J Appl Physiol 1999;86(6):1905–1913.

63. Irwin M. Psychoneuroimmunology of depression: clinical implications. Brain Behav Immunol 2002;16:1–16.

64. Nieman DC, Nehlsen-Cannarella SL, Henson DA, et al. Immune response to exercise training and/or energy restriction in obese women. Med Sci Sports Exerc 1998;30:679–686.

65. Bruunsgaard H, Pedersen BK. Effect of exercise on the immune system in the elderly population. Immunol Cell Biol 2000;78:523–531.

66. Courneya KS, Mackey JR, Quinney HA. Neoplasms. In: Myers JN, Herbert WG, Humphrey R, eds. ACSM's Resources for Clinical Exercise Physiology: Musculoskeletal, Neuromuscular, Neoplastic, Immunologic, and Hematologic Conditions. Baltimore: Lippincott Williams & Wilkins, 2002:179–191.
67. National Institutes of Health. Osteoporosis prevention, diagnosis and therapy. NIH Consensus Statement 2000;17:1–45.
68. Liu-Ambrose T, Khan K, McKay H. The role of exercise in preventing and treating osteoporosis. Int Sport Med J 2001;2(4):1–13.
69. Bloomfield SA, Smith SS. Osteoporosis. In: Durstine JL, Moore GE, eds. ACSM's Exercise Management for Persons with Chronic Diseases and Disabilities, 2nd ed. Champaign, IL: Human Kinetics, 2003:222–229.
70. American College of Sports Medicine. Position Stand: Osteoporosis and exercise. Med Sci Sports Exerc 1995;27:i–vii.
71. Hellekson KL. NIH releases statement on osteoporosis prevention, diagnosis, and therapy. Am Fam Phys 2002;66:161–162.
72. Hiatt WR, Hoag S, Hamman RF. Effect of diagnostic criteria on the prevalence of peripheral arterial disease. The San Luis Valley Diabetes Study. Circulation 1995;91:1472–1479.
73. Criqui MH. Peripheral arterial disease(epidemiological aspects. Vasc Med 2001;6:3–7.
74. Hirsch AT, Criqui MH, Treat-Jacobson D, et al. Peripheral arterial disease detection, awareness, and treatment in primary care. JAMA 2001;286:1317–1324.
75. Treat-Jacobson D, Halverson SL, Ratchford A, et al. A patient-derived perspective of health-related quality of life with peripheral arterial disease. J Nurs Scholarship 2002;34:55–60.
76. Hiatt WR. Medical treatment of peripheral arterial disease and claudication. N Engl J Med 2001;344:1608–1621.
77. Gardner AW, Skinner JS, Cantwell BW, et al. Progressive vs single-stage treadmill tests for evaluation of claudication. Med Sci Sports Exerc 1991;23:402–408.
78. Regensteiner JG, Steiner JF, Hiatt WR. Exercise training improves functional status in patients with peripheral arterial disease. J Vasc Surg 1996;23:104–115.
79. Ware JE Jr, Sherbourne CD. The MOS 36-item short-form health survey (SF-36). I. Conceptual framework and item selection. Med Care 1992;30:473–483.
80. Stewart KJ, Hiatt WR, Regensteiner JG, et al. Exercise training for claudication. N Engl J Med 2002;347:1941–1951.
81. Hiatt WR, Nawaz D, Regensteiner JG, et al. The evaluation of exercise performance in patients with peripheral vascular disease. J Cardiopulm Rehabil 1988;12:525–532.
82. Hiatt WR, Wolfel EE, Meier RH, et al. Superiority of treadmill walking exercise versus strength training for patients with peripheral arterial disease. Implications for the mechanism of the training response. Circulation 1994;90:1866–1874.
83. Berry MJ, Rejeski W, Adair N, et al. A randomized, controlled trial comparing long-term and short-term exercise in patients with chronic obstructive pulmonary disease. J Cardiopulm Rehabil 2003;23:60–68.
84. Ries AL, Kaplan RM, Limberg TM, et al. Effects of pulmonary rehabilitation on physiologic and psychosocial outcomes in patients with chronic obstructive pulmonary disease. Ann Intern Med 1995;122:823–832.
85. American College of Chest Physicians/American Association of Cardiovascular and Pulmonary Rehabilitation Guidelines Panel. Pulmonary rehabilitation: Joint ACCP/AACVPR evidence-based guidelines. Chest 1997;112:1363–1396.
86. Lacasse Y, Wong E, Guyatt GH, et al. Meta-analysis of respiratory rehabilitation in chronic obstructive pulmonary disease. Lancet 1996;347:1115–1119.
87. Celli BR, Rassulo J, Make BJ. Dyssynchronous breathing during arm but not leg exercise in patients with chronic airflow obstruction. N Engl J Med 1986;314:1485–1490.
88. Normandin EA, McCusker C, Connors M, et al. An evaluation of two approaches to exercise conditioning in pulmonary rehabilitation. Chest 2002;121:1085–1091.
89. Ries AL, Archibald CJ. Endurance exercise training at maximal targets in patients with chronic obstructive pulmonary disease. J Cardiac Rehab 1987;7:594–601.
90. Horowitz MB, Littenberg B, Mahler DA. Dyspnea ratings for prescribing exercise intensity in patients with COPD. Chest 1996;109:1169–1175.
91. Stewart TW, Stewart LA, Berry MJ. Exercise training in patients with chronic obstructive pulmonary disease using ratings of perceived dyspnea. Clin Exerc Physiol 2000;2:125–130.

92. American Thoracic Society and American College of Chest Physicians. ATS/ACCP Statement on cardiopulmonary exercise testing. Am J Respir Crit Care Med 2003;167:211–277.

93. American Thoracic Society and European Respiratory Society. Skeletal muscle dysfunction in chronic obstructive pulmonary disease. Am J Respir Crit Care Med 1999;159:S1–S40.

94. Lake FR, Henderson K, Briffa T, et al. Upper-limb and lower-limb exercise training in patients with chronic airflow obstruction. Chest 1990;97:1077–1082.

95. Simpson K, Killian K, McCartney N, et al. Randomised controlled trial of weightlifting exercise in patients with chronic airflow limitation. Thorax 1992;47:70–75.

96. Spruit MA, Gosselin R, Troosters T, et al. Resistance versus endurance training in patients with COPD and peripheral muscle weakness. Eur Respir J 2002;19:1072–1078.

97. Killian KJ, Jones NL. Respiratory muscles and dyspnea. Clin Chest Med 1988;9:237–248.

98. Mahler DA, Wells CK. Evaluation of clinical methods for rating dyspnea. Chest 1988;93:580–586.

99. Lotters F, van Tol B, Kwakkel G, et al. Effects of controlled inspiratory muscle training in patients with COPD: a meta-analysis. Eur Respir J 2002;20:570–576.

100. Nocturnal Oxygen Therapy Trial Group. Continuous or nocturnal oxygen therapy in hypoxemic chronic obstructive lung disease: a clinical trial. Nocturnal Oxygen Therapy Trial Group. Ann Intern Med 1980;93:391–398.

101. American College of Obstetricians and Gynecologists. Exercise during pregnancy and the postpartum period, ACOG Committee Opinion No. 267. Obstet Gynecol 2002;99:171–173.

102. Hale RW, Milne L. The elite athlete and exercise in pregnancy. Semin Perinatol 1996;20:277–284.

103. Wolf LA, Brenner IK, Mottola MF. Maternal exercise, fetal well-bring and pregnancy outcome. In: Holloszy JO, ed. Exercise & Sports Sciences Reviews. Baltimore: Williams & Wilkins, 1994: 145–194.

104. The Trials of Hypertension Prevention Collaborative Research Group. Effects of weight loss and sodium reduction intervention on blood pressure and hypertension incidence in overweight people with high-normal blood pressure. Arch Int Med 1997;157:657–667.

105. He J, Whelton P, Appel L, et al. Long-term effects of weight loss and dietary sodium reduction on incidence of hypertension. Hypertension 2000;35:544–549.

106. Sacks F, Svetkey L, Vollmer W, et al. Effects on blood pressure of reduced dietary sodium and the Dietary Approaches to Stop Hypertension (DASH) diet. DASH-Sodium Collaborative Research Group. N Engl J Med 2001;344:3–10.

107. Vollmer W, Sacks F, Ard J, et al. Effects of diet and sodium intake on blood pressure: Subgroup analysis of the DASH-sodium trial. Ann Intern Med 2001;135:1019–1028.

108. Chobanian A, Hill M. National Heart, Lung, and Blood Institute Workshop on Sodium and Blood Pressure: A critical review of the current scientific evidence. Hypertension 2000;35:858–863.

109. Kelley GA, Kelley KS. Progressive resistance exercise and resting blood pressure: a meta-analysis of randomized controlled trials. Hypertension 2000;35:838–843.

110. Xin X, He J, Frontini MG, et al. Effects of alcohol reduction on blood pressure: a meta-analysis of randomized, controlled trials. Hypertension 2001;38:1112–1117.

Exercise Testing and Prescription for Children and Elderly People

Children

A number of issues have prompted specific interest in physical activity and fitness in the pediatric population, including: 1) recognition of the role of regular exercise in the present and future health of youth, especially childhood obesity; 2) the growing number of children participating in elite-level sports competition; and 3) a growing awareness of the role of exercise testing and intervention in children and adolescents with chronic diseases. The growing body of research information surrounding these issues has identified a number of biological responses to exercise that are unique to physically immature individuals (Table 10-1). These have provided evidence that, physiologically, children are not simply small adults. It is important that these features be considered when performing clinical exercise testing or physical fitness testing in children as well as in designing exercise programs for young subjects.

CLINICAL LABORATORY TESTING

The basic premise for treadmill or cycle testing of young persons is not different than that for adults—to assess symptoms, tolerance, and cardiopulmonary responses to high-intensity exercise in a controlled setting. In general, satisfactory testing of children can be conducted equally well as in adults, even in subjects as young as 3 to 4 years. However, a number of particular features need to be appreciated when dealing with this age group.[1] Most importantly, children are emotionally immature and need encouragement and positive support by an experienced testing staff to achieve an adequate exercise effort.

The indications for exercise testing of children and adolescents are more diverse than for adults. Experience in pediatric exercise testing laboratories indicates that tests are most commonly performed for: 1) evaluating individuals who experience symptoms (e.g., chest pain, shortness of breath, syncope, palpitations) during sports or physical activity, 2) assessing cardiopulmonary functional capacity, 3) identifying myocardial ischemia (most commonly in patients with aortic valve stenosis or Kawasaki disease), 4) examining responses of heart rate, and rhythm (changes in ventricular ectopy, rate increases with complete heart block), and 5) assessing response to cardiac and pulmonary rehabilitation programs.

Both cycle and treadmill protocols have been used for exercise testing of children. However, use of the treadmill is more appropriate when testing very young

TABLE 10-1. Unique Physiologic Responses of Children Relative to Adults*†

Variable	Submaximal Exercise‡	Maximal Exercise
$\dot{V}O_2$ (L·min^{-1})	Lower	Lower
$\dot{V}O_2$ (mL·kg^{-1}·min^{-1})	Higher	Higher or equal
Heart rate	Higher	Higher
Cardiac output	Lower	Lower
Stroke volume	Lower	Lower
Lactate concentration	Lower	Lower
Tidal volume	Lower	Lower
Ventilation	Lower	Lower
RER	Lower	Lower
$\dot{V}_E/\dot{V}O_2$	Higher	Higher

*See references 1, 31, 32, and 33: Developed from Rowland TW. Aerobic exercise testing protocols. In: Rowland TW, ed. Pediatric Laboratory Exercise Testing: Clinical Guidelines. Champaign, IL: Human Kinetics, 1993:19–42; Bar-Or O. Pediatric Sports Medicine for the Practitioner. New York: Springer-Verlag, 1983:315–338; Rowland TW, Straub JS, Unnithan VB, et al. Mechanical efficiency during cycling in prepubertal and adult males. Int J Sports Med 1990;11:452–455; Washington RL. Measurement of cardiac output. In: Rowland TW, ed. Pediatric Laboratory Exercise Testing: Clinical Guidelines. Champaign, IL: Human Kinetics, 1993:133.

†Comparisons are based on exercise responses in a male child between 8 and 12 years of age compared with an apparently healthy young adult male.

‡Submaximal exercise responses are referenced to the same absolute work rate.

children, because this modality requires that the subject maintain the pace of the belt rather than provide the volitional effort to maintain a cycling cadence with increased workloads. Electronically braked cycle ergometers reduce the dependence on a specific cadence by allowing a range of cadence to achieve the same workload. However, appropriate small size cycle ergometers are not available in most laboratories. Seat height, handlebar height and position, and pedal crank length may have to be modified for cycle ergometer testing to accommodate children. Most children who are 125 cm (50 in.) tall or taller can be tested on a standard cycle ergometer. The greater potential for accidental falls on the treadmill requires greater attention by the testing staff. Regardless of the mode or protocol, children must be familiarized with all testing procedures to ensure the opportunity for a successful evaluation.

Because of the wide ranges of ages and testing indications, no single standard testing protocol has been used for children (Table 10-2). Most laboratories use the Bruce treadmill protocol for pediatric subjects, often modified to 2-minute work stages. In addition, various modifications of the Balke protocol commonly are employed in pediatric research studies and in some clinical laboratories. This protocol allows a constant comfortable speed (usually walking 3.0–3.5 mph or running at 5.0 mph), minimal slope elevation (2% per stage), and appropriate test duration (about 8–10 minutes). Its disadvantage is that, in contrast to the Bruce protocol, this protocol provides no standard norms for test duration to age as an indicator of physical fitness. Adjustments to the protocol speed may be necessary to accommodate for differences in stature and fitness levels. A number of different cycle testing protocols have been used for young subjects, most commonly the McMaster and James protocols. These are outlined in Table 10-2.

TABLE 10-2. Cycle Ergometer Protocols for Children*

Protocol	Cadence (RPM)	Body Size	Initial Load	Increment per Stage	Stage Duration (min)
McMaster	50	Height (cm)	Watts	Watts	
		<120	12.5	12.5	2
		120–140	12.5	25	2
		140–160	25	25	2
		>160	25	25 (female) 50 (male)	2
James	60–70	Body Surface Area (m^2)	$kg \cdot m \cdot min^{-1}$	$kg \cdot m \cdot min^{-1}$	
		<1.0	200	100	3
		1.0–1.2	200	200	3
		>1.2	200	300	3

*See references 31 and 34: Adapted from Bar-Or O. Pediatric Sports Medicine for the Practitioner. New York: Springer-Verlag, 1983:315–338; James F, Kaplan S, Glueck C, et al. Responses of normal children and young adults to controlled bicycle exercise. Circulation 1980;61:902–912

Abbreviations: RPM, revolutions per minute; cm, centimeters; min, minute.

Certain physiologic features can be anticipated during exercise testing of children.[2] The heart rate at rest, and both submaximal and maximal exercise are higher in young subjects compared with adults. Although the heart rate at rest and at a given workload progressively decreases as a child grows, maximal heart rate does not change. Heart rate at exhaustion in a progressive test remains stable for both boys and girls during the growing years, and does not begin to decline until about age 16 years. Consequently, formulae for estimating maximal heart rate (e.g., 220–age) are inappropriate for children and young adolescents. The achievable peak heart rate in young subjects depends on testing modality and protocol. During treadmill running the maximal rate is typically 200 bpm, whereas walking or cycling protocols usually elicit a peak rate of approximately 195 bpm. However, it should be recognized that wide interindividual variability exists in such values, and peak rates of 185 to 225 bpm are consistent with exhaustive exercise efforts in individual subjects.

Blood pressures at rest and during exercise are lower in children compared with adults.[3] At maximal exercise, a child with a body surface area (BSA) of 1.25 m^2 demonstrates a systolic blood pressure of about 140 mm Hg, whereas 160 mm Hg is expected in a subject with a BSA of 1.75 m^2.

Endurance time with a given exercise testing protocol progressively improves as a child ages. Mean duration times for males are greater than for females. Age-related norms for subjects during treadmill testing with the Bruce protocol have been published and used to assess cardiopulmonary fitness in children (Table 10-3).[4,5] However, it should be recognized that endurance time during exercise testing in children might differ between laboratories, even with the same protocol, because it is influenced by factors such as testing experience and level of encouragement by the testing staff.

TABLE 10-3. Endurance Time (Minutes) by Gender and Age Group with the Bruce Treadmill Protocol*

	Percentiles		
	10	50	90
Males			
Age (years)			
4–5	8.6	10.1	12.7
6–7	7.9	11.0	12.3
8–9	8.9	11.2	14.6
10–12	9.5	11.8	14.4
13–15	9.9	13.2	14.6
16–18	10.7	13.2	14.9
Females			
Age (years)			
4–5	5.9	9.5	11.2
6–7	8.2	10.2	12.0
8–9	8.6	10.5	13.6
10–12	9.2	11.0	13.8
13–15	8.2	10.8	13.0
16–18	8.1	10.0	11.4

*Treadmill times represent the average for a given gender-age group across two studies.[4,5] Data were derived from two pediatric cohorts referred for clinical exercise testing. Subjects were not allowed to use handrail support during the exercise test.

Electrocardiographic changes during exercise testing in children are similar to those observed in adults. An increase in R-wave voltage has been considered a marker of myocardial ischemia in adults but often is observed in healthy children. The traditional ST-segment indicators of myocardial ischemia in adults with coronary artery disease have been interpreted similarly in pediatric subjects. However, the validity of these changes as markers of coronary insufficiency in immature subjects is not certain.

Other physiologic features in children may not have a direct influence on clinical exercise testing but need to be appreciated by the testing staff. Children exhibit a much more rapid recovery of heart rate, blood pressure, and other physiologic variables after exercise testing compared with adults. The sweating rate of children is less than adults because of a decreased capacity per gland.[6] Young subjects have lower exercise economy during walking or running than adults, such that oxygen uptake (and heat production) per kg body mass at a given treadmill work rate is greater in children. Compensating for this, children have a larger ratio of body surface area to mass than adults. As a result, heat loss in a thermoneutral environment is comparable in the two populations. However, heat loss by the relatively greater body surface area of the child may be impaired at very high ambient temperatures.

FITNESS TESTING

Measurement of physical fitness and health in children and adolescents is a common practice in school-based physical education. Such testing also has been used in recreational programs, public health assessments, and clinical settings.

TABLE 10-4. Field Tests for Children

Health Fitness Component	Field Test
Cardiorespiratory fitness	1-mile walk/run
Muscular fitness	Curl-up test
	Pull-up/push-up test
Flexibility	Sit and reach test
Body composition	Body mass index or skin folds

Typically, a battery of simple field tests (generally four to six tests) are administered to evaluate different components of fitness and/or health.[7–9] Two of the most commonly administered test batteries are the FITNESSGRAM[7] and the President's Challenge Test.[8] Each provides criterion-referenced standards for interpretation of results. Table 10-4 provides a list of common field tests of physical fitness for children, with specific reference to the five components of physical fitness. Some communities, schools, and surveys develop their own battery of tests and standards of performance.[9] Questionnaires also have been used to assess physical activity patterns of young people.[10]

EXERCISE PRESCRIPTION

Regular exercise in children and adolescents can pay immediate health benefits (e.g., reduction of body fat, diminished mental stress), and, if persistent, can reduce the risk of future adult disorders such as atherosclerotic disease, osteoporosis, and systemic hypertension. For this reason, promotion of exercise in youth should be designed to introduce exercise habits that will serve as the basis for a long-term life style of regular physical activity. Although children are the most physically active age group, a significant minority is considered to have inadequate levels of regular exercise. Survey data suggest that only about 50% of American youth aged 12 to 21 are vigorously active on a regular basis. Daily enrollment in physical education classes also has declined in high school students from 42% in 1991 to 25% in 1995.[11] Physical activity typically declines through puberty, especially for girls, and the development of appropriate intervention strategies is important. Current research data do not allow recognition of a certain minimal level of daily physical activity in children necessary for long-term health benefits. However, a number of consensus groups have considered this issue and have concluded that a reasonable goal is for each child to engage in at least a moderate level of physical activity 30 to 60 minutes on most days of the week.[12,13] Such activity should include brief periods of rest and recovery as needed. Recently, the National Association for Sport and Physical Education released a position statement for children ages 5 to 12 that includes the following guidelines:[14]

- Children should accumulate at least 60 minutes, and up to several hours, of age-appropriate physical activity on all or most days of the week. This daily accumulation should include moderate and vigorous physical activity with the majority of the time being spent in activity that is intermittent in nature.
- Children should participate in several bouts of physical activity lasting 15 minutes or more each day.

- Children should participate in a variety of age-appropriate physical activities designed to achieve optimal health, wellness, fitness, and performance benefits.
- Extended periods (periods of 2 hours or more) of inactivity are discouraged for children, especially during the daytime hours.

Counseling efforts to improve level of activity have been applied to young persons who are identified as having a sedentary lifestyle. In addition, there are specific disease entities in which exercise intervention is considered an important component in management, including patients with familial hypercholesterolemia, type 2 diabetes, obesity, and essential hypertension. As in adults, the emphasis has shifted from improving physical fitness in youth to encouraging an increase in levels of habitual physical activity. Such activities should be well rounded, including those that tax the cardiovascular system (swimming, cycling), provide weight-bearing stress to bones (jumping, running), and improve muscle strength (calisthenics, lifting). Promotional efforts to maintain or improve habits of physical activity in children are most effective if multifactorial, including school physical education classes, community recreation programs, family-based activities, and counseling by health professionals.

Little research has been performed in the pediatric population to determine the most effective means of stimulating regular physical activity. For instance, it is not clear if psychosocial constructs used in programs designed to alter exercise behavior in adults, such as the transtheoretical model and social cognitive theory, are applicable to children. Studies examining the effect of physical activity interventions on youth in school and community settings indicate that motivational factors for exercise are likely to vary according to a child's developmental age.[15] However, certain components of a successful exercise intervention program for children seem evident, including the necessity for fun, lack of embarrassment, limited competition, peer and family support, and recognition of success. Unsafe neighborhoods, lack of proximity to playgrounds, and inability of parents to transport represent environmental barriers that also may modify the plan. The use of school recess and after school activities such as intramurals and activity-based latch-key programs may permit children to enhance physical activity.

At the present time there exists no evidence-based standard approach to improving the physical activity habits of children. The development of such standards is hampered by variations in age, motivation, and degree of parental support, as well as the varying influences of geographic location, socioeconomic level, and availability of recreational facilities. A number of different activity counseling models can be considered because no single exercise plan is likely to fit all children.

The Adult Prescription Model

By this traditional approach, a particular activity (usually walking) is recommended, to be performed by the child for a certain number of minutes (beginning at 15 minutes), three to five times per week, and then increasing duration and frequency to eventually reach the activity guidelines described previously. Walking can be done in interesting places to avoid boredom (e.g., at a zoo, museum, or mall) and in the company of family, friends, or pets. If the weather becomes inclement, the activity can be moved indoors (e.g., exercising on a stationary cycle while watching television).

This model has certain advantages for youth. It does not necessitate any athletic skill or special equipment, it requires no transportation by parents, it can be performed with or without company, and it is not physically taxing to the point of becoming uncomfortable. On the other hand, it might be expected to ultimately prove boring for an unmotivated child over an extended period of time.

The Exercise "Menu"

In this model, the child is presented with a list of possible activities to begin, which he or she can help compile, based on those feasible in a particular community. This widens the possibilities of exercise interventions to those involving team sports, recreational programs, and activity clubs. It offers the possibility of more social interaction and allows the child to select activities that are individually attractive; and, importantly, it permits the child a greater degree of autonomy in devising the exercise program. An exercise menu is only limited by one's imagination and resources, and may include activities such as soccer, dance, jump rope, karate, broom ball, skateboarding, hide and go seek, and pick-up basketball.

Increasing Lifestyle Activities

This approach does away with structured activities altogether and attempts to increase the child's caloric expenditure in his or her usual daily activities. This may be more attractive than a more formal schedule of regular exercise for young persons who are particularly sedentary or obese. The child can be instructed on specific ways of accomplishing this: Use stairs instead of the escalator, walk instead of riding in the car, do specific chores around the home, stand while talking on the telephone, don't stand still, or use a rocking chair while watching television. Activity lists can be checked as they are accomplished and signed by the parents, with a small reward (e.g., sports tickets, t-shirt) for a certain total.

Decreasing Sedentary Time

Recognizing the importance of regular exercise for the physical and emotional health of children has been coincident with concern that youth are spending an increasing amount of time in sedentary pursuits. In fact, sedentary habits may track or persist more as a child grows into adulthood than levels of physical activity. For this reason, reducing time spent watching television, in front of a computer, or playing video games can be a part of any prescription for sedentary youth.[16] Because physical activity experiences in childhood may be pivotal in terms of adult activity, health agencies have stepped up their efforts to encourage schools, families, and communities to promote *positive* childhood and youth physical activity experiences.[17-20]

Schools are encouraged to:

- Offer daily physical education classes at each grade.
- Increase time being physically active in physical education classes.
- Discuss health benefits of physical activity.
- Eliminate or sharply decrease exemptions for physical education.

Schools and communities should:

- Provide enjoyable, lifetime physical activities.
- Meet diverse ethnic and gender activity interests.
- Promote self-efficacy and skill development.
- Provide opportunities for all skill levels.
- Not limit activities exclusively to team-oriented sports.
- Provide safe facilities outside school hours.

Parents should:

- Set a good example by being physically active.
- Offer praise, interest, and encouragement.
- Get involved in school and/or community activity programs.
- Encourage children to be active around the home.
- Provide needed transportation.

Cardiorespiratory Training

Sustained cardiorespiratory endurance activities such as distance running, cycling, and swimming are not typical of the normal activity patterns of children. Still, issues of athletic training and responses to cardiac and pulmonary rehabilitation programs in youth have stimulated an interest in the aerobic characteristics of the pediatric age group.

Children have higher levels of maximal oxygen uptake ($\dot{V}O_{2max}$) relative to their body mass than at any other time in life. A typical $\dot{V}O_{2max}$ value in boys is ~52 mL·kg^{-1}·min^{-1}, which remains constant over the growing years. Little difference is seen in $\dot{V}O_{2max}$ between young boys and girls, but values in girls decline during childhood to ~40 mL·kg^{-1}·min^{-1} by age 16 years.[21] The $\dot{V}O_{2max}$ of a prepubertal child does not increase with endurance training to the same degree as is observed in young adults.[2] A previously sedentary adult placed in a program of endurance exercise of sufficient intensity, frequency, and duration typically demonstrates an improvement in $\dot{V}O_{2max}$ of approximately 15% to 30%. Children, on the other hand, are unlikely to increase their $\dot{V}O_{2max}$ in similar programs by more than 10%. The mean value of increase in maximal aerobic power in a meta-analysis of training programs in children was 5%,[22] and in some reports no change at all is observed. No gender differences have been observed in aerobic trainability in the pediatric age group. It appears that any aerobic training adaptations that occur in children can be elicited by the same frequency and duration training criteria as those recommended in adult programs. To improve $\dot{V}O_{2max}$, training intensity in children should produce a heart rate of 170 to 180 bpm.

The explanation for the limited rise in maximal aerobic power in children following endurance training is not known, but may result from a high innate level of activity and/or less effective training regimens. However, it is more likely that biological factors, possibly related to hormonal changes at puberty, are responsible. It is currently not clear if the dampened response of physiologic aerobic trainability in children also reflects a blunted improvement with training in performance in endurance events.

In young children, emphasis should be directed at active play (instead of exercise) and other activities of intermittent bouts of physical activity.[14] In older children, 20 to 30 minutes of vigorous exercise at least 3 d·wk^{-1} is recommended.[13] Increased duration (i.e., 30–60 minutes) and frequency (i.e., 6–7 d·wk^{-1}) of exercise are recommended to reduce overweight and obesity. Children do not generally require heart rate monitoring because of their low cardiac risk and their ability to adjust exercise through rating of perceived exertion and/or tolerance.

Resistance Training

Previously it was assumed that muscular strength could not be improved with resistance training in prepubertal subjects because of their lack of circulating testosterone. However, a series of recent studies has indicated clearly that strength can be effectively increased with training in both boys and girls before the age of puberty.[23] In fact, the relative magnitude of these increases in strength has been similar to that observed in training programs in adult subjects. Moreover, these reports indicate that age-appropriate, supervised resistance training programs can be conducted safely in children. Most studies have demonstrated that improvements in strength from resistance training in children are not accompanied by increases in muscle bulk. This observation has lent credence to the concept that neural adaptations can play a key role in the development of muscle strength with resistance training.

The role of resistance training in young subjects remains to be clarified. Whether strength improvements in children and adolescents can serve to protect against athletic injury, improve performance in strength-related sports, or have a long-term salutary influence on infirmities such as back disease and osteoporosis currently is being studied. Guidelines for resistance training in children are similar to those for adults (see Chapter 7); however, specific guidelines are noted:[13]

- The intermittent nature of resistance training is compatible with a child's natural physical activity patterns.
- Resistance training should be carefully supervised by a competent instructor.
- Avoid overly intense or maximal (1RM) resistance training. Gradual progression is important to avoid excessively demanding programs, which may discourage young subjects.
- Training equipment should be varied and appropriate to the size, strength, and degree of maturity of the child.
- Training should be a comprehensive program to increase motor skill and fitness level.
- The child should perform 8 to 15 repetitions per exercise. Resistance or weight should be increased only when the child can perform the desired number of repetitions with good form.
- Focus on participation and proper technique rather than the amount of resistance.
- If a prepubescent child cannot perform a minimum of eight repetitions in good form, the resistance is too heavy and should be reduced.
- A repetition range below eight should be reserved for adolescents (Tanner stage 5) of sufficient maturity.

Elderly People

There is increasing recognition that the term "elderly" is an inadequate generalization that obscures the variability of a broad age group. Physiologic aging does not occur uniformly across the population. Therefore, it is not satisfactory to define "elderly" by any specific chronologic age or set of ages. Individuals of the same chronologic age can differ dramatically in their physiologic age and response to an exercise stimulus. In addition, it is difficult to distinguish the effects of aging *per se* on physiologic function from that resulting from deconditioning and/or disease. Although aging is inevitable, both the rate and magnitude of decline in physiologic function may be amenable to, and even reversible with, exercise/activity intervention. Importantly, the possibility that an active or latent disease process may be present in the elderly individual always should be considered.

The safe and effective performance of exercise testing and the development of a sound exercise prescription requires a thorough knowledge of the effects of aging on physiologic function at rest and during graded exercise.[24,25] It should be noted that exercise training may attenuate some of the observed changes in aging. A list of key changes is provided in Table 10-5.

EXERCISE TESTING

The prevalence of coronary heart disease increases with advancing age; thus, the justification for exercise testing in elderly people may be even greater than that of the general adult population.[26] In accordance with Tables 2-1 and 2-4, medical clearance of older adults is advised before maximal exercise testing or prior to their participation in vigorous exercise. The assessment of cardiorespiratory function for elderly adults may require subtle differences in protocol, methodology, and dosage than that used for younger and middle-aged persons.

TABLE 10-5. Effects of the Aging Process on Selected Physiologic and Health-Related Variables

Variable	Change
Resting heart rate	Unchanged
Maximal heart rate	Lower
Maximal cardiac output	Lower
Resting and exercise blood pressures	Higher
Maximal $\dot{V}O_2$ (L·min^{-1} and mL·kg^{-1}·min^{-1})	Lower
Residual volume	Higher
Vital capacity	Lower
Reaction time	Slower
Muscular strength	Lower
Flexibility	Lower
Bone mass	Lower
Fat-free body mass	Lower
Percent body fat	Higher
Glucose tolerance	Lower
Recovery time	Longer

There is a wide selection of test protocols using a variety of modalities that have been used for testing the elderly population, either in their standard form or with slight modifications. Protocols are available for those who are highly deconditioned or physically limited. The following are special considerations for testing elderly people:[26]

- The initial workload should be low (2–3 metabolic equivalents [METs]) and workload increments should be small (0.5–1.0 METs) (e.g., Naughton protocol) for those with expected low work capacities.
- A cycle ergometer may be preferable to a treadmill for those with poor balance, poor neuromuscular coordination, impaired vision, senile gait patterns, weight-bearing limitations, and/or foot problems.
- Added treadmill handrail support may be required because of reduced balance, decreased muscular strength, poor neuromuscular coordination, or fear. However, handrail support for gait abnormalities can reduce the accuracy of estimating peak MET capacity based on exercise duration or peak workload achieved.
- Treadmill speed may need to be adapted according to walking ability.
- For those who have difficulty adjusting to the exercise equipment, the initial stage may need to be extended, the test restarted, or the test repeated.
- Exercise-induced dysrhythmias are more frequent in elderly people than in people in other age groups.
- Prescribed medications are common and may influence the electrocardiographic and hemodynamic responses to exercise.
- The exercise electrocardiogram has higher sensitivity (~84%) and lower specificity (~70%) than in younger age groups. The higher rate of false-positive outcomes may be related to the greater frequency occurrence of left ventricular hypertrophy and the presence of conduction disturbances.

There are no specific exercise test termination criteria that are necessary for the elderly population beyond those previously presented (see Box 5-2). However, the probable attainment of a lower peak VO_2 and/or the increased prevalence of cardiovascular, metabolic, and orthopedic problems[25] in elderly people often leads to an earlier test termination than in the young adult population. To avoid underestimating the level of stress imposed during graded exercise testing, it should be understood that many elderly subjects exceed the maximal heart rate predicted from the 220-age formula during a maximal exercise test.[27]

EXERCISE PRESCRIPTION

The general principles of exercise prescription (see Chapter 7) apply to adults of all ages. The relative adaptations to exercise also are similar to other age groups. The percent improvement in VO_{2max} in elderly persons can be comparable to that reported in younger populations. Unfortunately, low functional capacity, muscle weakness, and deconditioning are more common in elderly persons than in any other age group and can contribute to loss of independence in advanced age.[17] The particularly important components of the exercise prescription include cardiorespiratory fitness, resistance training, and flexibility.

Cardiorespiratory Fitness

Elderly people should be encouraged, whenever possible, to meet the population-wide recommendation to accumulate at least 30 minutes of moderate-intensity physical activity on most and preferably all days of the week. This can be accomplished with activities such as brisk walking, gardening, yard work, housework, climbing stairs, and active recreational pursuits (see Fig. 7-1, The Activity Pyramid). For those achieving this level, additional benefits may be obtained with longer-duration, moderate-intensity physical activity or by substituting moderate- with higher-intensity physical activity. Importantly, activities performed at a given MET value represent greater relative effort in elderly than young people because of the decrease in peak METs with age (Table 1-1). Elderly people should consult a physician before progressing to a vigorous exercise program.

The optimal mode of exercise for elderly persons can be influenced by physiologic and psychosocial variables, such as work capacity, orthopedic problems, poor balance, and travel limitations.

Mode

- The exercise modality should be one that does not impose excessive orthopedic stress.
- Walking is an excellent mode of exercise for many elderly people.
- Aquatic exercise and stationary cycle exercise may be especially advantageous for those with reduced ability to tolerate weight-bearing activity.
- The activity should be accessible, convenient, and enjoyable to the participant, all factors directly related to exercise adherence.
- A group setting may provide important social reinforcement to adherence.
- The wide range of health and fitness levels observed among older adults may require special considerations in terms of integrating intensity, frequency, and duration into an exercise plan.[17]

Intensity

- The intensity guidelines and precautions established for adults (see Chapter 7) for aerobic exercise training generally apply to elderly people.
- To minimize medical problems and promote long-term compliance, exercise intensity for inactive elderly people should start low and individually progress according to tolerance and preference. Initiating a program at less than 40% $\dot{V}O_2R$ or HRR is not unusual.
- Many older persons suffer from a variety of medical conditions; thus, a conservative approach to increasing exercise intensity may be warranted initially.
- Exercise need not be vigorous and continuous to be beneficial; a daily accumulation of 30 minutes of moderate-intensity physical activity can provide health benefits.
- Longer-duration or higher-aerobic intensity offers additional health and fitness benefits, although it can lead to greater risk of cardiovascular and musculoskeletal problems and lower compliance to a long-term exercise plan.
- A measured peak heart rate is preferable to an age-predicted peak heart rate when prescribing aerobic exercise because of the variability in peak heart rate

in persons more than 65 years of age and their greater risk of underlying coronary artery disease.

- Elderly persons are more likely than young persons to be taking medications that can influence heart rate.

Duration

- Exercise duration need not be continuous to produce benefits; thus, those who have difficulty sustaining exercise for 30 minutes or who prefer shorter bouts of exercise can be advised to exercise for 10-minute periods at different times throughout the day.
- To avoid injury and ensure safety, older individuals should initially increase exercise duration rather than intensity.

Frequency

- Physical activity performed at a moderate intensity should be performed most days of the week.
- If exercise is undertaken at a vigorous level, it should be performed at least 2 to 3 d·wk^{-1}, with exercise and no exercise or (low- to moderate-intensity) exercise days alternated.

Resistance Training

Muscular strength declines with advancing age at least in part because of reductions in muscle mass.[25,28] The reduction in muscle strength contributes to a decline in functional capacity. Resistance training increases muscular strength, power, and endurance (muscular fitness) in elderly individuals[25,28,29] and, in turn, has the potential to deter the untoward effects of frailty by improving mobility and preventing falls and fractures. Importantly, improved muscular fitness may allow the elderly adult to perform activities of daily living with less effort[28] and extend their functional independence by living the latter years in a self-sufficient, dignified manner. Therefore, resistance training should be an important focus of any exercise program, particularly for elderly people. The guidelines for resistance training for adults found in Chapter 7 generally apply to the older adult; however, some common sense guidelines are specific to elderly people:[30]

- The first several resistance training sessions should be closely supervised and monitored by trained personnel who are sensitive to the special needs and capabilities of elderly people.
- Begin (the first 8 weeks) with minimal resistance to allow for adaptations of the connective tissue elements.
- Perform one set of 8 to 10 exercises that use all the major muscle groups.
- A set should involve 10 to 15 repetitions that elicit a perceived exertion rating of 12 to 13 (somewhat hard).
- As a training effect occurs, achieve an overload initially by increasing the number of repetitions, and then by increasing the resistance.
- When returning from a layoff of more than 3 weeks, start with resistances of 50% or less of previous training intensity, and then gradually increase the resistance. The major goal of the resistance-training program is to develop

sufficient muscular fitness to enhance an individual's ability to live a physically independent lifestyle.
- Instruct participants to maintain their normal breathing pattern while exercising.
- Stress that all exercises should be performed in a manner in which the momentum is controlled. Avoid explosive movements.
- Perform the exercises in a range of motion that is within a "pain-free arc" (i.e., the maximum range of motion that does not elicit pain or discomfort).
- Perform multi-joint (as opposed to single-joint) exercises.
- Given a choice, use machines to resistance train, as opposed to free weights. Machines generally require less skill to use. They also protect the back by stabilizing the user's body position, and allow the user to more easily control the exercise range of motion.
- Allow participants ample time to adjust to postural changes and balance during the transition between resistance training exercises.
- Discourage participation in strength training exercises during active periods of pain or inflammation for arthritic patients.
- Engage in a year-round resistance-training program.
- Routine activities (e.g., domestic work, gardening, walking) may help to maintain muscular strength.

Flexibility

An adequate range of motion in all body joints is important to maintaining an acceptable level of musculoskeletal function, balance, and agility in older adults. What is almost universally accepted, although not documented, is the fact that maintaining adequate levels of flexibility enhances an individual's functional capabilities (e.g., bending and twisting) and reduces injury potential (e.g., risk of muscle strains, low back problems, and falls) particularly for aged people. Exercises should be prescribed for every major joint (hip, back, shoulder, knee, upper trunk, and neck regions) in the body. A well-rounded program of stretching can counteract the usual decline in flexibility of elderly people and may improve balance and agility. Yoga and tai chi movements may be helpful in this regard. Therefore, it is critical that a sound stretching program be included as part of each exercise session for older adults. Consider devoting an entire exercise session to flexibility for deconditioned older adults who are beginning an exercise program. Older adults should follow the recommendations for flexibility training found in Chapter 7.

REFERENCES

1. Rowland TW. Aerobic exercise testing protocols. In: Rowland TW, ed. Pediatric Laboratory Exercise Testing: Clinical Guidelines. Champaign, IL: Human Kinetics, 1993:19–42.
2. Rowland TW. Developmental Exercise Physiology. Champaign, IL: Human Kinetics, 1997.
3. Riopel DA, Taylor AB, Hohn AR. Blood pressure, heart rate, pressure-rate product and electrocardiographic changes in healthy children during treadmill exercise. Am J Cardiol 1979;44:697–704.
4. Cumming GR, Everatt D, Hastman L. Bruce treadmill test in children: normal values in a clinic population. Am J Cardiol 1978;41:69–75.
5. Wessel HU, Strasburger JF, Mitchell BM. New standards for the Bruce treadmill protocol in children and adolescents. Pediatr Exerc Sci 2001;13:392–401.
6. Falk B. Temperature regulation. In: Armstrong N, van Mechelen W, eds. Paediatric Exercise Science and Medicine. Oxford, UK: Oxford University Press, 2000:223–239.

7. The Cooper Institute for Aerobics Research. FITNESSGRAM. Champaign, IL: Human Kinetics, 1999.
8. President's Council on Physical Fitness and Sports. Get Fit: A Handbook for Youth Ages 6–17. Washington, DC: President's Council on Physical Fitness and Sports, 1998.
9. Ross JG. Evaluating fitness and activity assessments from the National Children and Youth Fitness Studies I and II. In: Assessing Physical Fitness and Physical Activity in Population-based Surveys. Rockville, MD: United States Department of Health and Human Services, 1989.
10. Pereira MA, Fitzgerald SJ, Gregg EW, et al. A collection of physical activity questionnaires for health-related research. Med Sci Sports Exerc 1997;29:S170–189, S201–205.
11. Centers for Disease Control and Prevention. Youth risk behavior surveillance: United States, 1999. MMWR 2000;49:1–94.
12. Cavill N, Biddle S, Sallis JF. Health enhancing physical activity for young people. Statement of the United Kingdom Expert Consensus Conference. Pediatr Exerc Sci 2001;13:12–25.
13. Sallis JF, Patrick K. Physical activity guidelines for adolescents: consensus statement. Pediatr Exerc Sci 1994;6:302–314.
14. National Association for Sport and Physical Education. Physical activity for children: A statement of guidelines, 2nd ed. Reston, VA: NASPE, 2004.
15. Pender NJ. Motivation for physical activity among children and adolescents. Annu Rev Nurs Res 1998;16:139–172.
16. Gortmaker SL, Must A, Sobol AM, et al. Television viewing as a cause of increasing obesity among children in the United States: 1986–1990. Arch Pediatr Adolesc Med 1996;150:356–362.
17. Physical activity and health. A report of the Surgeon General. Washington, DC: United States Department of Health and Human Services, 1996.
18. Public Health Service. Healthy People 2000: National Health Promotion and Disease Prevention Objectives. Washington, DC: DHHS Publication (PHS) 91-50212, 1991.
19. Pate RR, Pratt M, Blair SN, et al. Physical activity and public health. A recommendation from the Centers for Disease Control and Prevention and the American College of Sports Medicine. JAMA 1995;273:402–407.
20. United States Department of Health and Human Services. Guidelines for school and community programs to promote lifelong physical activity among young people. MMWR 1997;46:1–46.
21. Armstrong N, Welsman JR. Aerobic fitness. In: Armstrong N, Van Mechelen W, eds. Paediatric Exercise Science and Medicine. Oxford, UK: Oxford University Press, 2000:173–182.
22. Payne VG, Morrow JR. The effect of physical training on prepubescent VO2max: a meta-analysis. Res Q Exerc Sport 1993;64:305–313.
23. Falk B, Tenenbaum G. The effectiveness of resistance training in children. A meta-analysis. Sports Med 1996;22:176–186.
24. American College of Sports Medicine. Position Stand: Exercise and physical activity for older adults. Med Sci Sports Exerc 1998;30:992–1008.
25. Masoro E. Aging. In: Handbook of Physiology. American Physiological Society, Masoro E, ed. New York: Oxford University Press, 1995:681.
26. Gibbons RJ, Balady GJ, Bricker J, et al. ACC/AHA 2002 guideline update for exercise testing: a report of the American College of Cardiology/American Heart Association Task Force on Practice Guidelines (Committee on Exercise Testing). American College of Cardiology, 2002. Website available at: www.acc.org/clinical/guidelines/exercise/dirIndex.htm
27. Tanaka H, Monahan KD, Seals DR. Age-predicted maximal heart rate revisited. J Am Coll Cardiol 2001;37:153–156.
28. Roubenoff R. Sarcopenia and its implications for the elderly. Eur J Clin Nutr 2000;54(suppl 3):S40–47.
29. Fiatarone MA, O'Neill EF, Ryan ND, et al. Exercise training and nutritional supplementation for physical frailty in very elderly people. N Engl J Med 1994;330:1769–1775.
30. American College of Sports Medicine. Position Stand: The recommended quantity and quality of exercise for developing and maintaining cardiorespiratory and muscular fitness, and flexibility in healthy adults. Med Sci Sports Exerc 1998;30:975–991.
31. Bar-Or O. Pediatric Sports Medicine for the Practitioner. New York: Springer-Verlag, 1983:315–338.
32. Rowland TW, Straub JS, Unnithan VB, et al. Mechanical efficiency during cycling in prepubertal and adult males. Int J Sports Med 1990;11:452–455.
33. Washington RL. Measurement of cardiac output. In: Rowland TW, ed. Pediatric Laboratory Exercise Testing: Clinical Guidelines. Champaign, IL: Human Kinetics, 1993:133.
34. James F, Kaplan S, Glueck C, et al. Responses of normal children and young adults to controlled bicycle exercise. Circulation 1980;61:902–912.

Appendices

Common Medications

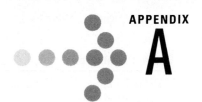

TABLE A-1. Generic and Brand Names of Common Drugs by Class

GENERIC NAME	BRAND NAME*
β-Blockers	
Acebutolol**	Sectral**
Atenolol	Tenormin
Betaxolol	Kerlone
Bisoprolol	Zebeta
Esmolol	Brevibloc
Metoprolol	Lopressor SR, Toprol XL
Nadolol	Corgard
Penbutolol**	Levatol**
Pindolol**	Visken**
Propranolol	Inderal
Sotalol	Betapace
Timolol	Blocadren

**β-Blockers with intrinsic sympathomimetic activity.

β-Blockers in Combination With Diuretics	
Atenolol + chlorthalidone	Tenoretic
Bisoprolol + hydrochlorothiazide	Ziac
Propranolol LA + hydrochlorothiazide	Inderide
Metoprolol + hydrochlorothiazide	Lopressor HCT
Nadolol + bendroflumethiazide	Corzide
Timolol + hydrochlorothiazide	Timolide
α- and β-Adrenergic Blocking Agents	
Carvedilol	Coreg
Labetalol	Normodyne, Trandate
α₁-Adrenergic Blocking Agents	
Doxazosin	Cardura
Prazosin	Minipress, Minizide
Terazosin	Hytrin
Central α₂-Agonists and Other Centrally Acting Drugs	
Clonidine	Catapres, Catapres-TTS (patch)
Guanfacine	Tenex
Methyldopa	Aldomet
Reserpine	Serpasil
Central α₂-Agonists in Combination With Diuretics	
Methyldopa + hydrochlorothiazide	Aldoril
Reserpine + chlorothiazide	Diupres
Reserpine + hydrochlorothiazide	Hydropres

continued

TABLE A-1. continued

GENERIC NAME	BRAND NAME*
Nitrates and Nitroglycerin	
Amyl nitrite	Amyl nitrite
Isosorbide mononitrate	Ismo, Monoket, Imdur
Isosorbide dinitrate	Isordil, Sorbitrate, Dilatrate
Nitroglycerin, sublingual	Nitrostat, NitroQuick
Nitroglycerin, translingual	Nitrolingual
Nitroglycerin, transmucosal	Nitrogard
Nitroglycerin, sustained release	Nitrong, Nitrocine, Nitroglyn, Nitro-Bid
Nitroglycerin, transdermal	Minitran, Nitro-Dur, Transderm-Nitro, Deponit, Nitrodisc, Nitro-Derm
Nitroglycerin, topical	Nitro-Bid, Nitrol
Calcium Channel Blockers (Nondihydropyridines)	
Diltiazem Extended Release	Cardizem CD, Cardizem LA, Dilacor XR, Tiazac
Verapamil Immediate Release	Calan, Isoptin
Verapamil Long Acting	Calan SR, Isoptin SR,
Verapamil-Coer	Covera HS, Verelan PM
Calcium Channel Blockers (Dihydropyridines)	
Amlodipine	Norvasc
Felodipine	Plendil
Isradipine	DynaCirc CR
Nicardipine Sustained Release	Cardene SR
Nifedipine Long-Acting	Adalat, Procardia XL
Nimodipine	Nimotop
Nisoldipine	Sular
Cardiac Glycosides	
Digoxin	Lanoxin, Lanoxicaps
Direct Peripheral Vasodilators	
Hydralazine	Apresoline
Minoxidil	Loniten
Angiotensin-Converting Enzyme (ACE) Inhibitors	
Benazepril	Lotensin
Captopril	Capoten
Cilazapril	Inhibace
Enalapril	Vasotec
Fosinopril	Monopril
Lisinopril	Zestril, Prinivil
Moexipril	Univasc
Perindopril	Aceon
Quinapril	Accupril
Ramipril	Altace
Trandolapril	Mavik

continued

TABLE A-1. continued

GENERIC NAME	BRAND NAME*
ACE Inhibitors in Combination With Diuretic	
Benazepril +hydrochlorothiazide	Lotensin HCT
Captopril + hydrochlorothiazide	Capozide
Enalapril + hydrochlorothiazide	Vaseretic
Lisinopril + hydrochlorothiazide	Prinzide, Zestoretic
Moexipril + hydrochlorothiazide	Uniretic
Quinapril + hydrochlorothiazide	Accuretic
ACE Inhibitors in Combination With Calcium Channel Blockers	
Benazepril + Amlodipine	Lotrel
Enalapril + felodipine	Lexxel
Trandolapril + verapamil	Tarka
Angiotensin II Receptor Antagonists	
Candesartan	Atacand
Eprosartan	Tevetan
Irbesartan	Avapro
Losartan	Cozaar
Olmesartan	Benicar
Telmisartan	Micardis
Valsartan	Diovan
Angiotensin II Receptor Antagonists in Combination With Diuretics	
Candesartan + hydrochlorothiazide	Atacand HCT
Eprosartan + hydrochlorothiazide	Teveten HCT
Irbesartan + hydrochlorothiazide	Avalide
Losartan + hydrochlorothiazide	Hyzaar
Telmisartan + hydrochlorothiazide	Micardis HCT
Valsartan + hydrochlorothiazide	Diovan HCT
Diuretics	
Thiazides	
Chlorothiazide	Diuril
Hydrochlorothiazide (HCTZ)	Microzide, HydroDiuril, Oretic
Polythiazide	Renese
Indapamide	Lozol
Metolazone	Mykron, Zaroxolyn
"Loop" Diuretics	
Bumetanide	Bumex
Ethacrynic Acid	Edecrin
Furosemide	Lasix
Torsemide	Demadex
Potassium-Sparing Diuretics	
Amiloride	Midamor
Triamterene	Dyrenium
Aldosterone Receptor Blockers	
Eplerenone	Inspra
Spironolactone	Aldactone

continued

TABLE A-1. continued

GENERIC NAME	BRAND NAME*
Diuretic Combined With Diuretic	
Triamterene + hydrochlorothiazide	Dyazide, Maxzide
Amiloride + hydrochlorothiazide	Moduretic

<table>
<tr><td colspan="2" align="center">*Antiarrhythmic Agents*</td></tr>
<tr><td colspan="2">***Class I***</td></tr>
<tr><td colspan="2">IA</td></tr>
<tr><td>Disopyramide</td><td>Norpace</td></tr>
<tr><td>Moricizine</td><td>Ethmozine</td></tr>
<tr><td>Procainamide</td><td>Pronestyl, Procan SR</td></tr>
<tr><td>Quinidine</td><td>Quinora, Quinidex, Quinaglute, Quinalan, Cardioquin</td></tr>
</table>

Class I	
IB	
Lidocaine	Xylocaine, Xylocard
Mexiletine	Mexitil
Phenytoin	Dilantin
Tocainide	Tonocard
IC	
Flecainide	Tambocor
Propafenone	Rythmol

Class II	
β-Blockers	see page 255

Class III	
Amiodarone	Cordarone, Pacerone
Bretylium	Bretylol
Sotalol	Betapace
Dofetilide	Tikosyn

Class IV	
Calcium channel blockers	see page 256

<table>
<tr><td colspan="2" align="center">*Antilipemic Agents*</td></tr>
<tr><td colspan="2">***Bile Acid Sequestrants***</td></tr>
<tr><td>Cholestyramine</td><td>Questran, Cholybar, Prevalite</td></tr>
<tr><td>Colesevelam</td><td>Welchol</td></tr>
<tr><td>Colestipol</td><td>Colestid</td></tr>
</table>

Fibric Acid Derivatives	
Clofibrate	Atromid
Gemfibrozil	Lopid
Fenofibrate	Tricor, Lofibra

continued

TABLE A-1. continued

GENERIC NAME	BRAND NAME*
HMG-CoA Reductase Inhibitors	
Atorvastatin	Lipitor
Fluvastatin	Lescol
Lovastatin	Mevacor
Pravastatin	Pravachol
Simvastatin	Zocor
Rosuvastatin	Crestor
Lovastatin + Niacin	Advicor
Nicotinic Acid	
Niacin	Niaspan, Nicobid, Slo-Niacin
Cholesterol Absorption Inhibitor	
Ezetimibe	Zeta
Ezetimibe + Simvasatin	Vytorin
Blood Modifiers (Anticoagulant or Antiplatelet)	
Clopidogrel	Plavix
Dipyridamole	Persantine
Pentoxifylline	Trental
Ticlopidine	Ticlid
Cilostazol	Pletal
Warfarin	Coumadin
Respiratory Agents	
Steroidal Antiinflammatory Agents	
Flunisolide	AeroBid
Triamcinolone	Azmacort
Beclomethasone	Beclovent, Qvar
Fluticasone	Flovent
Fluticasone and salmeterol (β_2 receptor agonist)	Advair Diskus
Budesonide	Pulmicort
Bronchodilators	
Anticholinergics (Acetylcholine Receptor Antagonist)	
Ipratropium	Atrovent
Anticholinergics with Sympathomimetics (β_2-Receptor Agonists)	
Ipratropium and Albuterol	Combivent
Sympathomimetics (β_2-Receptor Agonists)	
Salmeterol	Serevent
Metaproterenol	Alupent
Terbutaline	Brethine
Pirbuterol	Maxair
Albuterol	Proventil, Ventolin
Salmeterol and Fluticasone (steroid)	Advair
Xanthine Derivatives	
Theophyline	Theo-Dur, Uniphyl

continued

TABLE A-1. continued

GENERIC NAME	BRAND NAME*
Leukotriene Antagonists and Formation Inhibitors	
Zafirlukast	Accolate
Montelukast	Singulair
Zileuton	Zyflo

Mast Cell Stabilizers	
Cromolyn Inhaled	Intal
Nedocromil	Tilade
Omalizumab	Xolair

Antidiabetic Agents

Biguanides (Decrease hepatic glucose production and intestinal glucose absorption)	
Metformin	Glucophage, Riomet
Metformin and Glyburide	Glucovance

Glucosidase Inhibitors (Inhibit intestinal glucose absorption)	
Miglitol	Glyset

Insulins

Rapid-acting	Intermediate-acting	Intermediate- and rapid-acting combination	Long-Acting
Humalog	Humulin L	Humalog Mix	Humulin U
Humulin R	Humulin N	Humalog 50/50	Lantus Injection
Novolin R	Iletin II Lente	Humalog 70/30	
Iletin II R	Iletin II NPH	Novolin 70/30	
	Novolin L		
	Nivalin N		

Meglitinides (Stimulate pancreatic islet β cells)	
Nateglinide	Starlix
Repaglinide	Prandin, Gluconorm

Sulfonylureas (Stimulate pancreatic islet β cells)	
Glyburide	DiaBeta, Glynase, Micronase
Glipizide	Glucotrol
Gliclazide	Diamicron
Glimepiride	Amaryl
Tolazamide	Tolinase
Tolbutamide	Orinase
Chlorpropamide	Diabinese

Thiazolidinediones (Increase insulin sensitivity)	
Pioglitazone	Actos
Rosiglitazone	Avandia

Obesity Management

Appetite Suppressants	
Sibutramine	Meridia

Lipase Inhibitors	
Orlistat	Xenical

*Represent selected brands; these are not necessarily all inclusive.

TABLE A-2. Effects of Medications on Heart Rate, Blood Pressure, the Electrocardiogram (ECG), and Exercise Capacity

Medications	Heart Rate	Blood Pressure	ECG	Exercise Capacity
I. β-Blockers (including carvedilol and labetalol)	↓* (R and E)	↓ (R and E)	↓ HR* (R) ↓ ischemia† (E)	↑ in patients with angina; ↓ or ↔ in patients without angina
II. Nitrates	↑ (R) ↑ or ↔ (E)	↓ (R) ↓ or ↔ (E)	↑ HR (R) ↑ or ↔ HR (E) ↓ ischemia† (E)	↑ in patients with angina; ↔ in patients without angina; ↑ or ↔ in patients with congestive heart failure (CHF)
III. Calcium channel blockers				
Amlodipine Felodipine Isradipine Nicardipine Nifedipine Nimodipine Nisoldipine	↑ or ↔ (R and E)	↓ (R and E)	↑ or ↔ HR (R and E) ↓ ischemia† (E)	↑ in patients with angina; ↔ in patients without angina
Diltiazem Verapamil	↓ (R and E)		↓ HR (R and E) ↓ ischemia† (E)	
IV. Digitalis	↓ in patients with atrial fibrillation and possibly CHF Not significantly altered in patients with sinus rhythm	↔ (R and E)	May produce non-specific ST-T wave changes (R) May produce ST segment depression (E)	Improved only in patients with atrial fibrillation or in patients with CHF

*β-Blockers with ISA lower resting HR only slightly.

TABLE A-2. continued

Medications	Heart Rate	Blood Pressure	ECG	Exercise Capacity
V. Diuretics	↔ (R and E)	↔ or ↓ (R and E)	↔ or PVCs (R) May cause PVCs and "false-positive" test results if hypokalemia occurs May cause PVCs if hypomagnesemia occurs (E)	↔, except possibly in patients with CHF
VI. Vasodilators, nonadrenergic	↑ or ↔ (R and E)	↓ (R and E)	↑ or ↔ HR (R and E)	↔, except ↑ or ↔ in patients with CHF
ACE inhibitors and Angiotensin II receptor blockers	↔ (R and E)	↓ (R and E)	↔ (R and E)	↔, except ↑ or ↔ in patients with CHF
α-Adrenergic blockers	↔ (R and E)	↓ (R and E)	↔ (R and E)	↔
Antiadrenergic agents without selective blockade	↓ or ↔ (R and E)	↓ (R and E)	↓ or ↔ HR (R and E)	↔
VII. Antiarrhythmic agents	All antiarrhythmic agents may cause new or worsened arrhythmias (proarrhythmic effect)			
Class I				
Quinidine	↑ or ↔ (R and E)	↓ or ↔ (R)	↑ or ↔ HR (R)	↔
Disopyramide		↔ (E)	May prolong QRS and QT intervals (R) Quinidine may result in "false-negative" test results (E)	

continued

Procainamide	↔ (R and E)	↔ (R and E)	May prolong QRS and QT intervals (R) May result in "false-positive" test results (E)	↕
Phenytoin ⎫ Tocainide ⎬ Mexiletine ⎭	↔ (R and E)	↔ (R and E)		↕
Moricizine	↔ (R and E)	↔ (R and E)	May prolong QRS and QT intervals (R) ↔ (E)	↕
Propafenone	↓ (R) ↓ or ↔ (E)	↔ (R and E)	↓ HR (R) ↓ or ↔ HR (E)	↕
Class II β-Blockers (see I.)				
Class III Amiodarone Sotalol	↓ (R and E)	↔ (R and E)	↓ HR (R) ↔ (E)	↕
Class IV Calcium channel blockers (see III.)				

TABLE A-2. continued

Medications	Heart Rate	Blood Pressure	ECG	Exercise Capacity
VIII. Bronchodilators	↔ (R and E)	↔ (R and E)	↔ (R and E)	Bronchodilators ↑ exercise capacity in patients limited by bronchospasm
Anticholinergic agents	↑ or ↔ (R and E)	↔	↑ or ↔ HR May produce PVCs (R and E)	
Xanthine derivatives				
Sympathomimetic agents	↑ or ↔ (R and E)	↑, ↔, or ↓ (R and E)	↑ or ↔ HR (R and E)	↔
Cromolyn sodium	↔ (R and E)	↔ (R and E)	↔ (R and E)	↔
Steroidal Anti-inflamatory Agents	↔ (R and E)	↔ (R and E)	↔ (R and E)	↔
IX. Antilipemic agents	Clofibrate may provoke arrhythmias, angina in patients with prior myocardial infarction Nicotinic acid may ↓ BP All other hyperlipidemic agents have no effect on HR, BP, and ECG			↔
X. Psychotropic medications				
Minor tranquilizers	May ↓ HR and BP by controlling anxiety; no other effects			
Antidepressants	↑ or ↔ (R and E)	↓ or ↔ (R and E)	Variable (R) May result in "false-positive" test results (E)	
Major tranquilizers	↑ or ↔ (R and E)	↓ or ↔ (R and E)	Variable (R) May result in "false-positive" or "false-negative" test results (E)	

continued

Medication				
Lithium	↔ (R and E)	↔ (R and E)	May result in T wave changes and arrhythmias (R and E)	
XI. Nicotine	↑ or ↔ (R and E)	↑ (R and E)	↑ or ↔ HR May provoke ischemia, arrhythmias (R and E)	↔, except ↓ or ↔ in patients with angina
XII. Antihistamines	↔ (R and E)	↔ (R and E)	↔ (R and E)	↔
XIII. Cold medications with sympathomimetic agents	Effects similar to those described in sympathomimetic agents, although magnitude of effects is usually smaller			↔
XIV. Thyroid medications	↑ (R and E)	↑ (R and E)	↑ HR May provoke arrhythmias ↑ ischemia (R and E)	↔, unless angina worsened
Only levothyroxine				
XV. Alcohol	↔ (R and E)	Chronic use may have role in ↑ BP (R and E)	May provoke arrhythmias (R and E)	↔

TABLE A-2. continued

Medications	Heart Rate	Blood Pressure	ECG	Exercise Capacity
XVI. Hypoglycemic agents Insulin and oral agents	↔ (R and E)	↔ (R and E)	↔ (R and E)	↔
XVII. Blood Modifiers (Anticoagulants and Antiplatelets)	↔ (R and E)	↔ (R and E)	↔ (R and E)	↔
XVIII. Pentoxifylline	↔ (R and E)	↔ (R and E)	↔ (R and E)	↑ or ↔ in patients limited by intermittent claudication
XIX. Antigout medications	↔ (R and E)	↔ (R and E)	↔ (R and E)	↔
XX. Caffeine	Variable effects depending on previous use Variable effects on exercise capacity May provoke arrhythmias			
XXI. Anorexiants/diet pills	↑ or ↔ (R and E)	↑ or ↔ (R and E)	↑ or ↔ HR (R and E)	

*β-Blockers with ISA lower resting HR only slightly.

†May prevent or delay myocardial ischemia (see text).

Abbreviations: PVCs, premature ventricular contractions; ↑ = increase; ↔ = no effect; ↓ = decrease; R, rest; E, exercise; HR, heart rate.

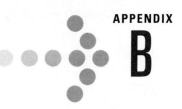

Emergency Management

The following key points are essential components of all emergency medical plans:

- All personnel involved with exercise testing and supervision should be trained in basic cardiopulmonary resuscitation (CPR) and preferably advanced cardiac life support (ACLS).
- There should be at least one, and preferably two trained ACLS personnel and a physician immediately available at all times when maximal sign- or symptom-limited exercise testing is performed.
- Telephone numbers for emergency assistance should be posted clearly on all telephones. Emergency communication devices must be readily available and working properly.
- Emergency plans should be established and posted. Regular rehearsal of emergency plans and scenarios should be conducted and documented.
- Regular drills should be conducted at least quarterly for all personnel.
  - A specific person or persons should be assigned to the regular maintenance of the emergency equipment and regular surveillance of all pharmacologic substances.
  - Records should be kept documenting function of emergency equipment such as defibrillator, oxygen supply, and suction. In addition, expiration dates for pharmacologic agents and other supportive supplies (e.g., intravenous equipment and intravenous fluids) should be kept.
  - Hospital emergency departments (or code teams) and other sources of support such as paramedics (if exercise testing is performed outside of a hospital setting) should be advised as to the exercise testing laboratory location as well as the usual times of operation.

If a problem occurs during exercise testing, the nearest available physician or other licensed and trained ACLS provider (paramedic or code team) should be summoned immediately. The physician should decide whether to call for evacuation to the nearest hospital if testing is not carried out in the hospital. If a physician is not available and any question exists as to the status of the patient, then emergency transportation to the closest hospital should be summoned immediately.

Equipment and drugs that should be available in any area where maximal exercise testing is performed are listed in Table B-1. Only those personnel

TABLE B-1. Emergency Equipment and Drugs

Equipment

- Portable, battery-operated defibrillator-monitor with hardcopy printout or memory, cardioversion capability, direct-current capability in case of battery failure (equipment must have battery low-light indicator). Defibrillator should be able to perform hard wire monitoring in case of exercise testing monitor failure. An automated external defibrillator (AED) is an acceptable alternative to a manual defibrillator in most settings.
- Sphygmomanometer, including aneroid cuff and stethoscope
- Airway supplies, including oral, nasopharyngeal, and/or intubation equipment (only in situations where licensed and trained personnel are available for use)
- Oxygen, available by nasal cannula and mask
- AMBU bag with pressure release valve
- Suction equipment
- Intravenous fluids and stand
- Intravenous access equipment in varying sizes including butterfly intravenous supplies
- Syringes and needles in multiple sizes
- Tourniquets
- Adhesive tape, alcohol wipes, gauze pads
- Emergency documentation forms (incident/accident form or code charting form)

Drugs (IV Form Unless Otherwise Indicated)

- American Heart Association ACLS, 2001[1]
  - Pharmacologic agents used to treat ventricular fibrillation/pulseless ventricular Tachycardia
    - Epinephrine
    - Vasopressin
  - Antiarrhythmics
    - Amiodarone
    - Lidocaine
    - Magnesium
    - Procainamide
  - Pharmacologic agents used to treat pulseless electrical activity and asystole
    - Epinephrine
    - Atropine
  - Pharmacologic agents used to treat acute coronary syndromes: acute ischemia chest pain
    - Oxygen (mask or nasal cannula)
    - Aspirin (oral)
    - Nitroglycerin (oral or IV)
    - Morphine (if pain not relieved with nitroglycerin)
      - MONA (morphine, oxygen, nitroglycerin, aspirin) greets all patients
    - β-Adrenergic blockers (see Appendix A for list)
    - Heparin

continued

TABLE B-1. continued

Drugs (IV Form Unless Otherwise Indicated)

- ○ ACE inhibitors (see Appendix A for list)
- ○ Glycoprotein IIb/IIIa receptor inhibitors
- ○ Fibrinolytic agents
  - Tissue plasminogen activator (tPA): Alteplase
  - Streptokinase
  - Reteplase: Retavase
  - Anisoylated plasminogen activator complex (APSAC): Eminase
  - TNKase: Tenecteplase
- • Pharmacologic agents used to treat bradycardias
  - ○ Atropine
  - ○ Dopamine
  - ○ Epinephrine
  - ○ Isoproterenol
- • Pharmacologic agents used to treat unstable and stable tachycardias

Most commonly used:
  - ○ Adenosine
  - ○ β-Adrenergic blockers (esmolol, atenolol, metoprolol)
  - ○ Calcium channel blockers (diltiazem, verapamil)
  - ○ Digoxin
  - ○ Procainamide
  - ○ Amiodarone
  - ○ Lidocaine
  - ○ Ibutilide
  - ○ Magnesium sulfate

Less commonly used:
  - ○ Flecainide
  - ○ Propafenone
  - ○ Sotalol (not approved for use in United States)

*Drugs in parentheses are used most frequently for tachycardias within a class of agents

The reader is encouraged to review ACLS algorithms, where the pharmacologic agents described in this table are used in the context of the ABCDs (Airway, opening and maintaining the airway; Breathing, providing positive-pressure ventilations; Circulation, chest compressions; Defibrillation, transcutaneous electrical pacing, or synchronized cardioversion).

authorized by law to use certain equipment (e.g., defibrillators, syringes, needles) and dispense drugs can lawfully do so. It is mandatory that such personnel be immediately available during maximal exercise testing of persons with known coronary artery disease.

Automated External Defibrillators

Early defibrillation continues to be the critical element for successful resuscitation of a life-threatening cardiac arrest. There is growing use and support for automated external defibrillators (AEDs) in medical and nonmedical settings (e.g., airports, during flights, casinos). Recent guidelines from the American Heart Association[1] indicate that for a witnessed cardiac arrest, immediate bystander CPR and early use of an AED can achieve outcomes equivalent to those achieved with the full ACLS armamentarium. Special conditions that may change how you use the AED are:

- Do not use AED on child less than 8 years of age
- Do not use on victim in standing water
- Do not place AED electrode directly over implanted cardioverter defibrillator (ICD)
- Do not place AED electrode over transdermal medication patch (nicotine, nitroglycerin)

For more detailed explanations on the expanding role of AEDs and management of various cardiovascular emergencies, the reader is encouraged to obtain the American Heart Association's 2000 Handbook of Emergency Cardiovascular Care (ECC) and/or Advanced Cardiovascular Life Support textbook.

Tables B-2 through B-4 provide sample plans for nonemergency situations (see Table B-2) and emergency situations (see Tables B-3 and B-4). These plans are provided only as examples, and specific plans must be tailored to individual program needs and local standards.

TABLE B-2. Plan for Nonemergency Situations

Level: Basic	Intermediate	High
At a field, pool, or park without emergency equipment	At a gymnasium or outside facility with basic equipment plus **manual defibrillator (or automated external defibrillator [AED])** and possibly a small "start-up" kit with drugs	Hospital or hospital adjunct with all the equipment of intermediate level plus a "code cart" containing emergency drugs and equipment for intravenous drug administration, intubation, drawing arterial blood gas samples and suctioning. Victim may be inpatient or outpatient

Level: Basic First Rescuer	Intermediate First Rescuer	High First Rescuer

1. Instruct victim to stop activity
2. Remain with victim until symptoms subside
  a. If symptoms worsen, use basic first aid
  b. If symptoms do not subside, bring victim to ER or physician's office for evaluation
3. Advise victim to seek medical advice before further activity
4. Document event
	Same as Basic Level Nos. 1 to 4
	Add:
	5. Take vital signs
	6. Monitor and record ECG rhythm **(or apply AED)**
	7. Bring record of vital signs and ECG rhythm strip to ER/physician's office if symptoms do not subside and visit is necessary
		Inpatient facility
		Same as Intermediate Level No. 1 to 6
		Add:
		7. Call for medical personnel on duty
		8. Notify primary physician
		9. Request new consult from physician to resume exercise if more than three consecutive exercise sessions are interrupted for same complaint

TABLE B-2. continued

Level: Basic Second Rescuer	Intermediate Second Rescuer	High Second Rescuer
1. Assist first rescuer, drive victim to ER or physician's office, if necessary	Same as Basic Level No. 1 Add: 2. Bring blood pressure cuff and ECG monitor to site 3. Assist with taking and monitoring vital signs	Same as Intermediate Level Nos. 1 to 3

Abbreviations: ECG, electrocardiogram; ER, emergency room; IV, intravenous.

TABLE B-3. Plan for Potentially Life-Threatening Situations

Level: Basic	Intermediate	High
At a field, pool, or park without emergency equipment	At a gymnasium or outside facility with basic equipment plus **manual defibrillator (or AED)** and possibly a small "start-up" kit with drugs	Hospital or hospital adjunct with all the equipment of intermediate level plus a "code cart" containing emergency drugs and equipment for oxygen, intravenous drug administration, intubation, drawing arterial blood gas samples, and suctioning Victim may be inpatient or outpatient

Level: Basic First Rescuer	Intermediate First Rescuer	High First Rescuer
1. Establish responsiveness a. Responsive: Instruct victim to sit Activate EMS Direct second rescuer to call EMS Stay with victim until EMS team arrives Note time of incident Apply pressure to any bleeding Note if victim takes any medication (i.e., nitroglycerin) Take pulse	Same as Basic Level Nos. 1 and 2 Add: 3. Apply monitor to victim and record rhythm **(or apply AED)**. Monitor continuously 4. Take vital signs every 1 to 5 minutes 5. Document vital signs and rhythm. Note time, and victim signs and symptoms	Same as Intermediate Level Nos. 1 to 5 Also may adapt/add: 1. Call nurse on ward 2. Call nurse if physician is off ward 3. Notify primary physician as soon as possible

TABLE B-3. continued

    b. Unresponsive:
       Activate EMS
       Place victim supine
       Open airway
       Check respiration. If absent, follow
         directions in Table B-4
       Maintain open airway
       Check pulse. If absent follow directions
         in Table B-4
       Direct second rescuer to call EMS
       Stay with victim; continue to monitor
         respiration and pulse
  2. Other considerations
    a. If bleeding, compress area to
       decrease/stop bleeding
    b. Suspected neck fracture: open airway
       with a jaw-thrust maneuver; do not
       hyperextend neck
    c. If seizing: prevent injury by removing
       harmful objects; place something under
       head if possible
    d. Turn victim on side, once seizure activity
       stops, to help drain secretions

TABLE B-3. continued

Level: Basic Second Rescuer	Intermediate Second Rescuer	High Second Rescuer

1. Call EMS
2. Wait to direct emergency team to scene
3. Return to scene to assist
	Same as Basic Level Nos. 1 to 3
	Add:
	4. Bring all emergency equipment and
	   a. Place victim on monitor
	   b. Run ECG rhythm strips
	     (or apply AED)_
	   c. Take vital signs
		Same as Intermediate
		Level Nos. 1 to 4

LEVEL: BASIC THIRD RESCUER	INTERMEDIATE THIRD RESCUER	HIGH THIRD RESCUER
1. Direct emergency team to scene or 2. Assist first rescuer	Same as Basic Level	Same as Basic Level

ECG, electrocardiogram; EMS, emergency medical services.

TABLE B-4. Plan for Life-Threatening Situations

Level: Basic	Intermediate	High
At a field, pool, or park without emergency equipment	At a gymnasium or outside facility with basic equipment plus manual defibrillator (or AED) and possibly a small "start-up" kit with drugs	Hospital or hospital adjunct with all the equipment of intermediate level plus a "code cart" containing emergency drugs and equipment for intravenous drug administration, intubation, oxygenation, drawing arterial blood gas samples, and suctioning Victim may be inpatient or outpatient

Level: Basic First Rescuer	Intermediate First Rescuer	High First Rescuer
1. Position victim (pull from pool if necessary) and place supine, determine unresponsiveness 2. Call for help (911 or local EMS number) 3. Open airway; look, listen, and feel for the air 4. Give two ventilations if no respirations 5. Check pulse (carotid artery) 6. Administer 15:2 compression/ventilation if no pulse 7. Continue ventilation if no respiration	Step Nos. 1 to 7 for Basic Level	Step Nos. 1 to 7 for Basic Level

TABLE B-4. continued

Level: Basic Second Rescuer	Intermediate Second Rescuer	High Second Rescuer

1. Locate nearest phone and call EMS
2. Return to scene and help with two-person CPR, or
3. Remain at designated area and direct emergency team to location
	Step Basic Level Nos. 1 to 3
	Add:
	4. Return to scene, bringing defibrillator: take "quick look" at rhythm Document rhythm (do not defibrillate unless certified to do so and this activity is part of your clinical privileges for the facility in which the work is being completed) (or apply AED)
	5. Place monitor leads on patient and monitor rhythm during CPR
	6. Bring emergency drug kit if available
	  a. Open oxygen equipment and use AMBU bag with oxygen at 10 L/min (i.e., 100%)[2] (if trained to do so)
	  b. Open drug kit and prepare intravenous line and drug administration (must only be done by trained, licensed professionals)
	  c. Keep equipment at scene for use by emergency personnel
		Step Intermediate Level Nos. 1 to 6

Level: Basic Third Rescuer	Intermediate Third Rescuer	High Third Rescuer
1. Assist with two-person CPR or 2. Help direct emergency team to site 3. Help clear area	Same as Basic Level	Same as Basic Level

EMS, emergency medical services.

REFERENCES

1. ACLS Provider Manual. Greenville, TX: American Heart Association, 2001.
2. Basic Life Support for Health Care Providers. Greenville, TX: American Heart Association, 2001.

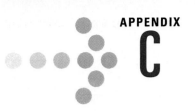

C

Electrocardiogram (ECG) Interpretation

The tables in this Appendix provide a quick reference source for electrocardiogram (ECG) recording and interpretation. Each of these tables should be used as part of the overall clinical picture when making diagnostic decisions about an individual.

TABLE C-1. Precordial (Chest Lead) Electrode Placement

Lead	Electrode Placement
V_1	4th intercostal space just to the right of the sternal border
V_2	4th intercostal space just to the left of the sternal border
V_3	At the midpoint of a straight line between V_2 and V_4
V_4	On the midclavicular line in the 5th intercostal space
V_5	On the anterior axillary line and horizontal to V_4
V_6	On the midaxillary line and horizontal to V_4 and V_5

TABLE C-2. Electrocardiogram Interpretation Steps

1. Check for correct calibration (1 mV = 10 mm) and paper speed (25 mm/sec)
2. Calculate the heart rate and determine the heart rhythm
3. Measure intervals (PR, QRS, QT)
4. Determine the mean QRS axis and mean T wave axis in the limb leads
5. Look for morphologic abnormalities of the P wave, QRS complex, ST segments, T waves and U waves (e.g., chamber enlargement, conduction delays, infarction, repolarization changes)
6. Interpret the present electrocardiogram (ECG)
7. Compare the present ECG with previous available ECGs
8. Conclusion, clinical correlation, and recommendations

TABLE C-3. Resting 12-Lead Electrocardiogram: Normal Limits

Parameter	Normal Limits	Abnormal If	Possible Interpretation(s)*
Heart rate	60–100 beats·min⁻¹	<60 >100	Bradycardia Tachycardia
PR interval	0.12–0.20 sec	<0.12 sec >0.20 sec	Preexcitation (i.e., WPW, LGL) First-degree AV block
QRS duration	Up to 0.10 sec	If ≥0.11 sec	Conduction abnormality (i.e., incomplete or complete bundle branch block, WPW, aberrant conduction)
QT interval	Rate dependent Normal QT = $K\sqrt{RR}$, where K = 0.37 for men and children and 0.40 for women	QTc long QTc short	Drug effects, electrolyte abnormalities, ischemia Digitalis effect, hypercalcemia
QRS axis	−30 to +110 degrees	<−30 degrees >+110 degree Indeterminate	Left axis deviation (i.e., chamber enlargement, hemiblock, infarction) Right axis deviation (i.e., RVH, pulmonary disease, infarction) All limb leads transitional

(continued)

TABLE C-3. continued

Parameter	Normal Limits	Abnormal If	Possible Interpretation(s)*
T axis	Generally same direction as QRS axis	The T axis (vector) is typically deviated away from the area of "mischief" (i.e., ischemia, bundle branch block, hypertrophy)	Chamber enlargement, ischemia, drug effects, electrolyte disturbances
ST segments	Generally at isoelectric line (PR segment) or within 1 mm. The ST may be elevated up to 3 mm in leads V_1–V_4.	Elevation of ST segment Depression of ST segment	Injury, ischemia, pericarditis, electrolyte abnormality, normal variant Injury, ischemia, electrolyte abnormality, drug effects, normal variant.
Q waves	<0.04 sec and <25% of R wave amplitude (exceptions lead III and V_1)	>0.04 sec and/or >25% of R wave amplitude except lead III (the lead of exceptions) and V_1	Infarction or pseudoinfarction (as from chamber enlargement, conduction abnormalities, WPW, chronic obstructive pulmonary disease, cardiomyopathy)
Transition zone	Usually between V_2–V_4	Before V_2 After V_4	Counterclockwise rotation Clockwise rotation

*If supported by other electrocardiograms (ECGs) and related clinical criteria.

Abbreviations: bpm, beats per minute; WPW, Wolff-Parkinson-White syndrome; LGL, Lown-Ganong-Levine syndrome; QTc, QT corrected for heart rate; COPD, chronic obstructive pulmonary disease.

TABLE C-4. Normal QT Interval as a Function of Heart Rate*†

Heart Rate	Age (Y)							
	18–29		30–39		40–49		50–60	
	L	U	L	U	L	U	L	U
115–84	0.30	0.37	0.30	0.37	0.31	0.37	0.31	0.37
83–72	0.32	0.39	0.33	0.39	0.33	0.40	0.33	0.40
71–63	0.34	0.41	0.35	0.41	0.35	0.41	0.35	0.42
62–56	0.36	0.42	0.36	0.43	0.37	0.43	0.37	0.43
55–45	0.39	0.45	0.39	0.45	0.39	0.46	0.39	0.46

*Adapted from Simonson E, Cady LD, Woodbury M. The normal QT interval. Am Heart J 1962;63:747, by permission of CV Mosby. Reproduced from Chou TC. Electrocardiography in Clinical Practice. Philadelphia: WB Saunders, 1996:16.
†A good rule of thumb for the QT interval is that at normal heart rates between 60 and 100 bpm, the T wave should be completely finished being inscribed before you get half way between the previous and subsequent R waves. In other words, if you bisect the RR interval, the T wave should end before you get to that bisecting line.
Abbreviations: L, lower limit in seconds; U, upper limit in seconds.

TABLE C-5. Localization of Transmural Infarcts*

Typical ECG Leads	Infarct Location
V_1-V_3	Anteroseptal
V_3-V_4	Localized anterior
V_4-V_6, I, aVL	Anterolateral
V_1-V_6	Extensive anterior
I, aVL	High lateral
II, III, aVF	Inferior
V_1-V_2	True posterior (R/S>1)
V_1, V_{3R}, V_{4R}	Right ventricular

*Based on abnormal Q waves except for true posterior myocardial infarction, which is reflected by abnormal R waves.

TABLE C-6. Supraventricular versus Ventricular Ectopic Beats*

Parameter		Supraventricular (Normal Conduction)	Supraventricular (Aberrant Conduction)	Ventricular
QRS complex	Duration	Up to 0.10 sec	≥0.11 sec	≥0.11 sec
	Configuration	Normal	Widened QRS usually with unchanged initial vector. P wave precedes QRS	Widened QRS often with abnormal initial vector. QRS usually not preceded by a P wave.
P wave		Present or absent but with relationship to QRS	Present or absent but with relationship to QRS	Present or absent but without relationship to QRS
Rhythm		Usually less than compensatory pause	Usually less than compensatory pause	Usually compensatory pause

*Numerous ECG criteria exist to try to distinguish premature ventricular contractions (PVCs) from aberrant conduction. Standard ECG texts review these. A major clinical problem is the patient with a wide QRS tachycardia. Such tachycardias can be ventricular or supraventricular with aberrant conduction. A good rule of thumb is that any wide QRS tachycardia in a patient with heart disease or a history of heart failure is likely to be ventricular tachycardia, especially if AV dissociation is identified.

TABLE C-7. Atrioventricular Block

Interpretation	P Wave Relationship to QRS	PR Interval	R-R Interval
1 degree Atrioventricular (AV) block	1:1	>0.20 sec	Regular or follows P-P interval
2 degree AV block: Mobitz I (Wenckebach)	>1:1	Progressively lengthens until a P-wave fails to conduct	Progressively shortens; pause less than two other cycles
2 degree AV block: Mobitz II	>1:1	Constant but with sudden dropping of QRS	Regular except for pause, which usually equals two other cycles
3 degree AV block	None	Variable but P-P interval constant	Usually regular (escape rhythm)

TABLE C-8. Atrioventricular Dissociation*

Type of Atrioventricular (AV) Dissociation	Electrophysiology	Example	Significance	Comment
AV dissociation resulting from complete AV block	AV block	Sinus rhythm with complete AV block	Pathologic	Unrelated P wave and QRS complexes. PP interval is shorter than RR interval
AV dissociation by default causing interference	Slowing of the primary or dominant pacemaker with escape of a subsidiary pacemaker	Sinus bradycardia with junctional escape rhythm	Physiologic	Unrelated P wave and QRS complexes. PP interval is longer than RR interval.
AV dissociation by usurpation	Acceleration of a subsidiary pacemaker usurping control of the ventricles	Sinus rhythm with either AV junctional or ventricular tachycardia	Physiologic	Unrelated P wave and QRS complexes. PP interval is longer than RR interval
Combination	AV block and interference	Atrial fibrillation with accelerated AV junctional pacemaker and block below this pacemaker	Pathologic	Unrelated P wave and QRS complexes

*What is meant by "AV dissociation"? When the atria and ventricles beat independently, their contractions are "dissociated" and AV dissociation exists. Thus, P waves and QRS complexes in the ECG are unrelated. AV dissociation may be complete or incomplete, transient or permanent. The causes of AV dissociation are "block" and "interference," and both may be present in the same ECG. "Block" is associated with a pathologic state of refractoriness, preventing the primary pacemaker's impulse from reaching the lower chamber. An example of this is sinus rhythm with complete AV block. "Interference" results from slowing of the primary pacemaker or acceleration of a subsidiary pacemaker. The lower chamber's impulse "interferes" with conduction by producing physiologic refractoriness, and AV dissociation results. An example of this is sinus rhythm with AV junctional or ventricular tachycardia and no retrograde conduction into the atria. A clear distinction must be made between block and interference. This table describes the four types of AV dissociation.

D Metabolic Calculations

The energy requirements of physical activity are calculated by measuring or estimating the oxygen requirements of the amount of exercise or activity being performed, commonly called the oxygen consumption ($\dot{V}O_2$). $\dot{V}O_2$ provides useful information for exercise professionals, such as the criterion measure of cardiorespiratory fitness ($\dot{V}O_{2max}$). Under steady-state conditions, $\dot{V}O_2$ provides a measure of the energy cost of exercise (kcal) and in combination with $\dot{V}CO_2$ can provide information about the fuels for exercise.

Measurement of $\dot{V}O_2$

The actual measurement of $\dot{V}O_2$ typically is performed in exercise laboratories or clinical settings using a procedure called *open-circuit spirometry*. During open-circuit spirometry the subject or patient uses a mouthpiece and nose clip (or mask), which directs the expired air to an integrated metabolic system and computer interface that measures the volume and percentage of O_2 and CO_2 of the expired air. Subsequently, oxygen consumption ($\dot{V}O_2$) and carbon dioxide output ($\dot{V}CO_2$) are calculated. In this notation for $\dot{V}O_2$:

- the V stands for volume
- the O_2 for oxygen
- the dot above the V denotes a rate, that is, the volume of oxygen per unit of time, typically per minute

Various expressions of $\dot{V}O_2$ are used depending on the purpose for its measurement:

- The **absolute** rate of $\dot{V}O_2$ is typically expressed by the unit liters per minute ($l \cdot min^{-1}$). In this form, $\dot{V}O_2$ can be converted to the overall rate of energy expenditure (kcal):
  - The consumption of 1 L of O_2 results in the liberation of approximately 5 kcal (i.e., 20.9 kJ; 1 kcal = 4.2 kj) of energy (i.e., 1 L $\dot{V}O_2$ = 5 kcal·min^{-1}).
  - The energy expenditure associated with a given level of $\dot{V}O_2$ varies slightly with the respiratory quotient (RQ). When the RQ, which is the ratio of $\dot{V}CO_2/\dot{V}O_2$, is 0.70, fats are the primary fuel source for energy metabolism and the kcal equivalent of a 1L $\dot{V}O_2$ is approximately 4.69. This increases to 5.05 kcal·L^{-1} $\dot{V}O_2$ when RQ is 1.0 and the primary fuel source for energy metabolism is carbohydrates. When RQ is not known, the value of 5.0 kcal·L^{-1} $\dot{V}O_2$ is used.

- The **relative** rate of $\dot{V}O_2$ (relative to body mass) is typically expressed by the units, milliliters per kilograms of body mass per minute ($mL \cdot kg^{-1} \cdot min^{-1}$). The relative rate is used when comparing the $\dot{V}O_2$ of individuals who vary in body mass, and is calculated by dividing the *absolute* $\dot{V}O_2$ ($mL \cdot min^{-1}$) by the individual's body weight (kg).

$$\dot{V}O_2 \ (mL \cdot min^{-1}) \div kg \ body \ mass = mL \cdot kg^{-1} \cdot min^{-1}$$

In some instances, one may express $\dot{V}O_2$ relative to kg of fat-free mass, to square meters of surface area, or to other indices of body size.

- The **gross** rate of oxygen uptake is the total $\dot{V}O_2$ including the resting oxygen requirements, expressed as either $L \cdot min^{-1}$ or $mL \cdot kg^{-1} \cdot min^{-1}$.
- The **net** rate of oxygen uptake is the $\dot{V}O_2$ associated with only the amount of exercise being performed exclusive of resting oxygen uptake, expressed as either $L \cdot min^{-1}$ or $mL \cdot kg^{-1} \cdot min^{-1}$.
- The **net $\dot{V}O_2$** is calculated by subtracting the resting $\dot{V}O_2$ from the gross $\dot{V}O_2$.

$$\textbf{Net } \dot{V}O_2 = Gross \ \dot{V}O_2 - resting \ \dot{V}O_2$$

Estimation of Energy Expenditure: Metabolic Calculations

Measuring $\dot{V}O_2$ requires equipment that is expensive and sophisticated and trained professional staff that can perform the test as well as interpret the data; it does not lend itself to large numbers of subjects or patients. Therefore, measuring $\dot{V}O_2$ is impractical in most nonlaboratory or fitness situations. When it is not possible or feasible to measure $\dot{V}O_2$, reasonable estimates of the $\dot{V}O_2$ during exercise can be made from regression equations derived from measured $\dot{V}O_2$ during steady-state exercise on ergometric devices and while walking and running. Moreover, for exercise prescription purposes, these equations may be used to determine the required exercise intensity associated with a desired level of energy expenditure.

For the greatest accuracy, several cautionary notes about the use of these "metabolic equations" are in order:

- The measured $\dot{V}O_2$ at a given work rate is highly reproducible for a given individual; that is, the $\dot{V}O_2$ at the same exercise intensity for the same individual is very similar every time he or she exercises. However, the inter-subject variability (variability between different subjects) in measured $\dot{V}O_2$ may have a standard error of estimate (SEE) as high as 7%.[1-3] Subsequently, the equations work well if tracking the same subject over time but are less accurate for comparing $\dot{V}O_2$ among different individuals and should be used with caution.
- These equations were derived during steady-state submaximal aerobic exercise; therefore, they are only appropriate for predicting $\dot{V}O_2$ during steady-state submaximal aerobic exercise. The $\dot{V}O_2$ is overestimated during non–steady-state exercise conditions, when the contribution from anaerobic metabolism is large.
- Although the accuracy of these equations is unaffected by most environmental influences (heat and cold), variables that change the mechanical efficiency (e.g., gait abnormalities, wind, snow, sand) result in a loss of accuracy.

- The use of the prediction equations presupposes that ergometers are calibrated properly and used appropriately (e.g., no rail holding during treadmill exercise).
- The equations are most accurate at the stated speeds and power outputs. There is a range of walking speeds for which neither the walking nor the running equations are applicable. These speeds (3.7–5.0 mph) are in the range of the transition from a walking to running motion. The degree of transition varies depending on the individual's size, leg length, stride length, and normal walking pace; therefore, interindividual variability in $\dot{V}O_2$ is very wide within this speed range.[4]

Despite these caveats, the proper and judicious use of metabolic calculations provides valuable information to the exercise professional.

DERIVATION OF METABOLIC EQUATIONS

Table D-1 presents the metabolic equations for the gross or total oxygen cost of walking, running, leg ergometry, arm ergometry, and stepping. For each prediction equation, there are some essential known physiologic constants, such as how much oxygen is required to move the body horizontally (walking on the flat) and vertically (walking up a grade or hill) or the oxygen costs of pedaling at no resistance.

Walking and Running

Constants

- Horizontal Component (Walking): During walking, approximately 0.1 mL O_2 is needed for transporting each kg of body mass a horizontal distance of 1 meter (m). ($0.1 \text{ mL·kg}^{-1}\text{·min}^{-1}$).[5]
- Horizontal Component (Running): The oxygen demand of running the same distance (1 m) is twice as great ($0.2 \text{ mL·kg}^{-1}\text{·min}^{-1}$).[6,7] Running on a level surface is more costly than walking because of the greater vertical displacement that occurs between each step and the greater need to overcome inertia to maintain the greater speed.
- Vertical Component (Walking): The oxygen demand of raising one's body mass against gravity at sea level for walking on the treadmill or ground is approximately 1.8 mL per kg of body mass for each meter (m) of vertical distance ($1.8 \text{ mL·kg}^{-1}\text{·min}^{-1}$).[8–10]
- Vertical Component (Running): During running on a treadmill or over ground, the oxygen cost of vertical ascent is half that of walking or 0.9 $\text{mL·kg}^{-1}\text{·min}^{-1}$.[7,11]
- Resting $\dot{V}O_2 = 3.5 \text{ mL·kg}^{-1}\text{·min}^{-1} = 1$ MET (metabolic equivalent)

Walking Equation

- Conversion: 1 mph = 26.8 m·min^{-1}
- Most accurate for speeds of 50 to 100 m·min^{-1} (1.9–3.7 mph)

TABLE D-1. Metabolic Equations for Gross $\dot{V}O_2$ in Metric Units*

Walking

$\dot{V}O_2$ (mL·kg^{-1}·min^{-1}) = (0.1·S) + (1.8·S·G) + 3.5 mL·kg^{-1}·min^{-1}

$\dot{V}O_2$ (mL·kg^{-1}·min^{-1}) = [0.1 mL·kg^{-1}·meter^{-1}·S (m·min^{-1})]
+ [1.8 mL·kg^{-1}·meter^{-1}·S (m·min^{-1})·G] + 3.5 mL·kg^{-1}·min^{-1}

Running

$\dot{V}O_2$ (mL·kg^{-1}·min^{-1}) = (0.2·S) + (0.9·S·G) + 3.5 mL·kg^{-1}·min^{-1}

$\dot{V}O_2$ (mL·kg^{-1}·min^{-1}) = [0.2 mL·kg^{-1}·meter^{-1}·S (m·min^{-1})]
+ [0.9 mL·kg^{-1}·meter^{-1}·S (m·min^{-1})·G] + 3.5 mL·kg^{-1}·min^{-1}

Leg Cycling

$\dot{V}O_2$ (mL·kg^{-1}·min^{-1}) = 1.8 (work rate)/(BM) + 3.5 mL·kg^{-1}·min^{-1}
+ 3.5 mL·kg^{-1}·min^{-1}

$\dot{V}O_2$ (mL·kg^{-1}·min^{-1}) = (1.8 mL·kg^{-1}·min^{-1})
× (work rate in kg·m·min^{-1}) (body mass in kg)
+ 3.5 mL·kg^{-1}·min^{-1} + 3.5 mL·kg^{-1}·min^{-1}

Arm Cycling

$\dot{V}O_2$ (mL·kg^{-1}·min^{-1}) = 3 (work rate)/(BM) + 3.5 mL·kg^{-1}·min^{-1}

$\dot{V}O_2$ (mL·kg^{-1}·min^{-1}) = (3 mL·kg^{-1}·meter^{-1})
× (work rate in kg·m·min^{-1}) (body mass in kg) + 3.5 mL·kg^{-1}·min^{-1}

Stepping

$\dot{V}O_2$ (mL·kg^{-1}·min^{-1}) = (0.2·f) + (1.33·1.8·H·f) + 3.5 mL·kg^{-1}·min^{-1}

$\dot{V}O_2$ (mL·kg^{-1}·min^{-1}) = 0.2 (steps·min^{-1})
+ (1.33 mL·kg^{-1}·meter^{-1}) (1.8 mL·kg^{-1}·meter^{-1})
× (step height in meters) (steps·min^{-1}) + 3.5 mL·kg^{-1}·min^{-1}

$\dot{V}O_2$ is gross oxygen consumption in mL·kg^{-1}·min^{-1}; S is speed in m·min^{-1}; BM is body mass (kg); G is the percent grade expressed as a fraction; work rate (kg·m·min^{-1}); f is stepping frequency in minutes; H is step height in meters.

- $\dot{V}O_2$ (mL·kg^{-1}·min^{-1}) = 0.1 (speed) + 1.8 (speed) (fractional grade) + 3.5 mL·kg^{-1}·min^{-1}

  (speed = m·min^{-1}; 1 mph = 26.8 m·min^{-1} fractional grade is in decimal form, 5% grade is 0.05)

Running Equation

- Most accurate for speeds >134 m·min^{-1} (5.0 mph) but appropriate for speeds as low as 80 m·min^{-1} (3 mph) if the individual is truly jogging or running.
- $\dot{V}O_2$ (mL·kg^{-1}·min^{-1}) = 0.2 (speed) + 0.9 (speed) (fractional grade) + 3.5 mL·kg^{-1}·min^{-1}

speed = m·min^{-1}; 1 mph = 26.8 m·min^{-1}
fractional grade is in decimal form, 5% grade is 0.05

For speeds between 100 m·min^{-1} (3.7 mph) and 134 m·min^{-1} (5.0 mph) observations of the individuals gait pattern determine which equation (walking or running) may be most accurate. Use the walking equation if the individual assumes a walking pattern. Use the running equation if the individual has to assume a running gait.

Leg and Arm Ergometry

Constants

Power is expressed in kg·m·min^{-1} for the leg and arm ergometer equations. To determine the power output during leg or arm ergometry:

- Power (kg·m·min^{-1}) = R (kg)·D (m)·f (revolutions per minute)

  R = resistance setting in kg;
  D = distance in meters (m) the flywheel travels for each pedal revolution

  - 6 m for Monark leg ergometers
  - 3 m for Tunturi and BodyGuard ergometers
  - 2.4 m for Monark arm ergometers

  f = the pedaling frequency (revolutions per minute).

- In the scientific literature, power is most commonly expressed in watts [W] as opposed to kg·m·min^{-1}. Watts = kg·m·min^{-1} divided by 6 [or more accurately 6.12.

  The total oxygen demand of leg ergometry includes: 1) unloaded cycling (i.e., the movement of the legs), 2) the external load (amount of resistance), and 3) the resting oxygen uptake.

- At 50 to 60 rpm, the oxygen cost of unloaded cycling is approximately 3.5 mL·kg^{-1}·min^{-1} above rest.[12–14]
- The cost of cycling against the external load (resistance) is approximately 1.8 mL·kg^{-1}·min^{-1} per kg·m·min^{-1}.[9]

  However, the arms are less efficient than the legs during cycling, most likely because of the recruitment of accessory muscles needed to stabilize the torso.

- Therefore, the oxygen cost against the external load during arm ergometry is greater than that of leg ergometry, approximately 3 mL·kg^{-1}·min^{-1} per kg·m·min^{-1}.[15–17]

Leg Cycling Equation

- Most accurate for power outputs between 300 and 1,200 $kg \cdot m \cdot min^{-1}$ (50 and 200 W)
- $\dot{V}O_2$ $(mL \cdot kg^{-1} \cdot min^{-1})$ = 1.8 (work rate)/(BM) + Resting $\dot{V}O_2$ (3.5 $mL \cdot kg^{-1} \cdot min^{-1}$) + Unloaded cycling (3.5 $mL \cdot kg^{-1} \cdot min^{-1}$)

    (work rate = $kg \cdot m \cdot min^{-1}$; BM = body mass [kg])

Arm Cycling Equation

- Most accurate for power outputs between 150 and 750 $kg \cdot m \cdot min^{-1}$ (25 and 125 W)
- $\dot{V}O_2$ $(mL \cdot kg^{-1} \cdot min^{-1})$ = 3 (work rate)/(BM) + Resting $\dot{V}O_2$ (3.5 $mL \cdot kg^{-1} \cdot min^{-1}$)

    (work rate = $kg \cdot m \cdot min^{-1}$; BM = body mass [kg])

Stepping Ergometry

Constants

Stepping is performed traditionally in a four-part process of lifting one leg onto a box, fixed bench, or step; pushing with this leg to raise the body; placing the other leg on the box; and stepping down with the first and then second leg in a repetitive fashion. The oxygen cost of stepping has horizontal and vertical components because one moves forward and backward horizontally, as well as up and down.

- Horizontal Component: The oxygen demand of the horizontal movement is approximately 0.2 mL O_2 per four-cycle step (stepping up and down) per kg of body mass (0.2 $mL \cdot kg^{-1}$).
- Vertical Component: The O_2 demand of vertical ascent is 1.8 $mL \cdot kg^{-1} \cdot min^{-1}$, and an additional one-third of this (1.33) must be added to account for the O_2 cost of stepping down, the deceleration against gravity.[6]

Stepping Equation

- Conversion: 1 inch = 0.0254 meters (m).
- Most accurate for stepping rates between 12 and 30 $steps \cdot min^{-1}$ and step heights 0.04 to 0.40 m (1.6 to 15.7 in.)
- $\dot{V}O_2$ $(mL \cdot kg^{-1} \cdot min^{-1})$ = 0.2 (stepping rate) + 1.33·1.8 (step height) (stepping rate) + 3.5 $mL \cdot kg^{-1} \cdot min^{-1}$

    (Stepping rate = $steps \cdot min^{-1}$; step height = meters)

Practical Use of the Metabolic Calculations

Tables D-2 thru D-6 were calculated from the equations as a practical reference for the gross $\dot{V}O_2$ for the respective types of steady-state exercise. The $\dot{V}O_2$ in each of the Tables are presented in METs. METs express oxygen uptake relative to resting values. An oxygen uptake of 8 METs means that the oxygen require-

TABLE D-2. Approximate Energy Requirements in METs for Horizontal and Grade Walking

% Grade	mph m·min⁻¹	1.7 45.6	2.0 53.6	2.5 67.0	3.0 80.4	3.4 91.2	3.75 100.5
0		2.3	2.5	2.9	3.3	3.6	3.9
2.5		2.9	3.2	3.8	4.3	4.8	5.2
5.0		3.5	3.9	4.6	5.4	5.9	6.5
7.5		4.1	4.6	5.5	6.4	7.1	7.8
10.0		4.6	5.3	6.3	7.4	8.3	9.1
12.5		5.2	6.0	7.2	8.5	9.5	10.4
15.0		5.8	6.6	8.1	9.5	10.6	11.7
17.5		6.4	7.3	8.9	10.5	11.8	12.9
20.0		7.0	8.0	9.8	11.6	13.0	14.2
22.5		7.6	8.7	10.6	12.6	14.2	15.5
25.0		8.2	9.4	11.5	13.6	15.3	16.8

TABLE D-3. Approximate Energy Requirements in METs for Horizontal and Grade Jogging/Running

% Grade	mph m·min⁻¹	5 134	6 161	7 188	7.5 201	8 214	9 241	10 268
0		8.6	10.2	11.7	12.5	13.3	14.8	16.3
2.5		9.5	11.2	12.9	13.8	14.7	16.3	18.0
5.0		10.3	12.3	14.1	15.1	16.1	17.9	19.7
7.5		11.2	13.3	15.3	16.4	17.4	19.4	
10.0		12.0	14.3	16.5	17.7	18.8		
12.5		12.9	15.4	17.7	19.0			
15.0		13.8	16.4	18.9				

TABLE D-4. Approximate Energy Requirements in METs During Leg Cycle Ergometry

Body Wt.		Power Output (kg·m·min⁻¹ and W)						
kg	lb	300 50	450 75	600 100	750 125	900 150	1,050 175	1,200 (kg·m·min⁻¹) 200 (W)
50	110	5.1	6.6	8.2	9.7	11.3	12.8	14.3
60	132	4.6	5.9	7.1	8.4	9.7	11.0	12.3
70	154	4.2	5.3	6.4	7.5	8.6	9.7	10.8
80	176	3.9	4.9	5.9	6.8	7.8	8.8	9.7
90	198	3.7	4.6	5.4	6.3	7.1	8.0	8.9
100	220	3.5	4.3	5.1	5.9	6.6	7.4	8.2

TABLE D-5. Approximate Energy Requirements in METs During Arm Ergometry

Body Wt.		Power Output (kg·m·min^{-1} and W)					
kg	lb	150 25	300 50	450 75	600 100	750 125	900 (kg·m·min^{-1}) 150 (W)
50	110	3.6	6.1	8.7	11.3	13.9	16.4
60	132	3.1	5.3	7.4	9.6	11.7	13.9
70	154	2.8	4.7	6.5	8.3	10.2	12.0
80	176	2.6	4.2	5.8	7.4	9.0	10.6
90	198	2.4	3.9	5.3	6.7	8.1	9.6
100	220	2.3	3.6	4.9	6.1	7.4	8.7

ment of the task is eight times that of rest. Metabolic equivalents (METS) are calculated as METs = $\dot{V}O_2$ (mL·kg^{-1}·min^{-1})/3.5].

For purposes of prescribing exercise, another utility of the metabolic equations is to estimate a *target* work rate that will elicit a desired level of oxygen uptake or energy expenditure. The equations are solved for the unknown variable on the workload side of the equation. In the case of treadmill exercise, when there are two unknown variables (i.e., speed and fractional grade), it is best to select an appropriate speed based on the ability and comfort of the client, and then solve for the fractional grade.

If knowledge of the caloric cost of exercise is desired, the $\dot{V}O_2$ should first be expressed in *net* terms (gross $\dot{V}O_2$ minus resting $\dot{V}O_2$). Once the net $\dot{V}O_2$ is determined, convert the value to caloric expenditure per minute using either of the following methods.

Method #1:
1. Convert $\dot{V}O_2$ (mL·kg^{-1}·min^{-1} or METs) into the absolute unit of L·min^{-1}
2. If starting from mL·kg^{-1}·min^{-1}:
   a. Multiply the mL·kg^{-1}·min^{-1} by the kg body mass and divide by 1,000
   b. mL·kg^{-1}·min^{-1} kg body mass/1,000 (*i.e., 1,000 mL per Liter*).

TABLE D-6. Approximate Energy Requirements in METs During Stair Stepping

Step Height		Stepping Rate per Minute					
in	m	20	22	24	26	28	30
4	0.102	3.5	3.8	4.0	4.3	4.5	4.8
6	0.152	4.2	4.6	4.9	5.2	5.5	5.8
8	0.203	4.9	5.3	5.7	6.1	6.5	6.9
10	0.254	5.6	6.1	6.5	7.0	7.5	7.9
12	0.305	6.3	6.8	7.4	7.9	8.4	9.0
14	0.356	7.0	7.6	8.2	8.8	9.4	10.0
16	0.406	7.7	8.4	9.0	9.7	10.4	11.1
18	0.457	8.4	9.1	9.9	10.6	11.4	12.1

3. If starting from METs:
   a. Multiply the MET value by 3.5 to obtain $mL \cdot kg^{-1} \cdot min^{-1}$ and then complete step 2a.
4. Convert $\dot{V}O_2$ ($L \cdot min^{-1}$) to caloric expenditure ($kcal \cdot min^{-1}$) by multiplying by 5 (*i.e., approximately 5 kcal per L O_2 during steady-state exercise*)

   Method #2:
1. Convert the $\dot{V}O_2$ in METs directly to caloric expenditure using the equation below from Chapter 7.
   a. $Kcal \cdot min^{-1} = (METs \times 3.5 \times body\ weight\ in\ kg)/200$

CASE STUDY EXAMPLE

A 30-year-old man has a resting heart rate of 60 bpm, a maximal heart rate of 190 bpm, weighs 180 lb, and has a $\dot{V}O_{2max}$ of 48 $mL \cdot kg^{-1} \cdot min^{-1}$. He wishes to begin an exercise program including treadmill walking and leg cycling on a Monark ergometer. Using feedback from the subject, you estimate that a comfortable walking speed for him is 3.5 mph. Based on his physical activity history and aerobic capacity, you select 70% $\dot{V}O_{2max}$ as his initial training intensity. Answer the following questions:

Q: What is his target $\dot{V}O_2$ using his $\dot{V}O_2R$ and a straight percentage of $\dot{V}O_{2max}$?

A: First calculate the $\dot{V}O_{2max}$ reserve ($\dot{V}O_{2max}R$)

$$\dot{V}O_{2max} = 48\ mL \cdot kg^{-1} \cdot min^{-1}$$

$$\dot{V}O_2R = (\dot{V}O_{2max} - \dot{V}O_{2rest})$$

$$\dot{V}O_2R = (48\ mL \cdot kg^{-1} \cdot min^{-1} - 3.5\ mL \cdot kg^{-1} \cdot min^{-1})$$

$$\dot{V}O_2R = 44.5\ mL \cdot kg^{-1} \cdot min^{-1}$$

Then calculate the Target $\dot{V}O_2$ ($mL \cdot kg^{-1} \cdot min^{-1}$)

Target $\dot{V}O_2$ ($mL \cdot kg^{-1} \cdot min^{-1}$) = (exercise intensity as a decimal) $\times (\dot{V}O_2R) + \dot{V}O_{2rest}$

Target $\dot{V}O_2$ ($mL \cdot kg^{-1} \cdot min^{-1}$) = (0.70) (44.5 $mL \cdot kg^{-1} \cdot min^{-1}$) + 3.5 $mL \cdot kg^{-1} \cdot min^{-1}$

Target $\dot{V}O_2$ ($mL \cdot kg^{-1} \cdot min^{-1}$) = 31.2 $mL \cdot kg^{-1} \cdot min^{-1}$ + 3.5 $mL \cdot kg^{-1} \cdot min^{-1}$

Target $\dot{V}O_2$ = 34.7 $mL \cdot kg^{-1} \cdot min^{-1}$

If using a straight percentage of $\dot{V}O_{2max}$ as the target VO_2:

Target $\dot{V}O_2$ ($mL \cdot kg^{-1} \cdot min^{-1}$) = (exercise intensity) $\times (\dot{V}O_{2max})$

Target $\dot{V}O_2$ (mL·kg^{-1}·min^{-1}) = 0.70 × 48 mL·kg^{-1}·min^{-1}

Target $\dot{V}O_2$ = 33.6 mL·kg^{-1}·min^{-1}

The remainder of the questions will use 34.7 mL·kg^{-1}·min^{-1} as the target VO$_2$ (i.e., 70% of his $\dot{V}O_2R$)

Q: If he is walking at 3.5 mph, how steep should the treadmill grade be to elicit a $\dot{V}O_2$ of 34.7 mL·kg^{-1}·min^{-1}? *Remember: 3.5 mph ×* *26.8 = 93.8 m·min^{-1}*

A: Use the walking equation and solve for the unknown fractional grade.

$\dot{V}O_2$ (mL·kg^{-1}·min^{-1}) = 0.1 (speed) + 1.8 (speed) (fractional grade) + 3.5 mL·kg^{-1}·min^{-1}

34.7 = 0.1 (93.8 m·min^{-1}) + 1.8 (93.8 m·min^{-1}) (fractional grade) + 3.5

31.2 = 0.1 (93.8 m·min^{-1}) + 1.8 (93.8 m·min^{-1}) (fractional grade)

31.2 = 9.38 + 168.8 (fractional grade)

21.8 = 168.8 (fractional grade)

0.129 = fractional grade = **12.9% grade**

Q: What is the target work rate (kg·m·min^{-1}) on the Monark bike?

A: First determine his body mass: 180 lb/2.2 = 81.8 kg
Then, use the leg cycling equation and solve for the unknown work rate.

$\dot{V}O_2$ (mL·kg^{-1}·min^{-1}) = 7.0 mL·kg^{-1}·min^{-1} + 1.8 (work rate) / (body mass)

34.7 mL·kg^{-1}·min^{-1} = 7.0 + 1.8 (work rate) / 81.8 kg

27.7 mL·kg^{-1}·min^{-1} = 1.8 (work rate) / 81.8 kg

2266 = 1.8 (work rate)

1,259 kg·m·min^{-1} = work rate

Q: If he is comfortable pedaling at 60 rpm on a Monark cycle, what resistance setting would be required?

A: Work rate (kg·m·min^{-1}) = (resistance setting) (distance) (pedal cadence)

1,259 (kg·m·min^{-1}) = (resistance setting) (6) (60)

1,259 (kg·m·min^{-1}) = (resistance setting) 360

3.5 kg = resistance setting

Q: What will be his net caloric expenditure during 30 minutes of exercise?

A: Net $\dot{V}O_2$ = 34.7 mL·kg^{-1}·min^{-1} − 3.5 mL·kg^{-1}·min^{-1} = **31.2 mL·kg^{-1}·min^{-1}**

$\dot{V}O_2$ in L·min^{-1} = ($\dot{V}O_2$ in mL·kg^{-1}·min^{-1}) (body mass) / 1,000

$\dot{V}O_2$ in L·min^{-1} = (31.2) (81.8) / 1,000 = **2.55 L·min^{-1}**

Net caloric expenditure in kcal·min^{-1} = 2.55 L·min^{-1} × 5 = **12.8 kcal·min^{-1}**

Net caloric expenditure for 30 minutes = 12.8 kcal·min^{-1} × 30 min = **384 kcal**

Q: What is an appropriate target heart rate according to the heart rate reserve method?

A: Target HR = (exercise intensity as a decimal) (HR_{max} − HR_{rest}) + HR_{rest}

Target HR = (0.70) (190–60) + 60

Target HR = (0.70) (130) + 60

Target HR = 91 + 60

Target HR = **151 beats·min^{-1}**

PRACTICE METABOLIC CALCULATIONS (WITH ANSWERS)

1. A man weighing 176 lb runs at a pace of 9 minutes per mile outdoors, on level ground. What is his estimated gross $\dot{V}O_2$?
2. To match this exercise intensity (from #1 above) on a Tunturi cycle ergometer, what setting (kg) would you use at a pedaling rate of 60 rpm?
3. If this same man exercised at this intensity five times per week for 30 minutes each session, how long would it take him to lose 12 lb (assuming all calories expended in this exercise are in excess of food intake)? *Hint:* Use the net $\dot{V}O_2$ to calculate the exercise energy expenditure.
4. A 198-lb cardiac patient wishes to use an arm ergometer for part of his rehabilitation program. He works at a power output of 300 kg·m·min^{-1} for 15 minutes, then at 450 kg·m·min^{-1} for 15 minutes. What is his average *net* $\dot{V}O_2$ (in mL·kg^{-1}·min^{-1}) over this session?
5. If an individual reduces his or her dietary intake by 1,750 kcal·wk^{-1}, how much weight (in lb) would he or she lose in 6 months (26 weeks)?
6. If an 18-year-old girl steps up and down on a 12-inch step at a rate of 20 steps (complete up and down cycles) per minute, what would her gross $\dot{V}O_2$ be (in mL·kg^{-1}·min^{-1})?
7. A 71-year-old man weighing 180 lb walks on a motor-driven treadmill at 3.5 mph and a 15% grade. What is his gross MET level?

ANSWERS

1. $39.2 \text{ mL·kg}^{-1}\text{·min}^{-1}$
2. 7.9 kg (or kp)
3. About 20 weeks
4. $12.5 \text{ mL·kg}^{-1}\text{·min}^{-1}$
5. 13 lb
6. $22.1 \text{ mL·kg}^{-1}\text{·min}^{-1}$
7. 10.9 METs

ESTIMATING $\dot{V}O_{2MAX}$

The metabolic equations presented in Table D-1 were derived during steady-state exercise and are not applicable for estimating non–steady-state conditions, such as peak or maximal levels of exercise. Using equations derived during steady-state exercise overestimates the $\dot{V}O_2$ during non–steady-state conditions and should not be used. Other prediction equations have been derived for use during peak or maximal exercise. The available equations are either generalized equations that can be used across gender, age, and for different protocols, or they are protocol specific and are a function of the time of exercise completed for that specific protocol. Modifying the protocol invalidates the equation.

One such commonly used equation is based on the Bruce protocol:[1,18]

$$\dot{V}O_{2max} (\text{mL·kg}^{-1}\text{·min}^{-1}) = 14.8 - 1.379 \text{ (time in min)} + 0.451 \text{ (time}^2) - 0.012 \text{ (time}^3)$$

$$SEE = 3.35 \text{ mL·kg}^{-1}\text{·min}^{-1}$$

Ramp treadmill protocols are discussed in Chapter 5. $\dot{V}O_{2max}$ can be predicted using the following equation that adjusts for the use of a ramping treadmill protocol:[19]

$$\dot{V}O_{2max} (\text{mL·kg}^{-1}\text{·min}^{-1}) = 0.72x + 3.67$$

$$SEE = 4.4 \text{ mL·kg}^{-1}\text{·min}^{-1}$$

(x is the predicted $\dot{V}O_2$ calculated for the peak speed/grade using the ACSM walking equation)

Another validated equation for use with a Ramp Bruce Treadmill Protocol is:[20]

$$\dot{V}O_{2max} (\text{mL·kg}^{-1}\text{·min}^{-1}) = 3.9 \text{ (time in min)} - 7.0$$

$$SEE = 3.4 \text{ mL·kg}^{-1}\text{·min}^{-1}$$

All of the aforementioned treadmill prediction equations assume that the patient does not use handrail support. However, for patients who may be unsteady or have difficulty walking on a motorized treadmill, non–handrail-supported exercise may be impossible or result in early test termination because of anxiety on the part of the patient. For such instances, there is a validated equation for predicting $\dot{V}O_{2max}$ during handrail supported treadmill exercise using the Bruce protocol:[21]

$$\dot{V}O_{2max} (\text{mL·kg}^{-1}\text{·min}^{-1}) = 2.282 \text{ (time in min)} + 8.545$$

$$SEE = 4.92 \text{ mL·kg}^{-1}\text{·min}^{-1}$$

TABLE D-7. Common Field Test Equations to Estimate $\dot{V}O_{2max}$*

Rockport Walking Test (1-Mile Walk)

$\dot{V}O_{2max}$ (mL·kg^{-1}·min^{-1}) = 132.853 − 0.1692 (body mass in kg) − 0.3877 (age in years) + 6.315 (gender) − 3.2649 (time in minutes) − 0.1565 (HR);
(SEE = 5.0 mL·kg^{-1}·min^{-1})

(gender = 0 for female, 1 for male; heart rate (HR) is taken at end of walk)

1.5-Mile Run Test

$\dot{V}O_{2max}$ (mL·kg^{-1}·min^{-1}) = 3.5 + 483 / (time in minutes)

*See references 23 and 24: From Kline GM, Porcari JP, Hintermeister R, et al. Estimation of $\dot{V}O2max$ from a one-mile track walk, gender, age, and body weight. Med Sci Sports Exerc 1987;19:253–259; Dolgener FA, Hensely LD, March JJ, et al. Validation of the Rockport Fitness Walking Test in college males and females. Res Q Exerc Sport 1994;65:152–158.

For predicting $\dot{V}O_{2max}$ during cycle ergometry using 15 W per min increments:[22]

Males: $\dot{V}O_{2max}$ (mL·min^{-1}) = 10.51 (W) + 6.35 (kg) − 10.49 (years) + 519.3

SEE = 212 mL·min^{-1}

(W = final power output completed in watts; kg = body mass; years = age)

Females: $\dot{V}O_{2max}$ (mL·min^{-1}) = 9.39 (W) + 7.7 (kg) − 5.88 (years) + 136.7

SEE = 147 mL·min^{-1}

(W = final power output completed in watts; kg = body mass; years = age)

FIELD TEST EQUATIONS

Field tests are an efficient and economically feasible option for predicting $\dot{V}O_{2max}$ when large numbers of individuals are being tested or the use of standard ergometry is not possible. These tests involve walking or running over level terrain to either cover a fixed distance (e.g., 1 or 1.5 miles) as quickly as possible or cover the greatest distance possible in a fixed period of time (e.g., 12 or 15 minutes). Field equations may incorporate other independent variables, such as age, gender, or body weight for enhanced predictive accuracy. Commonly used field test equations for the 1-mile walk and 1.5-mile run are given in Table D-7.

REFERENCES

1. Bruce RA, Kusumi F, Hosmer D. Maximal oxygen intake and nomographic assessment of functional aerobic impairment in cardiovascular disease. Am Heart J 1973;85:546–562.
2. Myers J, Madhavan R. Exercise testing with gas exchange analysis. Cardiol Clin 2001;19:433–445.
3. Shephard RJ. Tests of maximum oxygen uptake. A critical review. Sports Med 1984;1:99–124.
4. Workman JM, Armstrong BW. Oxygen cost of treadmill walking. J Appl Physiol 1963;18:798–803.
5. Dill DB. Oxygen cost of horizontal and grade walking and running on the treadmill. J Appl Physiol 1965;20:19–22.

6. Balke B. A simplified field test for assessment of physical fitness. Civil Aeromedical Research Institute Report, Oklahoma City, 1963:63–66.
7. Margaria R, Cerretelli P, Aghemo P. Energy cost of running. J Appl Physiol 1963;18:367–370.
8. Balke B, Ware RW. An experimental study of "physical fitness" of air force personnel. US Armed Forces Med J 1959;10:675–688.
9. Nagle F, Balke B, Baptista G, et al. Compatibility of progressive treadmill, bicycle and step tests based on oxygen uptake responses. Med Sci Sports 1971;3:149–154.
10. Nagle FJ, Balke B, Naughton JP. Gradational step tests for assessing work capacity. J Appl Physiol 1965;20:745–748.
11. Bassett DR Jr, Giese MD, Nagle FJ, et al. Aerobic requirements of overground versus treadmill running. Med Sci Sports Exerc 1985;17:477–481.
12. Lang PB, Latin RW, Berg KE, et al. The accuracy of the ACSM cycle ergometry equation. Med Sci Sports Exerc 1992;24:272–276.
13. Latin RW, Berg KE. The accuracy of the ACSM and a new cycle ergometry equation for young women. Med Sci Sports Exerc 1994;26:642–646.
14. Londeree BR, Moffitt-Gerstenberger J, Padfield JA, et al. Oxygen consumption of cycle ergometry is nonlinearly related to work rate and pedal rate. Med Sci Sports Exerc 1997;29:775–780.
15. Franklin BA. Exercise testing, training and arm ergometry. Sports Med 1985;2:100–119.
16. Bevegard S, Freyschuss U, Strandell T. Circulatory adaptation to arm and leg exercise in supine and sitting position. J Appl Physiol 1966;21:37–46.
17. Stenberg J, Astrand PO, Ekblom B, et al. Hemodynamic response to work with different muscle groups, sitting and supine. J Appl Physiol 1967;22:61–70.
18. Foster C, Jackson AS, Pollock ML, et al. Generalized equations for predicting functional capacity from treadmill performance. Am Heart J 1984;107:1229–1234.
19. Myers J, Buchanan N, Smith D, et al. Individualized ramp treadmill. Observations on a new protocol. Chest 1992;101:236S–241S.
20. Kaminsky LA, Whaley MH. Evaluation of a new standardized ramp protocol: the BSU/Bruce Ramp protocol. J Cardiopulm Rehabil 1998;18:438–444.
21. McConnell TR, Clark BA. Prediction of maximal oxygen consumption during handrail supported treadmill exercise. J Cardiopulm Rehabil 1987;7:324–331.
22. Storer TW, Davis JA, Caiozzo VJ. Accurate prediction of $\dot{V}O_{2max}$ in cycle ergometry. Med Sci Sports Exerc 1990;22:704–712.
23. Kline GM, Porcari JP, Hintermeister R, et al. Estimation of $\dot{V}O_{2max}$ from a one-mile track walk, gender, age, and body weight. Med Sci Sports Exerc 1987;19:253–259.
24. Dolgener FA, Hensely LD, March JJ, et al. Validation of the Rockport Fitness Walking Test in college males and females. Res Q Exerc Sport 1994;65:152–158.

E Environmental Considerations

The human body constantly responds to changes in the surrounding environment to maintain health and performance. For example, heat, cold, and high altitude comprise the greatest concerns for people engaged in recreational, fitness, or competitive activities (and the clinicians and trainers advising them). These environmental conditions exacerbate the physiologic strain of exercise.

Heat and Humidity

Muscular contractions generate heat that must be released to the environment; if not, the temperature of internal organs increases, eventually reaching dangerous levels. High ambient temperature and humidity impede heat dissipation. Unfortunately, no single standard defines safe upper limits for temperature and humidity during exercise. However, the American College of Sports Medicine (ACSM) has published guidelines regarding competitive exercise in heat.[1] For example, Figure E-1 illustrates categories of risk for heat illness, based on air temperature and humidity. Other guidelines, for industrial and military populations, also may be applied to exercise environments.[2,3] These guidelines can help to prevent dangerous elevations in body temperature during exercise and mitigate the deleterious effects of dehydration.

In a hot environment, body core temperature is affected by air temperature, humidity, air movement (i.e., wind speed), and solar radiation from the sun. The wet-bulb globe temperature (WBGT) integrates the effects of all these factors into a single value, with the goals of quantifying heat stress and preventing heat illness. The WBGT index combines dry-bulb air temperature (T_b); natural wet-bulb temperature (T_{wb}), which is measured by placing a wet wick over a thermometer bulb exposed to natural air movement; and globe temperature (T_g), the temperature measured inside a 15-cm diameter copper globe painted flat black. The WBGT is determined with specialized instruments that are commercially available.

Outdoors, WBGT is calculated as follows:

$$WBGT = 0.7\, T_{wb} + 0.2\, T_g + 0.1\, T_b$$

Indoors, WBGT is calculated using this formula:

$$WBGT = 0.7\, T_{wb} + 0.3\, T_g$$

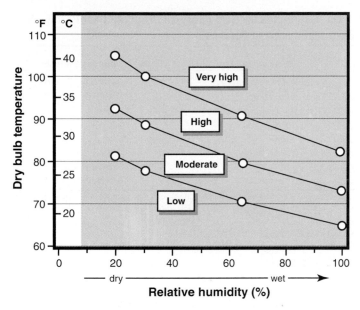

FIGURE E-1. Approximate risk of heatstroke or heat exhaustion during competitive distance running. Reprinted with permission from Armstrong LE, Epstein Y, Greenleaf JE, et al. American College of Sports Medicine position stand. Heat and cold illnesses during distance running. Med Sci Sports Exerc 1996;28:i–x.

The first use of WBGT occurred in the 1950s at military bases. Subsequently, other organizations promulgated similar WGBT guidelines[1–3] that have successfully reduced the incidence of heat illness during hot weather physical activity.[4] However, the WBGT index has limitations. For example, when relative humidity is high (>70%), the WBGT tends to underestimate the risk of heat illness.[4] Further, WBGT does not account for factors such as clothing insulation, exercise intensity, age, fitness, acclimatization, and illness that modify the physiologic strain imposed by a given environment.

The exertional heat illnesses (i.e., heatstroke, heat exhaustion, heat cramps, and heat syncope) are described in an ACSM position stand that focuses on competitive distance running.[1] For noncompetitive exercise, fitness professionals and clinicians can use industrial standards, established by the National Institute for Occupational Safety and Health (NIOSH),[2] as a convenient starting point. NIOSH standards define WBGT levels at which the risk of heat injury is increased, but exercise can be performed if preventive steps are taken. These steps include limiting the maximum duration of continuous exercise and requiring rest breaks between exercise periods. Table E-1 provides recommended exercise–rest intervals derived from NIOSH standards for moderate and vigorous exercise based on WBGT measurements.

TABLE E-1. Guidelines for Safe Exercise Duration: Rest Periods for Healthy Unacclimatized Persons*

WBGT (°F)	Moderate Exercise Work/Rest Periods (min·h^{-1})	Vigorous Exercise Work/Rest Periods (min·h^{-1})
70.0–72.9	No limitation	45/15
73.0–76.9	40/20	30/30
77.0–79.9	30/30	20/40
80.0–81.9	20/40	10/50
82.0–83.9	10/50	No work should be performed
84.0–86.0	No work should be performed	No work should be performed

*See reference 2: Adapted from National Institute for Occupational Safety and Health. Criteria for a recommended standard. Occupational exposure to hot environments. 1986. DHHS NIOSH Publ. No. 86-113.

Notes: Times indicate recommended maximum duration of intermittent exercise, followed by a rest period for cooling, before beginning another exercise bout. Rest means minimal physical activity (sitting or standing) in a shaded area if possible.

Other strategies to alleviate heat stress include:

- Wear clothing that allows heat loss and sweat evaporation.
- Reschedule exercise for a cooler time of day.
- Relocate exercise to a shady, breezy site or indoors with fans and air conditioning.
- Reduce exercise intensity and add rest breaks to maintain the same target heart rate as normally prescribed.

HEAT ACCLIMATIZATION

This process involves a series of physiologic adaptations that decrease the risk of heat illness and improve exercise performance in the heat. Following heat acclimatization, the heart rate, body temperature, rating of perceived exertion, and physiologic strain decrease for a given exercise intensity. Also, sweating rate increases and the sweat salt (i.e., sodium and chloride) concentration decreases. Thus, a person's water requirement increases but the salt requirement decreases. The best method of inducing heat acclimatization is to exercise in the heat, progressively increasing the duration and/or intensity of exercise for 10 to 14 days.

Individuals whose exercise prescription specifies a target heart rate (THR) should maintain the same exercise heart rate in the heat. This approach reduces the risk of heat illness while allowing acclimatization to develop. For example, in hot or humid weather, a reduced speed or resistance achieves the THR, even though the work of the heart (myocardial oxygen uptake) remains unchanged. As acclimatization occurs, progressively higher exercise intensity is tolerated and required to elicit the THR. The first exercise session in the heat may last as little as 10 to 15 minutes for safety reasons, but exercise duration can be increased gradually to its usual length. Most healthy people become fully acclimatized to the heat in 10 to 14 days, although illness or alcohol/drug abuse may slow this process.

DEHYDRATION

Maintaining proper hydration is a key to preventing heat illness and optimizing performance. Profuse sweating can lead to serious dehydration unless adequate fluid is consumed. Even mild dehydration impairs temperature regulation and compromises performance during exercise.[5] The scientific literature indicates that endurance performance begins to decline at approximately 3% body weight loss and strength/power performance begins to decline at about 5% body weight loss.[7] Exercise program organizers and leaders should ensure that replacement fluids are available and easily accessible. Program participants should be reminded to drink before, during, and after physical activity.[5] However, athletes who exercise for more than 3 hours continuously ought to realize that drinking too much fluid can lead to a serious medical condition known as hyponatremia, because of an excessive dilution of body fluids. Their goal ought to be to *optimize*, not *maximize*, fluid consumption.

In most people, especially those older than 60 years, drinking alleviates thirst sensations well before sufficient fluid is consumed to replace sweat losses. Generalized drinking recommendations are difficult to make. However, a simple suggestion involves drinking two cups of fluid 2 hours before exercise, and drinking during exercise at a rate that matches sweat losses.[5] Active individuals can weigh themselves before and after each exercise session to determine the amount of water that must be replaced, at a rate of 16 oz of fluid for each pound of weight lost.

Fluids should be chilled (59°F–72°F) and palatable to encourage consumption. For the vast majority of workout sessions, water is the replacement drink of choice. Unless the exercise bout lasts more than 50 to 60 minutes, there is little advantage in supplementing carbohydrates.[6] Electrolyte losses (e.g., sodium, potassium, calcium) usually are small during brief exercise sessions (20- to 40-minute duration) and persons consuming a normal diet easily replenish electrolytes when their next meal is eaten. Those who eat a low-salt diet should visit their physician to discuss the effects of exercise on their salt balance.

INCREASED RISK OF HEAT ILLNESS

Disease and the effects of some drugs may increase the risk of heat illness. For example, hypertension, cardiovascular disease, diabetes-associated neuropathies, and aging may impair cardiovascular, skin blood flow, or sweating responses and impair temperature regulation.[7] Drug therapies for these and other disorders (e.g., diuretics, β-blockers, α-agonists, vasodilators) as well as licit recreational drugs (e.g., alcohol), can alter blood flow and cardiovascular responses to heat stress, exacerbate dehydration, and interfere with the body's ability to dissipate heat. A prior history of heat illness or difficulty acclimatizing to heat also may forecast future problems. Obesity also impairs heat dissipation, exacerbating physiologic strain during exercise–heat stress, and increases the risk of heat illness.[8] Clinicians and exercise professionals should consider these limitations when recommending exercise programs for hot weather.

Fitness facilities and organizations that offer exercise programs must formulate a standardized heat stress management plan for hot or humid weather. A comprehensive heat stress management plan should establish procedures for the following:

- Screening and surveillance of at-risk participants
- Environmental assessment using the WBGT index
- WBGT criteria for modifying or canceling exercise
- Heat acclimatization of participants
- Providing easy access to fluids
- Increasing awareness of the signs and symptoms of heatstroke, heat exhaustion, heat cramps, and heat syncope
- Integrating heat illness into emergency procedures

Cold, Wind, and Rain

Although many people avoid cold exposure by exercising indoors during winter, those who choose to exercise outdoors usually are not at great risk because exercise generates heat. Health and fitness professionals are often asked, "Is it too cold to exercise?" Indeed, two cold illnesses are caused by excessive body heat loss during prolonged exposure to cold, hypothermia (core body temperature below 95°F [normal is 98.6°F]) and frostbite (freezing of skin and body tissues). Both cold air and wind favor body heat loss.[4] The wind chill index (WCI), which purports to integrate the potential stress arising from both factors, has achieved popular acceptance[9] and is presented in Table E-2. The reader should note that the color of each rectangle tells you the amount of time required for frostbite to occur in exposed skin (i.e., unshaded, little risk; light gray, 30 minutes; dark pink, 10 minutes; red, 5 minutes). Thus, if weather conditions are very severe, frostbite may occur in 5 minutes or less. Although the WCI provides useful guidance concerning the conduct or cancellation of outdoor activities, it has inherent limitations.[10] For example, wind chill tables provide no meaningful estimate of the risk of hypothermia. Also, the WCI estimates the risk of tissue freezing for sedentary persons only.

TABLE E-2. The Wind Chill Index*

Wind Speed (mph)	Air Temperature (°F)								
	40	30	20	10	0	−10	−20	−30	−40
0	40	30	20	10	0	−10	−20	−30	−40
10	34	21	9	−4	−16	−28	−41	−53	−66
20	30	17	4	−9	−22	−35	−48	−61	−74
30	28	15	1	−12	−26	−39	−53	−67	−80
40	27	13	−1	−15	−29	−43	−57	−71	−84
50	26	12	−3	−17	−31	−45	−60	−74	−88
60	25	10	−4	−19	−33	−48	−62	−76	−91

*See reference 11: From National Oceanic and Atmospheric Administration, 2003. Revised wind chill chart.
Color key:
□ = Little risk of frostbite
▨ = Frostbite occurs within 30 minutes
▦ = Frostbite occurs within 10 minutes
■ = Frostbite occurs within 5 minutes

Body heat production during moderate or strenuous exercise is sufficiently high to prevent hypothermia in air temperatures as low as −25°F. Once exercise stops and metabolic heat production declines, either wet clothing must be replaced or the individual must return indoors to maintain core body temperature. The insulation value of wet clothing is compromised, and wetting of the skin facilitates heat loss. During water immersion, conductive and convective heat transfer can be 70-fold greater than in air of the same temperature,[4] depending on the water depth and amount of body surface immersed. Thus, even when water temperatures are relatively mild (e.g., 75°F–80°F), long-distance swimmers, triathletes, and fishermen or hunters who wade in streams can lose considerable amounts of body heat and become hypothermic. Those who exercise in windproof clothing are at less risk of frostbite than the wind chill tables suggest. Indeed, proper clothing can reduce the risk of frostbite markedly. Active individuals should avoid restrictive garments because tight clothing restricts blood flow to the skin, which in turn increases the risk of frostbite.

Both fatigue and hypothermia negatively affect human performance in the following ways.[12] First, prolonged exercise leads to substrate (i.e., muscle glycogen) depletion that compromises further exercise and reduces the rate of heat production. Second, fatigue that does not deplete muscle glycogen still may impair constriction of skin blood vessels, allowing increased heat loss. Third, chronic fatigue that lasts many weeks may delay the onset of shivering at rest, until body temperature falls into a hypothermic state. Fourth, when chronic underfeeding results in significant loss of subcutaneous adipose tissue, body insulation may be compromised and the risk of hypothermia may increase.[12]

Health and fitness professionals also should consider the possible consequences of inhaling cold air during exercise. Fortunately, these effects are usually negligible. Upper airway temperatures, which remain unchanged during exercise under temperate conditions, fall substantially when extremely cold air (1°F–25°F) is breathed during strenuous exercise. In contrast, the temperature of the lower respiratory tract and the body's core are unaffected.[13] Pulmonary function during exercise is unaffected by breathing cold air, in healthy athletes[14] and nonathletes.[15] In allergy-prone athletes, breathing cold air during heavy exercise may cause bronchospasm. Interestingly, this bronchospasm is triggered by facial cooling rather than cooling of respiratory passages.[16] Chronic inhalation of cold air also can increase respiratory passage secretions and decrease mucociliary clearance; the resulting airway congestion may impair pulmonary mechanics during exercise.[17]

Older adults and persons who have cardiovascular and circulatory disorders may need to use greater caution. Cold exposure, even when mild, stimulates the sympathetic nervous system and elevates total peripheral resistance, arterial pressure, myocardial contractility, and cardiac work at rest and during exercise.[18] This likely explains why patients with coronary artery disease experience angina pectoris and ST-segment depression at low exercise intensities in cold weather.[18] Particular caution should be advised for chopping wood and snow shoveling,[19,20] which require significant upper body use, because these tasks exacerbate blood pressure responses greatly.[18] Fatalities resulting from coronary artery disease increase in winter, but the extent that this reflects the effects of cold exposure on untrained older adults remains unclear.[18]

High-Altitude Exposure

In mountainous areas, the wind, snow, and rain frequently contribute to cold stress, whereas strenuous activity, heavy clothing, and increased solar radiation can contribute to heat stress. However, hypoxia (i.e., low oxygen content of inspired air) is the unique physiologic stressor encountered at high altitudes. Because the fractional concentration of oxygen in the atmosphere (F_IO_2) remains constant at 0.2093, the decreasing barometric pressure with increasing altitude is associated with a decreasing pressure of oxygen in the inspired air (P_IO_2). Even in pressurized cabins, commercial airline passengers are exposed to barometric pressures that are equivalent to altitudes of 5,000 to 8,000 feet.

When low-altitude residents ascend to high altitude, they notice an increased pulmonary ventilation, particularly during exercise.[21] This accounts for the common sensation of breathlessness at high altitude. Although highly variable between individuals, this response becomes more pronounced after several days of residence at high altitude. Despite increased ventilation, arterial oxygenation (i.e., P_aO_2, and S_aO_2) usually falls when low-altitude residents ascend to 5,000 feet above sea level or higher.[21] The resulting decrease in blood oxygen content necessitates an increased cardiac output, which is achieved by tachycardia. Furthermore, $\dot{V}O_{2max}$ is lower at high altitude than at sea level. Thus, the increased cardiovascular strain of exercise, combined with the reduced $\dot{V}O_{2max}$ at high altitude, compromise work capacity and endurance. These impairments usually become noticeable at an elevation of about 5,000 feet (or lower for some very fit athletes) and worsen with increasing elevation. After 5 to 10 days of acclimatization at high altitude, cardiovascular adjustments lessen the physiologic strain of exercise, enabling some improvement in endurance and work capacity. This adaptation is not equivalent to full recovery to sea level performance, however.

Air temperature decreases 1°F per elevation increase of 300 feet and body water losses may be misjudged by climbers because the air temperature is cool on high peaks. Further, the possibility of acute dehydration increases because of inadequate drinking, increased urine production and increased water loss during breathing. A chronic body weight loss of 1 to 3 pounds per week is common at extreme altitude and results from factors such as loss of appetite and increased energy expenditure.[22] These facts emphasize the importance of wholesome nutrition in maintaining vigor and performance.

HIGH ALTITUDE ILLNESSES

When unacclimatized persons ascend rapidly to elevations above 8,000 feet, many experience high-altitude illnesses (Table E-3) and reduced exercise capacity.[23] The most common of these is acute mountain sickness (AMS), which is characterized by severe headache, nausea, gastrointestinal disturbances, and insomnia. In susceptible people these symptoms arise after 6 to 12 hours at altitude and usually abate after 3 to 7 days of residence. Less common, but much more serious and even life threatening, are high-altitude pulmonary edema (HAPE) and high-altitude cerebral edema (HACE). Exercise at altitude usually exacerbates the symptoms of these illnesses and may, at least in the case of

TABLE E-3. Three High-Altitude Illnesses

Condition	Symptoms
Acute mountain sickness (AMS)	Severe headache, fatigue, irritability, nausea, loss of appetite, indigestion, flatulence, constipation, vomiting, sleep disturbance
High-altitude pulmonary edema (HAPE)	Very rapid breathing and heart rate, breathlessness, cough producing pink frothy sputum, blue-colored skin because of low blood oxygen content
High-altitude cerebral edema (HACE)	Staggering gait, loss of upper body coordination, severe weakness, ashen skin color, confusion, drowsiness, mental impairment, loss of consciousness, coma

See reference 24: From Hackett PH, Roach RC. High-altitude medicine. In: Auerbach PS, ed. Wilderness Medicine. St. Louis: Mosby, 1995:1–37.

pulmonary edema, increase the likelihood that the illness will develop. Descent to a lower altitude constitutes the definitive treatment for these three illnesses.

The following six recommendations[22] reduce the risk of experiencing high-altitude illnesses:

- Ascend slowly.
- Conduct a climb in stages. If moving to 10,000 feet or higher, limit your rate of ascent to 1,000 feet per day.
- Climb with an experienced guide or team.
- Avoid dehydration, overexertion, and hypothermia.
- Eat a high-carbohydrate diet to reduce the symptoms of AMS.
- Ask a physician to prescribe medications (e.g., acetazolamide, dexamethasone) as a preventive measure.

High-altitude exposure increases cardiac output, cardiac work, and myocardial oxygen requirements, and necessitates an increase in coronary blood flow relative to sea level exercise.[18] These responses can induce angina and/or ischemic ST-segment depression, at lower exercise intensities than at sea level.[18] Hypertensive patients may experience a disproportionate elevation in blood pressure at high altitude, during both rest and exercise.[18] For the first 1 to 3 days after sea level residents ascend to high altitude, use of the same THR as prescribed for sea level exercise limits cardiac strain because it necessitates a reduction in exercise intensity. However, with the development of altitude acclimatization (e.g., longer than a 3-day visit to high altitude), tachycardia abates considerably. This effect of altitude acclimatization may require a downward adjustment in the prescribed THR for some individuals.

REFERENCES

1. Armstrong LE, Epstein Y, Greenleaf JE, et al. American College of Sports Medicine position stand. Heat and cold illnesses during distance running. Med Sci Sports Exerc 1996;28:i–x.
2. Criteria for a recommended standard. Occupational exposure to hot environments. DHHS NIOSH Publ. No. 86-113. Washington, DC: National Institute for Occupational Safety and Health, 1986.

3. TB Med 507. Prevention, treatment and control of heat injury. Washington, DC: Department of the Army, 1980.

4. Gonzalez RR. Biophysics of heat exchange and clothing: applications to sports physiology. Med Exerc Nutr Health 1995;4:290–305.

5. Convertino VA, Armstrong LE, Coyle EF, et al. American College of Sports Medicine position stand. Exercise and fluid replacement. Med Sci Sports Exerc 1996;28:i–vii.

6. Armstrong LE, Maresh CM, eds. Fluid replacement during exercise and recovery from exercise. In: Buskirk ER, Puhl SM, eds. Body Fluid Balance: Exercise and Sport. Boca Raton, FL: CRC Press, 1996:259–282.

7. Kenney WL. Thermoregulation at rest and during exercise in healthy older adults. Exerc Sport Sci Rev 1997;25:41–76.

8. Chung NK, Pin CH. Obesity and the occurrence of heat disorders. Mil Med 1996;161:739–742.

9. Siple PA, Passel CR. Measurements of dry atmospheric cooling in subfreezing temperatures. Proc Am Philosoph Soc 1945;89:177–199.

10. Danilesson U. Wind chill and the risk of tissue freezing. J Appl Physiol 1996;81:2666–2673.

11. National Oceanic and Atmospheric Administration, 2003. Revised wind chill chart.

12. Young AJ, Castellani JW. Exertion-induced fatigue and thermoregulation in the cold. Comp Biochem Physiol A Mol Integr Physiol 2001;128:769–776.

13. Jaeger JJ, Deal EC Jr, Roberts DE, et al. Cold air inhalation and esophageal temperature in exercising humans. Med Sci Sports Exerc 1980;12:365–369.

14. Helenius IJ, Tikkanen HO, Haahtela T. Exercise-induced bronchospasm at low temperature in elite runners. Thorax 1990;51:628–629.

15. Chapman KR, Allen LJ, Romet TT. Pulmonary function in normal subjects following exercise at cold ambient temperatures. Eur J Appl Physiol Occup Physiol 1990;60:228–232.

16. Koskela H, Tukiainen H. Facial cooling, but not nasal breathing of cold air, induces bronchoconstriction: a study in asthmatic and healthy subjects. Eur Respir J 1995;8:2088–2093.

17. Giesbrecht GG. The respiratory system in a cold environment. Aviat Space Environ Med 1995;66:890–902.

18. Pandolf KB, Young AJ. Altitude and cold. In: Pollock ML, Schmidt DH, eds. Heart Disease and Rehabilitation. Champaign, IL: Human Kinetics, 1995:309–326.

19. Franklin BA, Hogan P, Bonzheim K, et al. Cardiac demands of heavy snow shoveling. JAMA 1995;273:880–882.

20. Franklin BA, Bonzheim K, Gordon S, et al. Snow shoveling: a trigger for acute myocardial infarction and sudden coronary death. Am J Cardiol 1996;77:855–858.

21. Young AJ, Young PM. Human acclimatization to high terrestrial altitude. In: Pandolf KB, Sawka MN, Gonzalez RR, eds. Human Performance Physiology and Environmental Medicine at Terrestrial Extremes. Indianapolis: Benchmark, 1988:497–543.

22. Armstrong LE. Performing in Extreme Environments. Champaign, IL: Human Kinetics, 2000.

23. Malkonian MK, Rock PB. Medical problems related to altitude. In: Pandolf KB, Sawka MN, Gonzalez RR, eds. Human Performance Physiology and Environmental Medicine at Terrestrial Extremes. Indianapolis: Benchmark, 1988:545–563.

24. Hackett PH, Roach RC. High-altitude medicine. In: Auerbach PS, ed. Wilderness Medicine. St. Louis: Mosby, 1995:1–37.

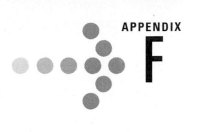

American College of Sports Medicine Certifications

This appendix details information about American College of Sports Medicine (ACSM) Certification and Registry Programs, as well as a complete listing of the current knowledge, skills, and abilities (KSAs) that comprise the foundations of these certification and registry examinations. The mission of the ACSM Committee on Certification and Registry Boards is to develop and provide high quality, accessible and affordable credentials and continuing education programs for health and exercise professionals who are responsible for preventive and rehabilitative programs that influence the health and well-being of all individuals.

ACSM Certifications and The Public

The first of the ACSM clinical certifications was initiated nearly 30 years ago in conjunction with publication of the first edition of the Guidelines for Exercise Testing and Prescription. That era was marked by rapid development of exercise programs for patients with stable coronary artery disease (CAD). ACSM sought a means to disseminate accurate information on this health care initiative through expression of consensus from its members in basic science, clinical practice, and education. Thus, these early clinical certifications were viewed as an aid to the establishment of safe and scientifically based exercise services within the framework of cardiac rehabilitation.

Over the past 30 years, exercise has gained widespread favor as an important component in programs of rehabilitative care or health maintenance for an expanding list of chronic diseases and disabling conditions. The growth of public interest in the role of exercise in health promotion has been equally impressive. In addition, federal government policy makers have revisited questions of medical efficacy and financing for exercise services in rehabilitative care of selected patients. Over the past several years, recommendations from the U.S. Public Health Service and the U.S. Surgeon General have acknowledged the central role for regular physical activity in the prevention of disease and promotion of health.

The development of the health/fitness certifications in the 1980s reflected ACSM's intent to increase the availability of qualified professionals to provide scientifically sound advice and supervision regarding appropriate physical activities for health maintenance in the apparently healthy adult population. Since 1975, more than 30,000 certificates have been awarded. With this consistent growth, ACSM has taken steps to ensure that its competency-based certifications will continue to be regarded as the premier program in the exercise field. For example, since 2002 ACSM has provided guidelines to assist colleges and universities with establishing standardized curricula that are focused on the knowledge, skills, and abilities (KSAs) requisite in the examinations for the ACSM Health/Fitness Instructor®, ACSM Exercise Specialist® and ACSM Registered Clinical Exercise Physiologist®.

Additionally, the ACSM University Connection Endorsement Program is designed to recognize institutions with educational programs that meet all of the KSAs specified by the ACSM Committee on Certification and Registry Boards (CCRB). Other examples include publishing a periodical addressing professional practice issues targeted to those who are certified, *ACSM's Certified News*, and oversight of continuing education requirements for maintenance of certification is another. Continuing education credits can be accrued through ACSM-sponsored educational programs such as ACSM workshops (Health/Fitness Instructor® and Exercise Specialist®), regional chapter and annual meetings, and other educational programs approved by the ACSM Professional Education Committee. These enhancements are intended to support the continued professional growth of those who have made a commitment to service in this rapidly growing health and fitness field.

Recently, ACSM, as a founder member of the multi-organizational Committee on Accreditation for the Exercise Sciences (CoAES), assisted with the development of Standards and Guidelines for educational programs seeking accreditation under the auspices of the Commission on Accreditation of Allied Health Education Programs (CAAHEP). Additional information on outcomes-based, programmatic accreditation can be obtained by visiting www.caahep.org, and specific information regarding the standards and guidelines can be obtained by visiting *www.coaes.org*. Because the standards and guidelines refer to the KSAs that follow, reference to specific KSAs as they relate to given sets of standards and guidelines will be noted when appropriate.

ACSM also acknowledges the expectation from successful candidates that the public will be informed of the high standards, values, and professionalism implicit in meeting these certification requirements. The College has formally organized its volunteer committee structure and national office staff to give added emphasis to informing the public, professionals, and government agencies about issues of critical importance to ACSM. Informing these constituencies about the meaning and value of ACSM certification is one important priority that will be given attention in this initiative.

ACSM Certification Programs

The ACSM certified Personal Trainer^SM is a fitness professional involved in developing and implementing an individualized approach to exercise leadership in healthy populations and/or those individuals with medical clearance to exercise. Using a variety of teaching techniques, the Personal Trainer is proficient in leading and demonstrating safe and effective methods of exercise by applying the fundamental principles of exercise science. The ACSM certified Personal Trainer^SM is familiar with forms of exercise used to improve, maintain, and/or optimize health-related components of physical fitness and performance. The ACSM certified Personal Trainer^SM is proficient in writing appropriate exercise recommendations, leading and demonstrating safe and effective methods of exercise, and motivating individuals to begin and to continue with their healthy behaviors.

The ACSM Health/Fitness Instructor® (HFI) is a professional qualified to assess, design, and implement individual and group exercise and fitness programs for low risk individuals and individuals with controlled disease. The HFI is skilled in evaluating health behaviors and risk factors, conducting fitness assessments, writing appropriate exercise prescriptions, and motivating individuals to modify negative health habits and maintain positive lifestyle behaviors for health promotion.

The ACSM Exercise Specialist® (ES) is a is a healthcare professional certified by ACSM to deliver a variety of exercise assessment, training, rehabilitation, risk factor identification and lifestyle management services to individuals with or at risk for cardiovascular, pulmonary, and metabolic disease(s). These services are typically delivered in cardiovascular/pulmonary rehabilitation programs, physicians' offices or medical fitness centers. The ACSM Exercise Specialist® is also competent to provide exercise-related consulting for research, public health, and other clinical and non-clinical services and programs.

The ACSM Registered Clinical Exercise Physiologist® (RCEP) is an allied health professional who works with persons with chronic diseases and conditions in which exercise has been shown to be beneficial. The RCEP performs health, physical activity, and fitness assessments, and prescribes exercise and physical activity primarily in hospitals or other health provider settings.

Certification at a given level requires the candidate to have a knowledge and skills base commensurate with that specific level of certification. In addition, the HFI level of certification incorporates the KSAs associated with the ACSM certified Personal Trainer™ certification, and the ES level of certification incorporates the KSAs associated with the HFI certification, as illustrated in Figure F-1. In addition, each level of certification has minimum requirements for experience, level of education, or other certifications.

How to Obtain Information and Application Materials

The certification programs of ACSM are subject to continuous review and revision. Content development is entrusted to a diverse committee of professional volunteers with expertise in exercise science, medicine, and program management. Expertise in design and procedures for competency assessment is also represented on this committee. Administration of certification is the responsibility of the ACSM National Center. Inquiries concerning certifications, application requirements, fees, and examination test sites and dates may be made to

ACSM Certification Resource Center
1-800-486-5643
Website: www.lww.com/acsmcrc
E-mail: certification@acsm.org

FIGURE F-1:

Level	Requirements	Recommended Competencies
ACSM certified Personal Trainer[SM]	*18 years of age or older *high school diploma or equivalent (GED) *Possess current Adult CPR certification that has a practical skills examination component (*such as the American Heart Association or the American Red Cross*).	*Demonstrate competence in the KSAs required of the ACSM certified Personal Trainer™ as listed in the current edition of the *ACSM's Guidelines for Exercise Testing and Prescription* *Adequate knowledge of and skill in risk factor and health status identification, fitness appraisal and exercise prescription *Demonstrate ability to incorporate suitable and innovative activities that will improve an individual's functional capacity Demonstrate the ability to effectively educate and/or communicate with individuals regarding lifestyle modification
ACSM Health/Fitness Instructor®	*An Associate's Degree or a Bachelor's degree in a health-related field from a regionally accredited college/university (one is eligible to sit for the exam if the candidate is in the last term of their degree program), AND *Possess current Adult CPR certification that has a practical skills examination component (*such as the American Heart Association or the American Red Cross*).	*Demonstrate competence in the KSAs required of the ACSM Health/Fitness Instructor® as listed in the current edition of the *ACSM's Guidelines for Exercise Testing and Prescription* *Work-related experience within the health and fitness field *Adequate knowledge of, and skill in, risk factor and health status identification, fitness appraisal, and exercise prescription *Demonstrate ability to incorporate suitable and innovative activities that will improve an individual's functional capacity *Demonstrate the ability to effectively educate and/or counsel individuals regarding lifestyle modification *Knowledge of exercise science including kinesiology, functional anatomy, exercise physiology, nutrition, program administration, psychology, and injury prevention

FIGURE F-1: continued

Level	Requirements	Recommended Competencies
ACSM Exercise Specialist®	*A Bachelor's Degree in an allied health field from a regionally accredited college of university (one is eligible to sit for the exam if the candidate is in the last term of their degree program); AND *Minimum of 600 hours of practical experience in a clinical exercise program (e.g. cardiac/pulmonary rehabilitation programs, exercise testing, exercise prescription, electrocardiography, patient education and counseling, disease management of cardiac, pulmonary, and metabolic diseases, and emergency management); AND *Current certification as a Basic Life Support Provider or CPR for the Professional Rescuer (*available through the American Heart Association or the American Red Cross*).	*Demonstrate competence in the KSAs required of the ACSM Exercise Specialist®, Health/Fitness Instructor®, as listed in the current edition of *ACSM's Guidelines for Exercise Testing and Prescription.* *Ability to demonstrate extensive knowledge of functional anatomy, exercise physiology, pathophysiology, electrocardiography, human behavior/psychology, gerontology, graded exercise testing for healthy and diseased populations, exercise supervision/leadership, patient counseling, and emergency procedures related to exercise testing and training situations.
ACSM Registered Clinical Exercise Physiologist®	*Master's Degree in exercise science, exercise physiology or kinesiology from a regionally accredited college or university * Current certification as a Basic Life Support Provider or CPR for the Professional Rescuer (*available through the American Heart Association or the American Red Cross*).	Demonstrate competence in the KSAs required of the ACSM Registered Clinical Exercise Physiologist® Exercise Specialist® and Health/Fitness Instructor® as listed in the current edition of *ACSM's Guidelines for Exercise Testing and Prescription.* The RCEP is an allied health professional who uses exercise and physical activity to assess and treat patients at risk of or with chronic diseases or conditions where exercise has been shown

continues

FIGURE F-1: continued

Level	Requirements	Scope of Practice
	*Minimum of 600 clinical hours are required with hours in each of the clinical practice areas, which may be completed as part of a formal degree program in exercise physiology. cardiovascular-200; pulmonary-100 ; metabolic-120; orthopedic/musculoskel etal-100; neuromuscular-40; immunological/hematological-40; These hours may be obtained with patients with co-morbid conditions. For example, time spent working with a patient who has Coronary Heart Disease and Parkinson's Disease may be counted in two practice areas IF you were providing exercise evaluation or programming specific to each of the conditions.	to provide therapeutic and/or functional benefit. Patients for whom RCEP services are appropriate may include, but are not limited to, persons with cardiovascular, pulmonary, metabolic, cancerous, immunologic, inflammatory, orthopedic, musculoskeletal, neuromuscular, gynecological, and obstetrical diseases and conditions. The RCEP provides scientific, evidence-based primary and secondary preventive and rehabilitative exercise and physical activity services to populations ranging from children to older adults. The RCEP performs exercise screening, exercise testing, exercise prescription, exercise and physical activity counseling, exercise supervision, exercise and health education/promotion, and evaluation of exercise and physical activity outcome measures. The RCEP works individually and as part of an interdisciplinary team in clinical, community, and public health settings. The practice and supervision of the RCEP is guided by published professional guidelines, standards, and applicable state and federal regulations. The practice of clinical exercise physiology is restricted to patients who are referred by and are under the care of a licensed physician.

Knowledge, Skills, and Abilities (KSAs) Underlining ACSM Certifications

Minimal competencies for each certification level are outlined below. Certification examinations are constructed based upon these KSAs. Two companion ACSM publications, *ACSM's Resource Manual for Guidelines for Exercise Testing and Prescription, fifth edition,* and *ACSM's Certification Review Book, second edition,* may also be used to gain further insight pertaining to the topics identified here. However, neither the Guidelines for Exercise Testing and Prescription nor either of the above mentioned Resource Manuals provides all of the information upon which the ACSM Certification examinations are based. Each may prove to be beneficial as a review of specific topics and as a general outline of many of the integral concepts to be mastered by those seeking certification.

CLASSIFICATION/NUMBERING SYSTEM FOR KNOWLEDGE, SKILLS, AND ABILITIES (KSAS)

The system for classifying and numbering KSAs has been changed. It is designed to be easier to use for certification candidates, where all the KSAs for a given certification/credential are listed in their entirety across a given Practice area and/or Content Matter area for each level of certification. Within each certification's/credential's KSA set, the numbering of individual KSAs uses a **three-part number** as follows:

First number–denotes Practice Area (1.x.x)
Second number–denotes Content Area (x.1.x)
Third number–denotes the sequential number of each KSA (x.x.1), within each Content Area

The Practice Areas (the first number) are numbered as follows:
1.x.x	General Population/Core
2.x.x	Cardiovascular
3.x.x	Pulmonary
4.x.x	Metabolic
5.x.x	Orthopedic/Musculoskeletal
6.x.x	Neuromuscular
7.x.x	Immunologic

The Content Matter Areas (the second number) are numbered as follows:
x.1.x	Exercise Physiology and related Exercise Science
x.2.x	Pathophysiology and Risk Factors
x.3.x	Health Appraisal, Fitness and Clinical Exercise Testing
x.4.x	Electrocardiography and Diagnostic Techniques
x.5.x	Patient Management and Medications
x.6.x	Medical and Surgical Management
x.7.x	Exercise Prescription and Programming
x.8.x	Nutrition and Weight Management
x.9.x	Human Behavior and Counseling
x.10.x	Safety, Injury Prevention, and Emergency Procedures
x.11.x	Program Administration, Quality Assurance, and Outcome Assessment
x.12.x	Clinical and Medical Considerations (ACSM certified Personal Trainer™ only)

EXAMPLES by Level of Certification/Credential:

ACSM certified Personal Trainer[SM] KSAs:

1.1.10   Knowledge to describe the normal acute responses to cardiovascular exercise.

In this example, the **practice** area is <u>General Population/Core</u>; the **content matter** area is <u>Exercise Physiology and Related Exercise Science</u>; and this KSA is the **tenth** KSA within this content matter area.

ACSM Health/Fitness Instructor® KSAs:

1.3.8 Skill in accurately measuring heart rate, blood pressure, and obtaining rating of perceived exertion (RPE) at rest and during exercise according to established guidelines.

In this example, the **practice** area is <u>General Population/Core</u>; the **content** matter area is <u>Health Appraisal, Fitness and Clinical Exercise Testing</u>; and this KSA is the **eighth** KSA within this content matter area.

ACSM Exercise Specialist® KSAs°:

1.7.17 **Design strength and flexibility programs for individuals with cardiovascular, pulmonary and/or metabolic diseases, elderly, and children.**

In this example, the **practice** area is <u>General Population/Core</u>; the **content** matter area is <u>Exercise Prescription and Programming</u>; and this KSA is the **seventeenth** KSA within this content matter area. Furthermore, because this specific KSA appears in **bold**, it covers multiple practice areas and content areas.

°*A special note about ACSM Exercise Specialist® KSAs:*

Like the other certifications presented thus far, the ACSM Exercise Specialist® KSAs are categorized by content area. However, some ES KSAs cover multiple practices areas within each area of content. For example, a number of them describe a specific topic with respect to both exercise testing and training, which are two distinct content areas. Rather than write out each separately (which would have greatly expanded the KSA list length) they have been listed under a single content area. When reviewing these KSAs, please note that KSAs in **bold text** cover multiple content areas. Each ES KSA begins with a 'l' as the practice area. However, where appropriate, some KSAs mention specific patient populations (i.e., practice area). If a specific practice area is not mentioned within a given KSA, then it applies equally to each of the general population, cardiovascular, pulmonary and metabolic practice areas. Note that "metabolic patients" are defined as those with at least one of the following: overweight or obese, diabetes (type I or II), metabolic syndrome. Each KSA describes either a single or multiple knowledge (K), skill (S), or ability (A), or a combination of K, S or A, that an individual should have mastery of to be considered a competent ACSM Exercise Specialist®. Finally, as stated previously, the ACSM Exercise Specialist® candidate is also responsible for the mastery of both the ACSM Health/Fitness Instructor® and the ACSM certified Personal Trainer™ KSAs.

ACSM Registered Clinical Exercise Physiologist KSAs:

7.6.1 "List the drug classifications commonly used in the treatment of patients with a National Institutes of Health (NIH) disease, name common generic and brand names drugs within each class, and explain the purposes, indications, major side effects, and the effects, if any, on the exercising individual."

The **practice** area is <u>Immunologic</u>; the **content matter** area is <u>Medical and Surgical Management</u>; and this KSA is the **second** KSA within this content matter area.

ACSM certified Personal Trainer^{SM} Knowledge, Skills, and Abilities (KSAs):

EXERCISE PHYSIOLOGY AND RELATED EXERCISE SCIENCE

1.1.1 Knowledge of the basic structures of bone, skeletal muscle, and connective tissues.

1.1.2 Knowledge of the basic anatomy of the cardiovascular system and respiratory system.

1.1.3 Knowledge of the definition of the following terms: inferior, superior, medial, lateral, supination, pronation, flexion, extension, adduction, abduction, hyper-extension, rotation, circumduction, agonist, antagonist, and stabilizer.

1.1.4 Knowledge of the plane in which each muscle action occurs.

1.1.5 Knowledge of the interrelationships among center of gravity, base of support, balance, stability, and proper spinal alignment.

1.1.6 Knowledge of the following curvatures of the spine: lordosis, scoliosis, and kyphosis.

1.1.7 Knowledge to describe the myotatic stretch reflex.

1.1.8 Knowledge of the biomechanical principles for the performance of the following activities: walking, jogging, running, swimming, cycling, weight lifting, and carrying or moving objects.

1.1.9 Ability to define aerobic and anaerobic metabolism.

1.1.10 Knowledge to describe the normal acute responses to cardiovascular exercise.

1.1.11 Knowledge to describe the normal acute responses to resistance training.

1.1.12 Knowledge of the normal chronic physiological adaptations associated with cardiovascular exercise.

1.1.13 Knowledge of the normal chronic physiological adaptations associated with resistance training.

1.1.14 Knowledge of the physiological principles related to warm-up and cool-down.

1.1.15 Knowledge of the common theories of muscle fatigue and delayed onset muscle soreness (DOMS).

1.1.16 Knowledge of the physiological adaptations that occur at rest and during submaximal and maximal exercise following chronic aerobic and anaerobic exercise training.

1.1.17 Knowledge of the physiological principles involved in promoting gains in muscular strength and endurance.

1.1.18 Knowledge of blood pressure responses associated with acute exercise, including changes in body position.

1.1.19 Knowledge of how the principle of specificity relates to the components of fitness.

1.1.20 Knowledge of the concept of detraining or reversibility of conditioning and its implications in fitness programs.

1.1.21 Knowledge of the physical and psychological signs of overtraining and to provide recommendations for these problems.

1.1.22 Knowledge of the following terms: progressive resistance, isotonic/isometric, concentric, eccentric, atrophy, hypertrophy, sets, repetitions, plyometrics, Valsalva maneuver.

1.1.23 Ability to identify the major bones and muscles. Major muscles include, but are not limited to, the following: trapezius, pectoralis major, latissimus dorsi, biceps, triceps, rectus abdominis, internal and external obliques, erector spinae, gluteus maximus, quadriceps, hamstrings, adductors, abductors, and gastrocnemius.

1.1.24   Ability to identify the major bones. Major bones include, but are not limited to the clavicle, scapula, strrernum, humerus, carpals, ulna, radius, femur, fibia, tibia, and tarsals.
1.1.25   Ability to identify the joints of the body.
1.1.26   Knowledge of the primary action and joint range of motion for each major muscle group.
1.1.27   Ability to locate the anatomic landmarks for palpation of peripheral pulses.

HEALTH APPRAISAL, FITNESS AND CLINICAL EXERCISE TESTING

1.3.1   Knowledge of and ability to discuss the physiological basis of the major components of physical fitness: flexibility, cardiovascular fitness, muscular strength, muscular endurance, and body composition.
1.3.2   Knowledge of the importance of a health/medical history.
1.3.3   Knowledge of the value of a medical clearance prior to exercise participation.
1.3.4   Knowledge of the categories of participants who should receive medical clearance prior to administration of an exercise test or participation in an exercise program.
1.3.5   Knowledge of relative and absolute contraindications to exercise testing or participation.
1.3.6   Knowledge of the limitations of informed consent and medical clearance prior to exercise testing.
1.3.7   Knowledge of the advantages/disadvantages and limitations of the various body composition techniques including, but not limited to: air displacement, plethysmography, hydrostatic weighing, Bod Pod, bioelectrical impedence.
1.3.8   Skill in accurately measuring heart rate, and obtaining rating of perceived exertion (RPE) at rest and during exercise according to established guidelines.
1.3.9   Ability to locate common sites for measurement of skinfold thicknesses and circumferences (for determination of body composition and waist-hip ratio).
1.3.10   Ability to obtain a basic health history and risk appraisal and to stratify risk in accordance with ACSM Guidelines.
1.3.11   Ability to explain and obtain informed consent.
1.3.12   Ability to instruct participants in the use of equipment and test procedures.
1.3.13   Knowledge of the purpose and implementation of pre-activity fitness testing, including assessments of cardiovascular fitness, muscular strength, muscular endurance, and flexibility, and body composition.
1.3.14   Ability to identify appropriate criteria for terminating a fitness evaluation and demonstrate proper procedures to be followed after discontinuing such a test.

EXERCISE PRESCRIPTION AND PROGRAMMING

1.7.1   Knowledge of the benefits and risks associated with exercise training in pre-pubescent and postpubescent youth.
1.7.2   Knowledge of the benefits and precautions associated with resistance and endurance training in older adults.
1.7.3   Knowledge of specific leadership techniques appropriate for working with participants of all ages.
1.7.4   Knowledge of how to modify cardiovascular and resistance exercises based on age and physical condition.
1.7.5   Knowledge of and ability to describe the unique adaptations to exercise training with regard to strength, functional capacity, and motor skills.
1.7.6   Knowledge of common orthopedic and cardiovascular considerations for older participants and the ability to describe modifications in exercise prescription that are indicated.

1.7.7 Knowledge of selecting appropriate testing and training modalities according to the age and functional capacity of the individual.

1.7.8 Knowledge of the recommended intensity, duration, frequency, and type of physical activity necessary for development of cardiorespiratory fitness in an apparently healthy population.

1.7.9 Knowledge to describe, and the ability to demonstrate (such as technique and breathing), exercises designed to enhance muscular strength and/or endurance of specific major muscle groups.

1.7.10 Knowledge of the principles of overload, specificity, and progression and how they relate to exercise programming.

1.7.11 Knowledge of the components incorporated into an exercise session and the proper sequence (i.e., preexercise evaluation, warm-up, aerobic stimulus phase, cool-down, muscular strength and/or endurance, and flexibility).

1.7.12 Knowledge of special precautions and modifications of exercise programming for participation at altitude, different ambient temperatures, humidity, and environmental pollution.

1.7.13 Knowledge of the importance and ability to record exercise sessions and performing periodic evaluations to assess changes in fitness status.

1.7.14 Knowledge of the advantages and disadvantages of implementation of interval, continuous, and circuit training programs.

1.7.15 Knowledge of the concept of "Activities of Daily Living" (ADLs) and its importance in the overall health of the individual.

1.7.16 Knowledge of Progressive Adaptation in resistance training and it's implications on program design and periodization

1.7.17 Understanding of personal training client's "personal space" and how it plays into a trainer's interaction with their client.

1.7.18 Skill to teach and demonstrate the components of an exercise session (i.e., warm-up, aerobic stimulus phase, cool-down, muscular strength/endurance, flexibility).

1.7.19 Skill to teach and demonstrate appropriate modifications in specific exercises for the following groups: older adults, pregnant and postnatal women, obese persons, and persons with low back pain.

1.7.20 Skill to teach and demonstrate appropriate exercises for improving range of motion of all major joints.

1.7.21 Skill in the use of various methods for establishing and monitoring levels of exercise intensity, including heart rate, RPE, and METs.

1.7.22 Knowledge of and ability to apply methods used to monitor exercise intensity, including heart rate and rating of perceived exertion.

1.7.23 Ability to describe modifications in exercise prescriptions for individuals with functional disabilities and musculoskeletal injuries

1.7.24 Ability to differentiate between the amount of physical activity required for health benefits and the amount of exercise required for fitness development.

1.7.25 Ability to determine training heart rates using two methods: percent of age-predicted maximum heart rate and heart rate reserve (Karvonen).

1.7.26 Ability to identify proper and improper technique in the use of resistive equipment such as stability balls, weights, bands, resistance bars, and water exercise equipment.

1.7.27 Ability to identify proper and improper technique in the use of cardiovascular conditioning equipment (e.g., stairclimbers, stationary cycles, treadmills, elliptical trainers).

1.7.28 Ability to teach a progression of exercises for all major muscle groups to improve muscular strength and endurance.

1.7.29 Ability to modify exercises based on age and physical condition.
1.7.30 Ability to explain and implement exercise prescription guidelines for apparently healthy clients or those who have medical clearance to exercise
1.7.31 Ability to adapt frequency, intensity, duration, mode, progression, level of supervision, and monitoring techniques in exercise programs for apparently healthy clients or those who have medical clearance to exercise
1.7.32 Ability to design resistive exercise programs to increase or maintain muscular strength and/or endurance.
1.7.33 Ability to periodize a resistance training program for continued muscular strength development
1.7.34 Ability to evaluate, prescribe, and demonstrate appropriate flexibility exercises for all major muscle groups.
1.7.35 Ability to design training programs using interval, continuous, and circuit training programs.
1.7.36 Ability to describe the advantages and disadvantages of various commercial exercise equipment in developing cardiorespiratory fitness, muscular strength, and muscular endurance.

NUTRITION AND WEIGHT MANAGEMENT

1.8.1 Knowledge of the role of carbohydrates, fats, and proteins as fuels for aerobic and anaerobic metabolism.
1.8.2 Knowledge to define the following terms: obesity, overweight, percent fat, Body Mass Index, lean body mass, anorexia nervosa, bulimia nervosa, and body fat distribution.
1.8.3 Knowledge of the relationship between body composition and health.
1.8.4 Knowledge of the effects of diet plus exercise, diet alone, and exercise alone as methods for modifying body composition.
1.8.5 Knowledge of the importance of an adequate daily energy intake for healthy weight management.
1.8.6 Knowledge of the importance of maintaining normal hydration before, during, and after exercise.
1.8.7 Knowledge of the USDA Food Pyramid.
1.8.8 Knowledge of the female athlete triad
1.8.9 Knowledge of the myths and consequences associated with inappropriate weight loss methods (e.g., saunas, vibrating belts, body wraps, electric simulators, sweat suits, fad diets).
1.8.10 Knowledge of the number of kilocalories in one gram of carbohydrate, fat, protein, and alcohol.
1.8.11 Knowledge of the number of kilocalories equivalent to losing 1 pound of body fat.
1.8.12 Knowledge of the guidelines for caloric intake for an individual desiring to lose or gain weight.
1.8.13 Knowledge of common nutritional ergogenic aids, the purported mechanism of action, and any risk and/or benefits (e.g., carbohydrates, protein/amino acids, vitamins, minerals, sodium bicarbonate, creatine, bee pollen, etc.)
1.8.14 Ability to describe the health implications of variation in body fat distribution patterns and the significance of the waist to hip ratio.

HUMAN BEHAVIOR AND COUNSELING

1.9.1 Knowledge of at least five behavioral strategies to enhance exercise and health behavior change (e.g., reinforcement, goal setting, social support).
1.9.2 Knowledge of the stages of motivational readiness.

1.9.3 Knowledge of the 3 stages of learning: Cognitive, Associative, Autonomous
1.9.4 Knowledge of specific techniques to enhance motivation (e.g., posters, recognition, bulletin boards, games, competitions). Define extrinsic and intrinsic reinforcement and give examples of each.
1.9.5 Knowledge of the different types of learners (Auditory, Visual, Kinesthetic) and how to apply teaching and training techniques to optimize a client's training session
1.9.6 Knowledge of the types of feedback and ability to use communication skills to optimize a client's training session.

SAFETY, INJURY PREVENTION, AND EMERGENCY PROCEDURES

1.10.1 Knowledge of and skill in obtaining basic life support and cardiopulmonary resuscitation certification.
1.10.2 Knowledge of appropriate emergency procedures (i.e., telephone procedures, written emergency procedures, personnel responsibilities) in a health and fitness setting.
1.10.3 Knowledge of basic first aid procedures for exercise-related injuries, such as bleeding, strains/sprains, fractures, and exercise intolerance (dizziness, syncope, heat injury).
1.10.4 Knowledge of basic precautions taken in an exercise setting to ensure participant safety.
1.10.5 Knowledge of the physical and physiological signs and symptoms of overtraining.
1.10.6 Knowledge of the effects of temperature, humidity, altitude, and pollution on the physiological response to exercise.
1.10.7 Knowledge of the following terms: shin splints, sprain, strain, tennis elbow, bursitis, stress fracture, tendonitis, patello-femoral pain syndrome, low back pain, plantar fasciitis, and rotator cuff tendonitis.
1.10.8 Knowledge of hypothetical concerns and potential risks that may be associated with the use of exercises such as straight leg sit-ups, double leg raises, full squats, hurdlers stretch, yoga plough, forceful back hyperextension, and standing bent-over toe touch.
1.10.9 Knowledge of safety plans, emergency procedures, and first aid techniques needed during fitness evaluations, exercise testing, and exercise training.
1.10.10 Knowledge of the cPT's responsibilities, limitations, and the legal implications of carrying out emergency procedures.
1.10.11 Knowledge of potential musculoskeletal injuries (e.g., contusions, sprains, strains, fractures), cardiovascular/pulmonary complications (e.g., tachycardia, bradycardia, hypotension/hypertension, tachypnea) and metabolic abnormalities (e.g., fainting/syncope, hypoglycemia/hyperglycemia, hypothermia/hyperthermia).
1.10.12 Knowledge of the initial management and first aid techniques associated with open wounds, musculoskeletal injuries, cardiovascular/pulmonary complications, and metabolic disorders.
1.10.13 Knowledge of the components of an equipment maintenance/repair program and how it may be used to evaluate the condition of exercise equipment to reduce the potential risk of injury.
1.10.14 Knowledge of the legal implications of documented safety procedures, the use of incident documents, and ongoing safety training.
1.10.15 Skill in demonstrating appropriate emergency procedures during exercise testing and/or training.
1.10.16 Ability to idenify the components that contribute to the maintenance of a safe environment.

1.10.17 Ability to assist or "spot" a client in a safe and effective manner during resistance exercise

PROGRAM ADMINISTRATION, QUALITY ASSURANCE, AND OUTCOME ASSESSMENT

1.11.1 Knowledge of the cPT's role in administration and program management within a health/fitness facility.

1.11.2 Knowledge of and the ability to use the documentation required when a client shows abnormal signs or symptoms during an exercise session and should be referred to a physician.

1.11.3 Knowledge of professional liability and most common types of negligence seen in training environments

1.11.4 Understand the practical and legal ramifications of the employee vs. independent contractor classifications as they relate to personal trainers

1.11.5 Knowledge of appropriate professional conduct, practice standards, and ethics in relationships dealing with clients, employers, and other allied health/medical/fitness professionals.

1.11.6 Knowledge of the types of exercise programs available in the community and how these programs are appropriate for various populations.

1.11.7 knowledge of and ability to implement effective, professional business practices and ethical promotion of personal training services

CLINICAL AND MEDICAL CONSIDERATIONS

1.12.1 Knowledge of cardiovascular, respiratory, metabolic, and musculoskeletal risk factors that may require further evaluation by medical or allied health professionals before participation in physical activity.

1.12.2 Knowledge of risk factors that may be favorably modified by physical activity habits.

1.12.3 Knowledge of the risk factor concept of Coronary Artery Disease (CAD) and the influence of heredity and lifestyle on the development of CAD.

1.12.4 Knowledge of how lifestyle factors, including nutrition, physical activity, and heredity, influence blood lipid and lipoprotein (i.e., cholesterol: high-density lipoprotein and low-density lipoprotein) profiles.

1.12.5 Knowledge of cardiovascular risk factors or conditions that may require consultation with medical personnel before testing or training, including inappropriate changes of resting or exercise heart rate and blood pressure, new onset discomfort in chest, neck, shoulder, or arm, changes in the pattern of discomfort during rest or exercise, fainting or dizzy spells, and claudication.

1.12.6 Knowledge of respiratory risk factors or conditions that may require consultation with medical personnel before testing or training, including asthma, exercise-induced bronchospasm, extreme breathlessness at rest or during exercise, bronchitis, and emphysema.

1.12.7 Knowledge of metabolic risk factors or conditions that may require consultation with medical personnel before testing or training, including body weight more than 20% above optimal, BMI> 30, thyroid disease, diabetes or glucose intolerance, and hypoglycemia.

1.12.8 Knowledge of musculoskeletal risk factors or conditions that may require consultation with medical personnel before testing or training, including acute or chronic back pain, osteoarthritis, rheumatoid arthritis, osteoporosis, tendonitis, and low back pain.

1.12.9 Knowledge of the basic principles of electrical conduction of the heart, it's phases of contraction, and it's implications.

1.12.10 Knowledge of common drugs from each of the following classes of medications and describe their effects on exercise: antianginals; antihypertensives; antiarrhythmics; bronchodilators; hypoglycemics; psychotropics; and vasodilators.
1.12.11 Knowledge of the effects of the following substances on exercise: antihistamines, tranquilizers, alcohol, diet pills, cold tablets, caffeine, and nicotine.

ACSM Health/Fitness Instructor® Knowledge, Skills, and Abilities (KSAs):

GENERAL POPULATION/CORE:
EXERCISE PHYSIOLOGY AND RELATED EXERCISE SCIENCE

1.1.1 Knowledge of the basic structures of bone, skeletal muscle, and connective tissues.
1.1.2 Knowledge of the basic anatomy of the cardiovascular system and respiratory system.
1.1.3 Knowledge of the definition of the following terms: inferior, superior, medial, lateral, supination, pronation, flexion, extension, adduction, abduction, hyperextension, rotation, circumduction, agonist, antagonist, and stabilizer.
1.1.4 Knowledge of the plane in which each muscle action occurs.
1.1.5 Knowledge of the interrelationships among center of gravity, base of support, balance, stability, and proper spinal alignment.
1.1.6 Knowledge of the following curvatures of the spine: lordosis, scoliosis, and kyphosis.
1.1.7 Knowledge to describe the myotatic stretch reflex.
1.1.8 Knowledge of fundamental biomechanical principles that underlie performance of the following activities: walking, jogging, running, swimming, cycling, weight lifting, and carrying or moving objects.
1.1.9 Ability to define aerobic and anaerobic metabolism.
1.1.10 Knowledge of the role of aerobic and anaerobic energy systems in the performance of various activities.
1.1.11 Knowledge of the following terms: ischemia, angina pectoris, tachycardia, bradycardia, arrhythmia, myocardial infarction, cardiac output, stroke volume, lactic acid, oxygen consumption, hyperventilation, systolic blood pressure, diastolic blood pressure, and anaerobic threshold.
1.1.12 Knowledge to describe normal cardiorespiratory responses to static and dynamic exercise in terms of heart rate, blood pressure, and oxygen consumption.
1.1.13 Knowledge of how heart rate, blood pressure, and oxygen consumption responses change with adaptation to chronic exercise training.
1.1.14 Knowledge of the physiological adaptations associated with strength training.
1.1.15 Knowledge of the physiological principles related to warm-up and cool-down.
1.1.16 Knowledge of the common theories of muscle fatigue and delayed onset muscle soreness (DOMS).
1.1.17 Knowledge of the physiological adaptations that occur at rest and during submaximal and maximal exercise following chronic aerobic and anaerobic exercise training.
1.1.18 Knowledge of the differences in cardiorespiratory response to acute graded exercise between conditioned and unconditioned individuals.
1.1.19 Knowledge of the structure of the skeletal muscle fiber and the basic mechanism of contraction.

1.1.20   Knowledge of the characteristics of fast and slow twitch fibers.

1.1.21   Knowledge of the sliding filament theory of muscle contraction.

1.1.22   Knowledge of twitch, summation, and tetanus with respect to muscle contraction.

1.1.23   Knowledge of the physiological principles involved in promoting gains in muscular strength and endurance.

1.1.24   Knowledge of muscle fatigue as it relates to mode, intensity, duration, and the accumulative effects of exercise.

1.1.25   Knowledge of the basic properties of cardiac muscle and the normal pathways of conduction in the heart.

1.1.26   Knowledge of the response of the following variables to acute static and dynamic exercise: heart rate, stroke volume, cardiac output, pulmonary ventilation, tidal volume, respiratory rate, and arteriovenous oxygen difference.

1.1.27   Knowledge of blood pressure responses associated with acute exercise, including changes in body position.

1.1.28   Knowledge of and ability to describe the implications of ventilatory threshold (anaerobic threshold) as it relates to exercise training and cardiorespiratory assessment.

1.1.29   Knowledge of and ability to describe the physiological adaptations of the respiratory system that occur at rest and during submaximal and maximal exercise following chronic aerobic and anaerobic training.

1.1.30   Knowledge of how each of the following differs from the normal condition: dyspnea, hypoxia, and hypoventilation.

1.1.31   Knowledge of how the principle of specificity relates to the components of fitness.

1.1.32   Knowledge of the concept of detraining or reversibility of conditioning and its implications in fitness programs.

1.1.33   Knowledge of the physical and psychological signs of overtraining and to provide recommendations for these problems.

1.1.34   Knowledge of and ability to describe the changes that occur in maturation from childhood to adulthood for the following: skeletal muscle, bone structure, reaction time, coordination, heat and cold tolerance, maximal oxygen consumption, strength, flexibility, body composition, resting and maximal heart rate, and resting and maximal blood pressure.

1.1.35   Knowledge of the effect of the aging process on the musculoskeletal and cardiovascular structure and function at rest, during exercise, and during recovery.

1.1.36   Knowledge of the following terms: progressive resistance, isotonic/isometric, concentric, eccentric, atrophy, hypertrophy, sets, repetitions, plyometrics, Valsalva maneuver.

1.1.37   Knowledge of and skill to demonstrate exercises designed to enhance muscular strength and/or endurance of specific major muscle groups.

1.1.38   Knowledge of and skill to demonstrate exercises for enhancing musculoskeletal flexibility.

1.1.39   Ability to identify the major bones and muscles. Major muscles include, but are not limited to, the following: trapezius, pectoralis major, latissimus dorsi, biceps, triceps, rectus abdominis, internal and external obliques, erector spinae, gluteus maximus, quadriceps, hamstrings, adductors, abductors, and gastrocnemius.

1.1.40   Ability to identify the major bones. Major bones include, but are not limited to the clavicle, scapula, strrernum, humerus, carpals, ulna, radius, femur, fibia, tibia, and tarsals.

1.1.41   Ability to identify the joints of the body.
1.1.42   Knowledge of the primary action and joint range of motion for each major muscle group.
1.1.43   Ability to locate the anatomic landmarks for palpation of peripheral pulses.

PATHOPHYSIOLOGY AND RISK FACTORS

1.2.1   Knowledge of the physiological and metabolic responses to exercise associated with chronic disease (heart disease, hypertension, diabetes mellitus, and pulmonary disease).
1.2.2   Knowledge of cardiovascular, respiratory, metabolic, and musculoskeletal risk factors that may require further evaluation by medical or allied health professionals before participation in physical activity.
1.2.3   Knowledge of risk factors that may be favorably modified by physical activity habits.
1.2.4   Knowledge to define the following terms: total cholesterol (TC), high-density lipoprotein cholesterol (HDL-C), TC/HDL-C ratio, low-density lipoprotein cholesterol (LDL-C), triglycerides, hypertension, and atherosclerosis.
1.2.5   Knowledge of plasma cholesterol levels for adults as recommended by the National Cholesterol Education Program.
1.2.6   Knowledge of the risk factor concept of CAD and the influence of heredity and lifestyle on the development of CAD.
1.2.7   Knowledge of the atherosclerotic process, the factors involved in its genesis and progression, and the potential role of exercise in treatment.
1.2.8   Knowledge of how lifestyle factors, including nutrition, physical activity, and heredity, influence lipid and lipoprotein profiles.

HEALTH APPRAISAL, FITNESS AND CLINICAL EXERCISE TESTING

1.3.1   Knowledge of and ability to discuss the physiological basis of the major components of physical fitness: flexibility, cardiovascular fitness, muscular strength, muscular endurance, and body composition.
1.3.2   Knowledge of the importance of a health/medical history.
1.3.3   Knowledge of the value of a medical clearance prior to exercise participation.
1.3.4   Knowledge of the categories of participants who should receive medical clearance prior to administration of an exercise test or participation in an exercise program.
1.3.5   Knowledge of relative and absolute contraindications to exercise testing or participation.
1.3.6   Knowledge of the limitations of informed consent and medical clearance prior to exercise testing.
1.3.7   Knowledge of the advantages/disadvantages and limitations of the various body composition techniques including air displacement, plethysmography, hydrostatic weighing, skinfolds and bioelectrical impedence.
1.3.8   Skill in accurately measuring heart rate, blood pressure, and obtaining rating of perceived exertion (RPE) at rest and during exercise according to established guidelines.
1.3.9   Skill in measuring skinfold sites, skeletal diameters, and girth measurements used for estimating body composition.
1.3.10 Skill in techniques for calibration of a cycle ergometer and a motor-driven treadmill.
1.3.11 Ability to locate the brachial artery and correctly place the cuff and stethoscope in position for blood pressure measurement.

1.3.12   Ability to locate common sites for measurement of skinfold thicknesses and circumferences (for determination of body composition and waist-hip ratio).

1.3.13   Ability to obtain a health history and risk appraisal that includes past and current medical history, family history of cardiac disease, orthopedic limitations, prescribed medications, activity patterns, nutritional habits, stress and anxiety levels, and smoking and alcohol use.

1.3.14   Ability to obtain informed consent.

1.3.15   Ability to explain the purpose and procedures for monitoring clients prior to, during, and after cardiorespiratory fitness testing.

1.3.16   Ability to instruct participants in the use of equipment and test procedures.

1.3.17   Ability to describe the purpose of testing, determine an appropriate submaximal or maximal protocol, and perform an assessment of cardiovascular fitness on the cycle ergometer or the treadmill.

1.3.18   Ability to describe the purpose of testing, determine appropriate protocols, and perform assessments of muscular strength, muscular endurance, and flexibility.

1.3.19   Ability to perform various techniques of assessing body composition, including the use of skinfold calipers.

1.3.20   Ability to analyze and interpret information obtained from the cardiorespiratory fitness test and the muscular strength and endurance, flexibility, and body composition assessments for apparently healthy individuals and those with stable disease.

1.3.21   Ability to identify appropriate criteria for terminating a fitness evaluation and demonstrate proper procedures to be followed after discontinuing such a test.

1.3.22   Ability to modify protocols and procedures for cardiorespiratory fitness tests in children, adolescents, and older adults.

1.3.23   Ability to identify individuals for whom physician supervision is recommended during maximal and submaximal exercise testing.

ELECTROCARDIOGRAPHY AND DIAGNOSTIC TECHNIQUES

1.4.1   Knowledge of how each of the following differs from the normal condition: premature atrial contractions and premature ventricular contractions.

1.4.2   Ability to locate the appropriate sites for the limb and chest leads for resting, standard, and exercise (Mason Likar) electrocardiograms (ECGs), as well as commonly used bipolar systems (e.g., CM-5).

PATIENT MANAGEMENT AND MEDICATIONS

1.5.1   Knowledge of common drugs from each of the following classes of medications and describe the principal action and the effects on exercise testing and prescription: antianginals; antihypertensives; antiarrhythmics; bronchodilators; hypoglycemics; psychotropics; and vasodilators.

1.5.2   Knowledge of the effects of the following substances on exercise response: antihistamines, tranquilizers, alcohol, diet pills, cold tablets, caffeine, and nicotine.

EXERCISE PRESCRIPTION AND PROGRAMMING

1.7.1   Knowledge of the relationship between the number of repetitions, intensity, number of sets, and rest with regard to strength training.

1.7.2   Knowledge of the benefits and risks associated with exercise training in prepubescent and postpubescent youth.

1.7.3   Knowledge of the benefits and precautions associated with resistance and endurance training in older adults.

1.7.4 Knowledge of specific leadership techniques appropriate for working with participants of all ages.

1.7.5 Knowledge of how to modify cardiovascular and resistance exercises based on age and physical condition.

1.7.6 Knowledge of the differences in the development of an exercise prescription for children, adolescents, and older participants.

1.7.7 Knowledge of and ability to describe the unique adaptations to exercise training in children, adolescents, and older participants with regard to strength, functional capacity, and motor skills.

1.7.8 Knowledge of common orthopedic and cardiovascular considerations for older participants and the ability to describe modifications in exercise prescription that are indicated.

1.7.9 Knowledge of selecting appropriate testing and training modalities according to the age and functional capacity of the individual.

1.7.10 Knowledge of the recommended intensity, duration, frequency, and type of physical activity necessary for development of cardiorespiratory fitness in an apparently healthy population.

1.7.11 Knowledge of and the ability to describe exercises designed to enhance muscular strength and/or endurance of specific major muscle groups.

1.7.12 Knowledge of the principles of overload, specificity, and progression and how they relate to exercise programming.

1.7.13 Knowledge of the various types of interval, continuous, and circuit training programs.

1.7.14 Knowledge of approximate METs for various sport, recreational, and work tasks.

1.7.15 Knowledge of the components incorporated into an exercise session and the proper sequence (i.e., preexercise evaluation, warm-up, aerobic stimulus phase, cool-down, muscular strength and/or endurance, and flexibility).

1.7.16 Knowledge of special precautions and modifications of exercise programming for participation at altitude, different ambient temperatures, humidity, and environmental pollution.

1.7.17 Knowledge of the importance of recording exercise sessions and performing periodic evaluations to assess changes in fitness status.

1.7.18 Knowledge of the advantages and disadvantages of implementation of interval, continuous, and circuit training programs.

1.7.19 Knowledge of the types of exercise programs available in the community and how these programs are appropriate for various populations.

1.7.20 Knowledge of the concept of "Activities of Daily Living" (ADLs) and its importance in the overall health of the individual.

1.7.21 Skill to teach and demonstrate the components of an exercise session (i.e., warm-up, aerobic stimulus phase, cool-down, muscular strength/endurance, flexibility).

1.7.22 Skill to teach and demonstrate appropriate modifications in specific exercises for the following groups: older adults, pregnant and postnatal women, obese persons, and persons with low back pain.

1.7.23 Skill to teach and demonstrate appropriate exercises for improving range of motion of all major joints.

1.7.24 Skill in the use of various methods for establishing and monitoring levels of exercise intensity, including heart rate, RPE, and METs.

1.7.25 Ability to identify and apply methods used to monitor exercise intensity, including heart rate and rating of perceived exertion.

1.7.26 Ability to describe modifications in exercise prescriptions for individuals with functional disabilities and musculoskeletal injuries

1.7.27   Ability to differentiate between the amount of physical activity required for health benefits and the amount of exercise required for fitness development.

1.7.28   Ability to determine training heart rates using two methods: percent of age-predicted maximum heart rate and heart rate reserve (Karvonen).

1.7.29   Ability to identify proper and improper technique in the use of resistive equipment such as stability balls, weights, bands, resistance bars, and water exercise equipment.

1.7.30   Ability to identify proper and improper technique in the use of cardiovascular conditioning equipment (e.g., stairclimbers, stationary cycles, treadmills, elliptical trainers).

1.7.31   Ability to teach a progression of exercises for all major muscle groups to improve muscular strength and endurance.

1.7.32   Ability to communicate effectively with exercise participants.

1.7.33   Ability to design, implement, and evaluate individualized and group exercise programs based on health history and physical fitness assessments.

1.7.34   Ability to modify exercises based on age and physical condition.

1.7.35   Knowledge and ability to determine energy cost, $\dot{V}O_2$, METs, and target heart rates and apply the information to an exercise prescription.

1.7.36   Ability to convert weights from pounds (lb) to kilograms (kg) and speed from miles per hour (mph) to meters per minute (m/min^{-1}).

1.7.37   Ability to convert METs to $\dot{V}O_2$ expressed as mL/kg^{-1}/min^{-1}, L/min^{-1}, and/or mL/kg FFW^{-1}/min^{-1}.

1.7.38   Ability to determine the energy cost in METs and kilocalories for given exercise intensities in stepping exercise, cycle ergometry, and during horizontal and graded walking and running.

1.7.39   Ability to prescribe exercise intensity based on $\dot{V}O_2$ data for different modes of exercise, including graded and horizontal running and walking, cycling, and stepping exercise.

1.7.40   Ability to explain and implement exercise prescription guidelines for apparently healthy clients, increased risk clients, and clients with controlled disease.

1.7.41   Ability to adapt frequency, intensity, duration, mode, progression, level of supervision, and monitoring techniques in exercise programs for patients with controlled chronic disease (e.g., heart disease, diabetes mellitus, obesity, hypertension), musculoskeletal problems, pregnancy and/or postpartum, and exercise-induced asthma.

1.7.42   Ability to design resistive exercise programs to increase or maintain muscular strength and/or endurance.

1.7.43   Ability to evaluate flexibility and prescribe appropriate flexibility exercises for all major muscle groups.

1.7.44   Ability to design training programs using interval, continuous, and circuit training programs.

1.7.45   Ability to describe the advantages and disadvantages of various commercial exercise equipment in developing cardiorespiratory fitness, muscular strength, and muscular endurance.

1.7.46   Ability to modify exercise programs based on age, physical condition, and current health status.

NUTRITION AND WEIGHT MANAGEMENT

1.8.1   Knowledge of the role of carbohydrates, fats, and proteins as fuels for aerobic and anaerobic metabolism.

1.8.2   Knowledge to define the following terms: obesity, overweight, percent fat, lean body mass, anorexia nervosa, bulimia, and body fat distribution.

1.8.3 Knowledge of the relationship between body composition and health.

1.8.4 Knowledge of the effects of diet plus exercise, diet alone, and exercise alone as methods for modifying body composition.

1.8.5 Knowledge of the importance of an adequate daily energy intake for healthy weight management.

1.8.6 Knowledge of the difference between fat-soluble and water-soluble vitamins.

1.8.7 Knowledge of the importance of maintaining normal hydration before, during, and after exercise.

1.8.8 Knowledge of the USDA Food Pyramid.

1.8.9 Knowledge of the importance of calcium and iron in women's health.

1.8.10 Knowledge of the myths and consequences associated with inappropriate weight loss methods (e.g., saunas, vibrating belts, body wraps, electric simulators, sweat suits, fad diets).

1.8.11 Knowledge of the number of kilocalories in one gram of carbohydrate, fat, protein, and alcohol.

1.8.12 Knowledge of the number of kilocalories equivalent to losing 1 pound of body fat.

1.8.13 Knowledge of the guidelines for caloric intake for an individual desiring to lose or gain weight.

1.8.14 Knowledge of common nutritional ergogenic aids, the purported mechanism of action, and any risk and/or benefits (e.g., carbohydrates, protein/amino acids, vitamins, minerals, sodium bicarbonate, creatine, bee pollen).

1.8.15 Knowledge of nutritional factors related to the female athlete triad syndrome (i.e., eating disorders, menstrual cycle abnormalities, and osteoporosis).

1.8.16 Knowledge of the NIH Consensus statement regarding health risks of obesity, Nutrition for Physical Fitness Position Paper of the American Dietetic Association, and the ACSM Position Stand on proper and improper weight loss programs.

1.8.17 Ability to describe the health implications of variation in body fat distribution patterns and the significance of the waist to hip ratio.

HUMAN BEHAVIOR AND COUNSELING

1.9.1 Knowledge of at least five behavioral strategies to enhance exercise and health behavior change (e.g., reinforcement, goal setting, social support).

1.9.2 Knowledge of the five important elements that should be included in each counseling session.

1.9.3 Knowledge of specific techniques to enhance motivation (e.g., posters, recognition, bulletin boards, games, competitions). Define extrinsic and intrinsic reinforcement and give examples of each.

1.9.4 Knowledge of extrinsic and intrinsic reinforcement and give examples of each.

1.9.5 Knowledge of the stages of motivational readiness.

1.9.6 Knowledge of three counseling approaches that may assist less motivated clients to increase their physical activity.

1.9.7 Knowledge of symptoms of anxiety and depression that may necessitate referral to a medical or mental health professional.

1.9.8 Knowledge of the potential symptoms and causal factors of test anxiety (i.e., performance, appraisal threat during exercise testing) and how it may affect physiological responses to testing.

SAFETY, INJURY PREVENTION, AND EMERGENCY PROCEDURES

1.10.1 Knowledge of and skill in obtaining basic life support and cardiopulmonary resuscitation certification.

1.10.2 Knowledge of appropriate emergency procedures (i.e., telephone procedures, written emergency procedures, personnel responsibilities) in a health and fitness setting.

1.10.3 Knowledge of basic first aid procedures for exercise-related injuries, such as bleeding, strains/sprains, fractures, and exercise intolerance (dizziness, syncope, heat injury).

1.10.4 Knowledge of basic precautions taken in an exercise setting to ensure participant safety.

1.10.5 Knowledge of the physical and physiological signs and symptoms of overtraining.

1.10.6 Knowledge of the effects of temperature, humidity, altitude, and pollution on the physiological response to exercise.

1.10.7 Knowledge of the following terms: shin splints, sprain, strain, tennis elbow, bursitis, stress fracture, tendonitis, patellar femoral pain syndrome, low back pain, plantar fasciitis, and rotator cuff tendonitis.

1.10.8 Knowledge of hypothetical concerns and potential risks that may be associated with the use of exercises such as straight leg sit-ups, double leg raises, full squats, hurdlers stretch, yoga plough, forceful back hyperextension, and standing bent-over toe touch.

1.10.9 Knowledge of safety plans, emergency procedures, and first aid techniques needed during fitness evaluations, exercise testing, and exercise training.

1.10.10 Knowledge of the health/fitness instructor's responsibilities, limitations, and the legal implications of carrying out emergency procedures.

1.10.11 Knowledge of potential musculoskeletal injuries (e.g., contusions, sprains, strains, fractures), cardiovascular/pulmonary complications (e.g., tachycardia, bradycardia, hypotension/hypertension, tachypnea) and metabolic abnormalities (e.g., fainting/syncope, hypoglycemia/hyperglycemia, hypothermia/hyperthermia).

1.10.12 Knowledge of the initial management and first aid techniques associated with open wounds, musculoskeletal injuries, cardiovascular/pulmonary complications, and metabolic disorders.

1.10.13 Knowledge of the components of an equipment maintenance/repair program and how it may be used to evaluate the condition of exercise equipment to reduce the potential risk of injury.

1.10.14 Knowledge of the legal implications of documented safety procedures, the use of incident documents, and ongoing safety training.

1.10.15 Skill to demonstrate exercises used for people with low back pain.

1.10.16 Skill in demonstrating appropriate emergency procedures during exercise testing and/or training.

1.10.17 Ability to identify the components that contribute to the maintenance of a safe environment.

PROGRAM ADMINISTRATION, QUALITY ASSURANCE, AND OUTCOME ASSESSMENT

1.11.1 Knowledge of the health/fitness instructor's role in administration and program management within a health/fitness facility.

1.11.2 Knowledge of and the ability to use the documentation required when a client shows signs or symptoms during an exercise session and should be referred to a physician.

1.11.3   Knowledge of how to manage of a fitness department (e.g., working within a budget, training exercise leaders, scheduling, running staff meetings).

1.11.4   Knowledge of the importance of tracking and evaluating member retention.

1.11.5

1.11.6   Ability to administer fitness-related programs within established budgetary guidelines.

1.11.7   Ability to develop marketing materials for the purpose of promoting fitness-related programs.

1.11.8   Ability to create and maintain records pertaining to participant exercise adherence, retention, and goal setting.

1.11.9   Ability to develop and administer educational programs (e.g., lectures, workshops) and educational materials.

CARDIOVASCULAR: PATHOPHYSIOLOGY AND RISK FACTORS

2.2.1   Knowledge of cardiovascular risk factors or conditions that may require consultation with medical personnel before testing or training, including inappropriate changes of resting or exercise heart rate and blood pressure, new onset discomfort in chest, neck, shoulder, or arm, changes in the pattern of discomfort during rest or exercise, fainting or dizzy spells, and claudication.

2.2.2   Knowledge of the causes of myocardial ischemia and infarction.

2.2.3   Knowledge the pathophysiology of hypertension, obesity, hyperlipidemia, diabetes, chronic obstructive pulmonary diseases, arthritis, osteoporosis, chronic diseases, and immunosuppressive disease.

2.2.4   Knowledge the effects of the above diseases and conditions on cardiorespiratory and metabolic function at rest and during exercise.

PULMONARY: PATHOPHYSIOLOGY AND RISK FACTORS

3.2.1   Knowledge of respiratory risk factors or conditions that may require consultation with medical personnel before testing or training, including asthma, exercise-induced bronchospasm, extreme breathlessness at rest or during exercise, bronchitis, and emphysema.

METABOLIC: PATHOPHYSIOLOGY AND RISK FACTORS

4.2.1   Knowledge of metabolic risk factors or conditions that may require consultation with medical personnel before testing or training, including body weight more than 20% above optimal, BMI> 30, thyroid disease, diabetes or glucose intolerance, and hypoglycemia.

ORTHOPEDIC/MUSCULOSKELETAL: PATHOPHYSIOLOGY AND RISK FACTORS

5.2.1   Knowledge of musculoskeletal risk factors or conditions that may require consultation with medical personnel before testing or training, including acute or chronic back pain, osteoarthritis, rheumatoid arthritis, osteoporosis, tendonitis, and low back pain.

NOTE: The KSAs listed above for the ACSM Health/Fitness Instructor® are the same KSAs for educational programs seeking undergraduate (bachelor's degree) academic accreditation through the CoAES. Specifically, these programs are typically Exercise Science, Kinesiology, and/or Physical Education departments with professional development tracks for those students interested in careers in the fitness industry. For more information, please visit www.coaes.org.

ACSM Exercise Specialist® Knowledge, Skills, and Abilities (KSAs):

EXERCISE PHYSIOLOGY AND RELATED EXERCISE SCIENCE

1.1.1   **Describe coronary anatomy.**

1.1.2   **Describe the physiological effects of bed rest and discuss the appropriate physical activities that might be used to counteract these changes.**

1.1.3   Identify the cardiorespiratory responses associated with postural changes.

1.1.4   Describe activities that are primarily aerobic and anaerobic.

1.1.5   Identify the metabolic equivalent (MET) requirements of various occupational, household, sport/exercise, and leisure time activities.

1.1.6   Knowledge of the unique hemodynamic responses of arm versus leg exercise and of static versus dynamic exercise.

1.1.7   Define the determinants of myocardial oxygen consumption and the effects of exercise training on those determinants.

1.1.8   Determine maximal oxygen (O_2) consumption and describe the methodology for measuring it.

1.1.9   Plot the normal resting and exercise values associated with increasing exercise intensity (and how they may differ for diseased populations) for the following: heart rate, stroke volume, cardiac output, double product, arteriovenous O_2 difference, O_2 consumption, systolic and diastolic blood pressure, minute ventilation, tidal volume, breathing frequency, Vd/Vt, $\dot{V}_E/\dot{V}O_2$, and $\dot{V}_E/\dot{V}CO_2$.

1.1.10   **Discuss the effects of isometric exercise in individuals with cardiovascular, pulmonary, and/or metabolic diseases or with low functional capacity.**

1.1.11   **Knowledge of acute and chronic adaptations to exercise for apparently healthy individuals (low risk) and for those with cardiovascular, pulmonary, and metabolic diseases.**

1.1.12   **Describe the effects of variation in environmental factors (e.g. temperature, humidity, altitude) for normal individuals and those with cardiovascular, pulmonary, and metabolic diseases.**

PATHOPHYSIOLOGY AND RISK FACTORS

1.2.1   Summarize the atherosclerotic process, including current hypotheses regarding onset and rate of progression and/or regression.

1.2.2   Compare and contrast the differences between typical, atypical, and vasospastic angina.

1.2.3   Describe the pathophysiology of the healing myocardium and the potential complications after acute myocardial infarction (MI) (extension, expansion, rupture)

1.2.4   Describe silent ischemia and its implications for exercise testing and training.

1.2.5   **Examine the role of diet on cardiovascular risk factors such as hypertension, blood lipids and body weight.**

1.2.6   **Describe the lipoprotein classifications and define their relationship to atherosclerosis or other diseases.**

1.2.7   **Describe the cardiorespiratory and metabolic responses that accompany or result from pulmonary diseases at rest and during exercise.**

1.2.8   **Describe the influence of exercise on cardiovascular risk factors.**

1.2.9   **Describe the normal and abnormal cardiorespiratory responses at rest and exercise.**

1.2.10   **Identify the mechanisms by which functional capacity and cardiovascular, pulmonary, metabolic, and neuromuscular adaptations occur** in response to exercise testing and training in healthy and disease states.

1.2.11 **Describe the cardiorespiratory and metabolic responses in myocardial dysfunction and ischemia at rest and during exercise.**

HEALTH APPRAISAL, FITNESS AND CLINICAL EXERCISE TESTING

1.3.1 **Describe common procedures and apply knowledge of results from radionuclide imaging (e.g., thallium, technetium, sestamibi, single photon emission computed tomography (SPECT)).**

1.3.2 **Knowledge of exercise testing procedures for various clinical populations including those individuals with cardiovascular, pulmonary, and metabolic diseases in terms of exercise modality, protocol, physiological measurements, and expected outcomes.**

1.3.3 Describe anatomical landmarks as they relate to exercise testing and programming.

1.3.4 Locate and palpate anatomic landmarks of radial, brachial, carotid, femoral, popliteal, and tibialis arteries.

1.3.5 Select an appropriate test protocol according to the age and functional capacity of the individual.

1.3.6 Identify individuals for whom physician supervision is recommended during maximal and submaximal exercise testing.

1.3.7 Conduct pre-exercise test procedures.

1.3.8 Describe basic equipment and facility requirements for exercise testing.

1.3.9 Instruct the test participant in the use of the RPE scale and other appropriate subjective rating scales, such as the dyspnea and angina scales.

1.3.10 Obtain informed consent and describe its purpose.

1.3.11 Describe the importance of accurate and calibrated testing equipment (e.g., treadmill, ergometers, electrocardiograph, and sphygmomanometers).

1.3.12 Measure physiological and subjective responses (e.g., symptoms, ECG, blood pressure, heart rate, RPE and other scales, oxygen saturation, and oxygen consumption) at appropriate intervals during the test.

1.3.13 Describe the effects of age, weight, level of fitness, and health status on the selection of an exercise test protocol.

1.3.14 Ability to measure oxygen consumption during an exercise test.

1.3.15 Ability to provide testing procedures and protocol for children and the elderly with or without various clinical conditions.

1.3.16 **Obtain and interpret medical history and physical examination findings as they relate to health appraisal and exercise testing.**

1.3.17 **Accurately record and interpret right and left arm pre-exercise blood pressures in the supine and upright positions.**

1.3.18 **Describe and analyze the importance of the absolute and relative contraindications of an exercise test.**

1.3.19 **Select and perform appropriate procedures and protocols for the exercise test, including modes of exercise, starting levels, increments of work, ramping versus incremental protocols, length of stages, and frequency of data collection.**

1.3.20 **Describe and conduct immediate postexercise procedures and various approaches to cool-down.**

1.3.21 **Record, organize, perform, and interpret necessary calculations of test data.**

1.3.22 **Describe the differences in the physiological responses to various modes of ergometry (e.g., treadmill, cycle and arm ergometers) as they relate to exercise testing and training.**

1.3.23   Describe normal and abnormal chronotropic and inotropic responses to exercise testing and training.

1.3.24   Describe and apply Baye's theorem as it relates to pretest likelihood of CAD and the predictive value of positive or negative diagnostic exercise ECG results.

1.3.25   Compare and contrast obstructive and restrictive lung diseases and their effect on exercise testing and training.

1.3.26   Identify orthopedic limitations (e.g., gout, foot drop, specific joint problems) as they relate to modifications of exercise testing and programming.

1.3.27   Identify neuromuscular disorders (e.g., Parkinson's disease, multiple sclerosis) as they relate to modifications of exercise testing and programming.

1.3.28   Describe the aerobic and anaerobic metabolic demands of exercise testing and training in individuals with cardiovascular, pulmonary, and/or metabolic diseases undergoing exercise testing or training.

1.3.29   Identify the variables measured during cardiopulmonary exercise testing (e.g., heart rate, blood pressure, rate of perceived exertion, ventilation, oxygen consumption, ventilatory threshold, pulmonary circulation) and their potential relationship to cardiovascular, pulmonary, and metabolic disease.

1.3.30   Discuss the appropriate use of static and dynamic exercise for individuals with cardiovascular, pulmonary, and metabolic disease.

ELECTROCARDIOGRAPHY AND DIAGNOSTIC TECHNIQUES

1.4.1   Summarize the purpose of coronary angiography.

1.4.2   Describe myocardial ischemia and identify ischemic indicators of various cardiovascular diagnostic tests.

1.4.3   Describe the differences between Q-wave and non-Q-wave infarction.

1.4.4   Identify the ECG patterns at rest and responses to exercise in patients with pacemakers and ICDs.

1.4.5   Identify resting and exercise ECG changes associated with the following abnormalities:bundle branch blocks and bifascicular blocks; atrioventricular blocks; sinus bradycardia and tachycardia; sinus arrest; supraventricular premature contractions and tachycardia; ventricular premature contractions (including frequency, form, couplets, salvos, tachycardia); atrial flutter and fibrillation; ventricular fibrillation; myocardial ischemia, injury, and infarction.

1.4.6   Define the ECG criteria for initiating and/or terminating exercise testing or training.

1.4.7   Identify ECG changes that correspond to ischemia in various myocardial regions.

1.4.8   Describe potential causes of various cardiac arrhythmias.

1.4.9   Identify potentially hazardous arrhythmias or conduction defects observed on the ECG at rest, during exercise, and recovery.

1.4.10   Describe the diagnostic and prognostic significance of ischemic ECG responses and arrhythmias at rest, during exercise, or recovery.

1.4.11   Identify resting and exercise ECG changes associated with cardiovascular disease, hypertensive heart disease, cardiac chamber enlargement, pericarditis, pulmonary disease, and metabolic disorders.

1.4.12   Administer and interpret basic resting spirometric tests and measures including FEV1.0, FVC, and MVV.

1.4.13 Locate the appropriate sites for the limb and chest leads for resting, standard, and exercise (Mason Likar) electrocardiograms (ECGs), as well as commonly used bipolar systems (e.g., CM-5).

1.4.14 Obtain and interpret a pre-exercise standard and modified (Mason-Likar) 12-lead ECG on a participant in the supine and upright position.

1.4.15 Ability to minimize ECG artifact.

1.4.16 Describe the diagnostic and prognostic implications of the exercise test ECG and hemodynamic responses.

1.4.17 Identify ECG changes that typically occur due to hyperventilation, electrolyte abnormalities, and drug therapy.

1.4.18 Identify the causes of false positive and false negative exercise ECG responses and methods for optimizing sensitivity and specificity.

1.4.19 Identify and describe the significance of ECG abnormalities in designing the exercise prescription and in making activity recommendations.

1.4.20 Explain indications and procedures for combining exercise testing with radionuclide or echocardiographic imaging.

PATIENT MANAGEMENT AND MEDICATIONS

1.5.1 List indications for use of streptokinase, tissue plasminogen activase, and other thrombolytic agents.

1.5.2 Describe mechanisms and actions of medications that may affect exercise testing and prescription.

1.5.3 Recognize medications associated in the clinical setting, their indications for care, and their effects at rest and during exercise (e.g., antianginals, antihypertensives, antiarrythmics, bronchodilators, hypoglycemics, psychotropics, vasodilators, anticoagulant and antiplatelet drugs, and lipid-lowering agents).

MEDICAL AND SURGICAL MANAGEMENT

1.6.1 Describe percutaneous coronary and peripheral interventions (e.g., PTCA, stent) as an alternative to medical management or bypass surgery.

1.6.2 Describe indications and limitations for medical management and interventional techniques in different subsets of individuals with CAD and PAD.

EXERCISE PRESCRIPTION AND PROGRAMMING

1.7.1 Describe basic joint movements, muscle actions, and points of insertions as it relates to exercise programming.

1.7.2 Compare and contrast benefits and risks of exercise for individuals with CAD risk factors and for individuals with cardiovascular, pulmonary, and/or metabolic diseases.

1.7.3 Design appropriate exercise prescription in environmental extremes for normal individuals and those with cardiovascular, pulmonary, and metabolic diseases.

1.7.4 Design, implement and supervise individualized exercise prescriptions for people with chronic disease and disabling conditions.

1.7.5 Design a supervised exercise program beginning at hospital discharge and continuing for up to six months for the following conditions: MI; angina: LVAD; congestive heart failure; PCI; CABG; medical management of CAD; chronic pulmonary disease; weight management; diabetes; and cardiac transplants.

1.7.6 Knowledge of the concept of "Activities of Daily Living" (ADLs) and its importance in the overall rehabilitation of the individual.

1.7.7	**Prescribe exercise using nontraditional modalities (e.g., bench stepping, elastic bands, isodynamic exercise, water aerobics) for individuals with cardiovascular, pulmonary, or metabolic diseases.**
1.7.8	Discuss equipment adaptations necessary for different age groups.
1.7.9	Identify individuals who require exercise testing prior to exercise training.
1.7.10	Organize GXT and clinical data and counsel patients regarding issues such as ADL, return to work and physical activity.
1.7.11	Describe relative and absolute contraindications to exercise training.
1.7.12	Identify characteristics that correlate or predict poor compliance to exercise programs, and strategies to increase exercise adherence.
1.7.13	**Describe the importance of warm-up and cool-down sessions with specific reference to angina and ischemic ECG changes, and for overal patient safety.**
1.7.14	**Identify and explain the mechanisms by which exercise may contribute to preventing or rehabilitating individuals with cardiovascular, pulmonary, and metabolic diseases.**
1.7.15	**Describe common gait abnormalities as they relate to exercise testing and programming.**
1.7.16	**Describe the principle of specificity of training as it relates to the mode of exercise testing and training.**
1.7.17	**Design a strength and flexibility programs for individuals with cardiovascular, pulmonary and/or metabolic diseases, elderly, and children.**
1.7.18	**Determine appropriate testing and training modalities according to the age and functional capacity of the individual.**
1.7.19	**Describe the indications and methods for ECG monitoring during exercise testing and training.**
1.7.20	**Describe the importance of and appropriate methods for resistance training in older individuals.**
1.7.21	**Ability to modify exercise testing and training to the limitations of peripheral arterial disease (PAD).**

NUTRITION AND WEIGHT MANAGEMENT

1.8.1	**Describe and discuss dietary considerations for cardiovascular and pulmonary diseases, chronic heart failure, and diabetes that are recommended to minimize disease progression and optimize disease management.**
1.8.2	Compare and contrast dietary practices used for weight reduction and address the benefits, risks, and scientific support for each practice. Examples of dietary practices are high protein/low carbohydrate diets, Mediterranean diet, and low fat diets such as the American Heart Association recommended diet.
1.8.3	Calculate the effect of caloric intake and energy expenditure on weight management.

HUMAN BEHAVIOR AND COUNSELING

1.9.1	**List and apply five behavioral strategies as they apply to lifestyle modifications, such as exercise, diet, stress, and medication management.**
1.9.2	Describe signs and symptoms of maladjustment and/or failure to cope during an illness crisis and/or personal adjustment crisis (e.g., job loss) that might prompt a psychological consult or referral to other professional services.
1.9.3	Describe the general principles of crisis management and factors influencing coping and learning in illness states.

1.9.4   Identify the psychological stages involved with the acceptance of death and dying and ability to recognize when it is necessary for a psychological consult or referral to a professional resource.

1.9.5   Recognize observable signs and symptoms of anxiety or depressive symptoms and the need for a psychiatric referral.

1.9.6   Describe the psychological issues to be confronted by the patient and by family members of patients who have cardiovascular disease and/or who have had an acute MI or cardiac surgery.

1.9.7   Identify the psychological issues associated with an acute cardiac event versus those associated with chronic cardiac conditions.

SAFETY, INJURY PREVENTION, AND EMERGENCY PROCEDURES

1.10.1   Respond appropriately to emergency situations (e.g. cardiac arrest, hypoglecemia and hyperglycemia; bronchospasm; sudden onset hypotension; serious cardiac arrhythmias; implantable cardiac defibrillator (ICD) discharge; transient ischemic attack (TIA) or stroke; MI) which might arise before, during, and after administration of an exercise test and/or exercise session.

1.10.2   List medications that should be available for emergency situations in exercise testing and training sessions

1.10.3   Describe the emergency equipment and personnel that should be present in an exercise testing laboratory and rehabilitative exercise training setting.

1.10.4   Describe the appropriate procedures for maintaining emergency equipment and supplies.

1.10.5   Describe the effects of cardiovascular, pulmonary, and metabolic diseases on performance and safety during exercise testing and training.

1.10.6   Risk stratify individuals with cardiovascular, pulmonary, and metabolic diseases, using appropriate materials and understanding the prognostic indicators for high-risk individuals.

PROGRAM ADMINISTRATION, QUALITY ASSURANCE, AND OUTCOME ASSESSMENT

1.11.1   Discuss the role of outcome measures in chronic disease management programs such as cardiovascular and pulmonary rehabilitation programs.

1.11.2   Identify and discuss various outcome measurements that could be used in a cardiac or pulmonary rehabilitation program.

1.11.3   Identify and discuss specific outcome collection instruments that could be used to collect outcome data in a cardiac or pulmonary rehabilitation program.

ACSM Registered Clinical Exercise Physiologist Knowledge, Skills, and Abilities (KSAs):

GENERAL POPULATION/CORE:
KSA #   EXERCISE PHYSIOLOGY AND RELATED EXERCISE SCIENCE

1.1.1   Describe the acute responses to aerobic and resistance exercise training on the function of the cardiovascular, respiratory, musculoskeletal, neuromuscular, metabolic, endocrine, and immune systems.

1.1.2   Describe the chronic effects of aerobic, resistance, and flexibility exercise training on the structure and function of the cardiovascular, respiratory, musculoskeletal, neuromuscular, metabolic, endocrine, and immune systems.

1.1.3   List typical values in sedentary and trained persons for oxygen uptake, heart rate, mean arterial pressure, systolic and diastolic blood pressure, cardiac output, stroke volume, minute ventilation, respiratory rate, and tidal volume at rest and during submaximal and maximal exercise.

1.1.4   Describe the physiological determinants of VO2, MVO2, and mean arterial pressure and explain how these determinants may be altered with aerobic and resistance exercise training.

1.1.5   Explain how environmental factors may affect the physiological responses to exercise, including ambient temperature, humidity, air quality (e.g., CO, ozone, air pollution) and altitude, and describe appropriate alterations in exercise recommendations due to environmental conditions and patient health status.

1.1.6   Explain the health benefits of a physically active lifestyle, the hazards of sedentary behavior and summarize key recommendations of US national reports of physical activity (e.g. US Surgeon General, Institute of Medicine, ACSM, AHA)

1.1.7   Explain the physiological adaptations to exercise training that may result in improvement in or maintenance of health, including metabolic (i.e., Metabolic syndrome, glucose and lipid metabolism), cardiovascular (i.e., atherosclerosis), musculoskeletal (i.e. bone density), neuromuscular, pulmonary (i.e. lung function), and immune system (i.e. colds, acute illness) health.

1.1.8   Explain the mechanisms underlying the physiological adaptations to aerobic and resistance exercise training including those resulting in changes in or maintenance of maximal and submaximal oxygen consumption, lactate and ventilatory (anaerobic) threshold, myocardial oxygen consumption, heart rate, blood pressure, ventilation (including ventilatory (anaerobic) threshold), muscle structure, bioenergetics (e.g., substrate utilization), and immune function.

1.1.9   Explain the physiological effects of physical inactivity, including bed rest, and methods that may counteract these effects.

1.1.10   Recognize and respond to abnormal signs and symptoms during exercise.

GENERAL POPULATION/CORE:
HEALTH APPRAISAL, FITNESS AND CLINICAL EXERCISE TESTING

1.3.1   Conduct pre-test procedures including explaining test procedures to the patient and obtaining informed consent, obtaining a focused medical history and results of prior tests and physical exam, disease-specific risk factor assessment (i.e., CVD, Metabolic, Pulmonary diseases), presenting concise information to other health care providers and third party payers.

1.3.2   Conduct a brief physical examination including evaluation of peripheral edema, measuring blood pressure, peripheral pulses, respiratory rate, and ausculating heart and lung sounds.

1.3.3   Calibrate lab equipment used frequently in the practice of clinical exercise physiology (e.g. motorized/computerized treadmill, mechanical cycle ergometer and arm ergometer, electrocardiograph, spirometer, respiratory gas analyzer (Metabolic cart)).

1.3.4   Administer exercise tests consistent with US nationally accepted standards for testing (I.e., ACSM, AHA).

1.3.5   Identify contraindications to an exercise session

1.3.6   Appropriately select and administer functional tests to measure patient outcomes and functional status including the 6 minute walk, Get Up and Go, Berg Balance Scale, Physical Performance Test.

1.3.7   Evaluate patient outcomes from serial outcome data collected before, during and after exercise interventions.

1.3.8 Interpret the variables that may be assessed during clinical exercise testing including maximal oxygen consumption, resting Metabolic rate, ventilatory volumes and capacities, respiratory exchange ratio, ratings of perceived exertion and discomfort (chest pain, dyspnea, claudication), ECG, heart rate, blood pressure, rate pressure product, ventilatory (anaerobic) threshold, oxygen saturation, breathing reserve, muscular strength, and muscular endurance and other common measures employed for diagnosis and prognosis of disease.

1.3.9 Determine atrial and ventricular rate from rhythm strip and 12-lead ECG and explain the clinical significance of abnormal atrial or ventricular rate (e.g.. tachycardia, bradycardia).

1.3.10 Identify ECG changes associated with drug therapy, electrolyte abnormalities, subendocardial and transmural ischemia, myocardial injury, and infarction and explain the clinical significance of each.

1.3.11 Identify SA, AV, and bundle branch blocks from a rhythm strip & 12-lead ECG, and explain the clinical significance of each.

1.3.12 Identify sinus, atrial, functional, and ventricular dysrhythmias from a rhythm strip & 12-lead ECG, and explain the clinical significance of each.

1.3.13 Identify contraindications to exercise testing.

1.3.14 Determine an individual's pre-test and post-test probability of CHD, identify factors associated with test complications, and apply appropriate precautions to reduce risks to the patient.

1.3.15 Extract and interpret clinical information needed for safe exercise management of individuals with chronic disease.

1.3.16 Identify probable disease-specific endpoints for testing in a patient with chronic disease or disability.

1.3.17 Select and employ appropriate techniques for preparation and measurement of ECG, heart rate, blood pressure, oxygen saturation, RPE, symptoms (e.g., angina, dyspnea, claudication), expired gases, and other measures as needed before, during and following exercise, pharmacologic, echocardiography, and radionuclide tests.

1.3.18 Select and administer appropriate exercise tests to evaluate functional capacity, strength, and flexibility in patients with chronic disease.

1.3.19 Discuss strengths and limitations of various methods of measures and indices of body composition.

1.3.20 Appropriately select, apply, and interpret body composition tests and indices.

GENERAL POPULATION/CORE: EXERCISE PRESCRIPTION AND PROGRAMMING

1.7.1 Adapt Exercise Prescriptions for patients with comorbid conditions and disease complications.

1.7.2 Design and supervise comprehensive exercise programs for outpatients with chronic disease

1.7.3 Determine the appropriate level of supervision and monitoring recommended for individuals with known disease based on chronic disease risk stratification (e.g., cardiovascular, metabolic, musculoskeletal, etc), and current health status.

1.7.4 Develop and supervise an appropriate Exercise Prescription (e.g., aerobic, strength and flexibility training) for individuals with co-morbid disease.

1.7.5 Implement appropriate precautions prior to, during, and following exercise in patients with chronic disease according to health status, medical treatment, environmental conditions, and other relevant factors.

1.7.6 Instruct individuals with chronic disease in techniques for performing physical activities safely and effectively in an unsupervised exercise setting.

1.7.7   Modify the Exercise Prescription or discontinue exercise based upon patient symptoms, current health status, musculoskeletal limitations, and environmental considerations.

GENERAL POPULATION/CORE: HUMAN BEHAVIOR AND COUNSELING

1.9.1   Summarize contemporary theories of health behavior change including social cognitive theory, theory of reasoned action, theory of planned behavior, Transtheoretical model, health belief model and apply techniques to promote healthy behaviors including physical activity.

1.9.2   Describe characteristics associated with poor adherence to exercise programs.

1.9.3   Describe the psychological issues associated with acute and chronic illness such as depression, social isolation, hostility, aggression, and suicidal ideation.

1.9.4   Counsel patients with chronic diseases and conditions on topics such as disease processes, treatments, diagnostic techniques, and lifestyle management.

1.9.5   Select and apply behavioral techniques such as goal setting, relapse prevention, and social support, which enhance adoption of and adherence to healthy behaviors including exercise.

1.9.6   Explain factors that may increase anxiety prior to or during exercise testing and describe methods to reduce anxiety.

1.9.7   Recognize signs and symptoms of failure to cope during personal crises such as job loss, bereavement, and illness.

GENERAL POPULATION/CORE:
SAFETY, INJURY PREVENTION, AND EMERGENCY PROCEDURES

1.10.1   List routine emergency equipment, drugs, and supplies present in an exercise testing laboratory and therapeutic exercise session area.

1.10.2   Provide immediate responses to emergencies (I.e., first responder) including basic cardiac life support, AED, joint immobilization, activation of EMS.

1.10.3   Verify operating status of emergency equipment including defibrillator, laryngoscope, oxygen, etc.

1.10.4   Explain Universal Precautions procedures and apply as appropriate.

1.10.5   Develop and implement a plan for responding to emergencies.

GENERAL POPULATION/CORE: PROGRAM ADMINISTRATION,
QUALITY ASSURANCE AND OUTCOME ASSESSMENT

1.11.1   Describe appropriate staffing for exercise programs and exercise testing laboratories based on factors such as patient health status, facilities, and program goals.

1.11.2   List necessary equipment and supplies for exercise programs and exercise testing laboratories.

1.11.3   Select, document and report treatment outcomes using patient-relevant results of tests (e.g., exercise tests, physical work simulations, biomarkers, and other laboratory tests) and surveys (e.g., physical functioning and health-related quality of life).

1.11.4   Explain legal issues pertinent to health care delivery by licensed and non-licensed health care professionals providing rehabilitative services and exercise testing (e.g., torts, contracts, informed consent, negligence, malpractice, liability, standards of care) and legal risk management techniques.

1.11.5   Identify patients requiring referral to a physician or allied health services such as physical therapy, dietary counseling, stress management, weight management, psychosocial and social services.

1.11.6   Develop a plan for patient discharge from therapeutic exercise program, including community referrals.

CARDIOVASCULAR: EXERCISE PHYSIOLOGY AND RELATED EXERCISE SCIENCE

2.1.1   Describe the indications for, physiologic responses to, and potential complications of pharmacological and pacing stress testing in individuals with cardiovascular diseases.

2.1.2   Describe the potential benefits and hazards of aerobic, resistance, and flexibility exercise in individuals with cardiovascular diseases.

2.1.3   Explain how cardiovascular diseases may affect the physiological responses to exercise training on the ischemic cascade and the components of the Fick equation.

CARDIOVASCULAR: PATHOPHYSIOLOGY AND RISK FACTORS

2.2.1   Explain current hypotheses regarding the pathophysiology of atherosclerosis, including the etiology and rate of progression of disease.

2.2.2   Describe the epidemiology, pathophysiology, risk factors, and key clinical findings of cardiovascular diseases

2.2.3   Explain the ischemic cascade and its effect on myocardial function.

CARDIOVASCULAR: HEALTH APPRAISAL, FITNESS AND CLINICAL EXERCISE TESTING

2.3.1   Describe common techniques used to diagnose cardiovascular disease, including echocardiography, radionuclide imaging, angiography, pharmacologic testing, and biomarkers (e.g., Troponin, CK, etc) and explain the indications, limitations, risks and normal and abnormal results for each.

2.3.2   Explain how cardiovascular disease may affect physical examination findings.

2.3.3   List the key clinical findings during a physical exam of a patient with cardiovascular diseases.

2.3.4   Recognize and respond to abnormal signs and symptoms in individuals with cardiovascular diseases such as pain, peripheral edema, dyspnea, fatigue.

CARDIOVASCULAR: MEDICAL AND SURGICAL MANAGEMENT

2.6.2   Explain the common medical and surgical treatments of cardiovascular diseases including pharmacologic therapy, revascularization procedures, ICD, pacemakers, and transplant.

2.6.3   Summarize key recommendations current U.S. clinical practice guidelines for the prevention, treatment and management of cardiovascular diseases (e.g., AHA, ACC, NHLBI)

2.6.4   List the drug classifications commonly used in the treatment of individuals with cardiovascular diseases, name common generic and brand names drugs within each class, and explain the purposes, indications, major side effects, and the effects, if any, on the exercising individual.

2.6.5   Explain how treatments for cardiovascular disease, including preventive care, may affect the rate of progression of disease.

2.6.6   Apply current U.S. national guidelines for primary and secondary prevention of heart disease (e.g., lipoproteins, obesity, pharmacologic, behavioral) to identify and manage cardiovascular risk.

CARDIOVASCULAR: EXERCISE PRESCRIPTION AND PROGRAMMING

2.7.1   Develop an appropriate Exercise Prescription (e.g., aerobic, strength and flexibility training) for individuals with cardiovascular disease.

2.7.2   Design & adapt Exercise Prescriptions for individuals with cardiovascular disease to accomodate physical disabilities and complications due to cardiovascular diseases

2.7.3   Design and supervise comprehensive outpatient exercise programs for individuals with cardiovascular disorders.

2.7.4   Instruct an individual with cardiovascular diseases and disabilities in techniques for performing physical activities safely and effectively in an unsupervised exercise setting.

PULMONARY: EXERCISE PHYSIOLOGY AND RELATED EXERCISE SCIENCE

3.1.1   Describe the potential benefits and hazards of aerobic, resistance, and flexibility exercise in individuals with Pulmonary diseases.
3.1.2   Explain how Pulmonary diseases may affect the physiologic responses to aerobic, resistance, and flexibility exercise.
3.1.3   Explain how scheduling of exercise relative to meals can affect dyspnea.
3.1.4   Explain how Pulmonary diseases may affect range of motion, muscular strength and endurance.

PULMONARY: PATHOPHYSIOLOGY AND RISK FACTORS

3.2.1   Describe the epidemiology, pathophysiology, risk factors, and key clinical findings of Pulmonary diseases
3.2.2   Explain the common medical and surgical treatments of Pulmonary diseases including pharmacologic therapy, surgery, and transplant.

PULMONARY: HEALTH APPRAISAL, FITNESS AND CLINICAL EXERCISE TESTING

3.3.1   Explain how Pulmonary disease may affect physical examination findings
3.3.2   List the key clinical findings during a physical exam of a patient with Pulmonary disease
3.3.3   Have knowledge of lung volumes and capacities (e.g., tidal volume, residual volume, inspiratory volume, expiratory volume, total lung capacity, vital capacity, functional residual capacity, peak flow rate) and how they may differ between normals and patients with Pulmonary disease.
3.3.4   Recognize and respond to abnormal signs and symptoms in individuals with Pulmonary diseases such as wheezing, cough, sputum, edema, dyspnea, fatigue.

PULMONARY: MEDICAL AND SURGICAL MANAGEMENT

3.6.1   Describe the epidemiology, pathophysiology, risk factors, and key clinical findings of Pulmonary diseases
3.6.2   List the drug classifications commonly used in the treatment of individuals with Pulmonary diseases and disabilities, name common generic and brand names drugs within each class, and explain the purposes, indications, major side effects, and the effects, if any, on the exercising individual.
3.6.3   Explain how treatments for Pulmonary disease, including preventive care, may affect the rate of progression of disease.
3.6.4   List the risk factors for Pulmonary disease and explain methods of reducing risk.

PULMONARY: EXERCISE PRESCRIPTION AND PROGRAMMING

3.7.1   Develop an appropriate Exercise Prescription (e.g., aerobic, strength, flexibility training) for individuals with chronic Pulmonary diseases.
3.7.2   Design & adapt Exercise Prescriptions for individuals with chronic Pulmonary diseases to accommodate physical disabilities and complications due to Pulmonary diseases
3.7.3   Design and supervise comprehensive outpatient exercise programs for individuals with chronic Pulmonary disease.
3.7.4   Instruct an individual with Pulmonary diseases in proper breathing techniques and exercises and methods for performing physical activities safely and effectively in an unsupervised exercise setting.

METABOLIC: PATHOPHYSIOLOGY AND RISK FACTORS

4.2.1　Describe the epidemiology, pathophysiology, risk factors, and key clinical findings of Metabolic diseases (e.g. Renal Failure, Diabetes, Hyperlipidemia, Obesity, Frailty)

4.2.2　Explain current hypotheses regarding the pathophysiology of Metabolic diseases, including the etiology and rate of progression of disease.

4.2.3　Describe the potential benefits and hazards of aerobic, resistance, and flexibility exercise in individuals with Metabolic diseases.

4.2.4　Explain how Metabolic diseases may affect the physiologic responses to aerobic, resistance, and flexibility exercise.

4.2.5　Describe the probable effects of dialysis treatment on exercise performance, functional capacity, and safety, and explain methods for preventing adverse effects

4.2.6　Describe the probable effects of hypo/hyperglycemia on exercise performance, functional capacity, and safety, and explain methods for preventing adverse effect

METABOLIC: HEALTH APPRAISAL, FITNESS AND CLINICAL EXERCISE TESTING

4.3.1　Describe common techniques used to diagnose Metabolic diseases including biomarkers, glucose tolerance testing, GFR, and explain the indications, limitations, risks and normal and abnormal results for each.

4.3.2　List the key clinical findings during a physical exam of a patient with Metabolic disease(s).

4.3.3　Explain appropriate techniques for monitoring blood glucose before, during, and after an exercise session.

4.3.4　Recognize and respond to abnormal signs and symptoms in individuals with Metabolic diseases such as hypo/ hyperglycemia, peripheral neuropathies, fluid overload, loss of appetite, low hematocrit, and hypotension, and orthopedic problems.

METABOLIC: MEDICAL AND SURGICAL MANAGEMENT

4.6.2　Summarize key recommendations of current U.S. clinical practice guidelines (e.g. ADA, NIH, NHLBI) for the prevention, treatment and management of Metabolic diseases (e.g. Renal Failure, Diabetes, Hyperlipidemia, Obesity, Frailty)

4.6.3　Explain the common medical and surgical treatments of Metabolic diseases including pharmacologic therapy, surgery, and transplant.

4.6.4　List the drug classifications commonly used in the treatment of patients with Metabolic disease, name common generic and brand names drugs within each class, and explain the purposes, indications, major side effects, and the effects, if any, on the exercising individual.

4.6.5　Explain how treatments for Metabolic diseases, including preventive care, may affect the rate of progression of disease.

4.6.6　Apply current U.S. national guidelines for prevention of Metabolic diseases to identify and manage disease complications and reduce cardiovascular risk (i.e. ADA).

4.6.7　Apply current U.S. national guidelines for primary prevention of heart disease (e.g., lipoproteins, obesity, pharmacologic, behavioral) to identify and manage cardiovascular risk.

METABOLIC: EXERCISE PRESCRIPTION AND PROGRAMMING

4.7.1　Develop an appropriate Exercise Prescription (e.g., aerobic, strength, flexibility training) for individuals with Metabolic disease.

4.7.2   Design, adapt, and supervise an Exercise Prescription for patients with complications due to Metabolic diseases (e.g., amputations, retinopathy, autonomic neuropathies, vision impairment, hypotension, hypertension and during hemodialysis treatments)

4.7.3   Design and supervise comprehensive outpatient exercise programs for individuals with Metabolic diseases.

4.7.4   Instruct individuals with Metabolic diseases in techniques for performing physical activities safely and effectively in an unsupervised exercise setting.

ORTHOPEDIC/MUSCULOSKELETAL:
EXERCISE PHYSIOLOGY AND RELATED EXERCISE SCIENCE

5.1.1   Describe the potential benefits and hazards of aerobic, resistance, and flexibility exercise in individuals with musculoskeletal diseases and disabilities (e.g., low back pain, arthritis, osteoporosis/fibromyalgia, and tendinitis/impingement syndrome, amputation).

5.1.2   Explain how musculoskeletal diseases may affect the physiologic responses to aerobic, resistance, and flexibility exercise.

5.1.3   Describe the appropriate use of rest, spinal extension-flexion exercises vs. lumbar stabilization, and the appropriate dose of avoidance of physical activity in patients with back pain.

5.1.4   Explain how musculoskeletal diseases and disabilities may affect functional capacity, range of motion, balance, agility, muscular strength and endurance.

ORTHOPEDIC/MUSCULOSKELETAL: PATHOPHYSIOLOGY AND RISK FACTORS

5.2.1   Describe the epidemiology, pathophysiology, risk factors, and key clinical findings of orthopedic/musculoskeletal diseases & disabilities (e.g., low back pain, arthritis, osteoporosis, tendonitis/impingement syndrome, and amputation)

ORTHOPEDIC/MUSCULOSKELETAL: HEALTH APPRAISAL, FITNESS AND
CLINICAL EXERCISE TESTING

5.3.1   Recognize and respond to abnormal signs and symptoms in individuals with musculoskeletal diseases and disabilities such as pain, muscle weakness.

ORTHOPEDIC/MUSCULOSKELETAL: MEDICAL AND SURGICAL MANAGEMENT

5.6.1   List the drug classifications commonly used in the treatment of patients with musculoskeletal diseases and disabilities, name common generic and brand names drugs within each class, and explain the purposes, indications, major side effects, and the effects, if any, on the exercising individual.

5.6.2   Explain how treatments for musculoskeletal disease, including preventive care, may affect the rate of progression of disease.

ORTHOPEDIC/MUSCULOSKELETAL: EXERCISE PRESCRIPTION
AND PROGRAMMING

5.7.1   Explain exercise training concepts specific to industrial or occupational rehabilitation, which includes work hardening, work conditioning, work fitness, and job coaching.

5.7.2   Design, adapt, and supervise an Exercise Prescription (aerobic, strength, and flexibility training) to accommodate patients with complications due to musculoskeletal diseases & disabilities (e.g., low back pain, arthritis, osteoporosis, tendinitis/impingement syndrome and amputation)

5.7.3   Instruct an individual with musculoskeletal diseases and disabilities in techniques for performing physical activities safely and effectively in an unsupervised exercise setting.

NEUROMUSCULAR: EXERCISE PHYSIOLOGY AND RELATED EXERCISE SCIENCE

6.1.1   Describe the potential benefits and hazards of aerobic, resistance, and flexibility exercise in individuals with Neuromuscular diseases & disabilities (e.g., Multiple Sclerosis, Muscular Dystrophy, Parkinson's Disease, Polio and Post Polio Syndrome, Stroke and Head Injury, Cerebral Palsy, Amyotrophic Lateral Sclerosis, Peripheral Neuropathy, Spinal cord injury, Epilepsy)

6.1.2   Explain how Neuromuscular diseases may affect the physiologic responses to aerobic, resistance, and flexibility exercise.

6.1.3   Describe the effects of nonmotor complications, such as fatigue, on exercise performance in patients with Neuromuscular diseases and disabilities.

6.1.4   Explain how Neuromuscular diseases and disabilities may affect range of motion, balance, agility, muscular strength and endurance.

NEUROMUSCULAR: HEALTH APPRAISAL, FITNESS AND CLINICAL EXERCISE TESTING

6.3.1   Recognize and respond to abnormal signs and symptoms in individuals with Neuromuscular diseases and disabilities such as muscle weakness, cognitive deficit, fatigue.

NEUROMUSCULAR: EXERCISE PRESCRIPTION AND PROGRAMMING

6.7.1   Adapt the Exercise Prescription based on the functional limits and benefits of assistive devices (e.g. wheelchairs, crutches, and canes).

6.7.2   Develop an appropriate Exercise Prescription (e.g. aerobic, strength, flexibility training) for individuals with Neuromuscular diseases and disabilities including those treated with surgery.

6.7.3   Design, Adapt, and Supervise aerobic, strength training and flexibility exercise routines to accommodate patients with complications due to Neuromuscular diseases and disabilities (e.g., Multiple Sclerosis, Muscular Dystrophy, Parkinson's Disease, Polio and Post Polio Syndrome, Stroke and Head Injury, Cerebral Palsy, Amyotrophic Lateral Sclerosis, Peripheral Neuropathy, Spinal cord injury, Epilepsy)

6.7.4   Instruct an individual with Neuromuscular diseases and disabilities in techniques for performing physical activities safely and effectively in an unsupervised exercise setting.

IMMUNOLOGIC: EXERCISE PHYSIOLOGY AND RELATED EXERCISE SCIENCE

7.1.1   Describe the immediate and long-term influence of medical therapies for NIH on Cardiopulmonary and musculoskeletal responses to exercise training.

7.1.2   Describe the potential benefits and hazards of aerobic, resistance, and flexibility exercise in individuals with NIH disease (e.g. cancer, anemia, bleeding disorders, AIDS, organ transplant, Chronic Fatigue Syndrome)

7.1.3   Explain how NIH diseases may affect the physiologic responses to aerobic, resistance, and flexibility exercise.

7.1.4   Explain how cancer therapy (e.g., surgery, radiation, and chemotherapy) may affect functional capacity, range of motion, and the physiological responses to exercise.

7.1.5   Apply current U.S. national guidelines for primary and secondary prevention of NIH disease (e.g. ACS, NIH).

IMMUNOLOGIC: PATHOPHYSIOLOGY AND RISK FACTORS

7.2.1 Describe the epidemiology, pathophysiology, risk factors, and key clinical findings of NIH diseases (e.g. cancer, anemia, bleeding disorders, AIDS, organ transplant, Chronic Fatigue Syndrome)

IMMUNOLOGIC: HEALTH APPRAISAL, FITNESS AND CLINICAL EXERCISE TESTING

7.3.1 Recognize and respond to abnormal signs and symptoms in individuals with NIH diseases such as fatigue, dyspnea, tachycardia.

IMMUNOLOGIC: MEDICAL AND SURGICAL MANAGEMENT

7.6.1 List the drug classifications commonly used in the treatment of patients with NIH disease, name common generic and brand names drugs within each class, and explain the purposes, indications, major side effects, and the effects, if any, on the exercising individual.

7.6.2 Summarize key recommendations of current U.S. clinical practice guidelines (e.g. ACS, NIH) for the prevention, treatment and management of NIH diseases (e.g. cancer, anemia, bleeding disorders, AIDS, organ transplant, Chronic Fatigue Syndrome)

7.6.3 Explain the common medical and surgical treatments of NIH diseases including pharmacologic therapy, and surgery.

IMMUNOLOGIC: EXERCISE PRESCRIPTION AND PROGRAMMING

7.7.1 Develop an appropriate Exercise Prescription (e.g. aerobic, strength, flexibility training) for individuals with NIH disorders (e.g. cancer, anemia, bleeding disorders, AIDS, organ transplant, Chronic Fatigue Syndrome)

7.7.2 Design, adapt, and supervise the Exercise Prescription to accommodate patients with physical disabilities and complications due to NIH diseases

7.7.3 Design and supervise comprehensive outpatient exercise programs for individuals with immunologic/hematological disorders (e.g. cancer, anemia, bleeding disorders, AIDS, organ transplant, Chronic Fatigue Syndrome)

7.7.4 Instruct an individual with immunologic/hematological diseases and disabilities in techniques for performing physical activities safely and effectively in an unsupervised exercise setting.

NOTE: The KSAs listed above for the ACSM Registered Clinical Exercise Specialist® are the same KSAs for educational programs in Clinical Exercise Physiology seeking graduate (master's degree) academic accreditation through the CoAES. For more information, please visit www.coaes.org.

Additional KSAs required (in addition to the ACSM Health/Fitness Instructor® KSAs) for programs seeking academic accreditation in Applied Exercise Physiology

The KSAs that follow, IN ADDITION TO the ACSM Health/Fitness Instructor® KSAs above, represent the KSAs for educational programs in Applied Exercise Physiology seeking graduate (master's degree) academic accreditation through the CoAES. For more information, please visit www.coaes.org.

GENERAL POPULATION/CORE:
KSA #   **EXERCISE PHYSIOLOGY AND RELATED EXERCISE SCIENCE**

1.1.1 Ability to describe modifications in exercise prescription for individuals with functional disabilities and musculoskeletal injuries.

1.1.2   Ability to describe the relationship between biomechanical efficiency, oxygen cost of activity (economy), and performance of physical activity.

1.1.3   Knowledge of the muscular, cardiorespiratory, and metabolic responses to decreased exercise intensity.

GENERAL POPULATION/CORE: PATHOPHYSIOLOGY AND RISK FACTORS

1.2.1   Ability to define atherosclerosis, the factors causing it, and the interventions that may potentially delay or reverse the atherosclerotic process.

1.2.2   Ability to describe the causes of myocardial ischemia and infarction.

1.2.3   Ability to describe the pathophysiology of hypertension, obesity, hyperlipidemia, diabetes, chronic obstructive pulmonary diseases, arthritis, osteoporosis, chronic diseases, and immunosuppressive disease.

1.2.4   Ability to describe the effects of the above diseases and conditions on cardiorespiratory and metabolic function at rest and during exercise.

GENERAL POPULATION/CORE: HEALTH APPRAISAL, FITNESS AND CLINICAL EXERCISE TESTING

1.3.1   Knowledge of the selection of an appropriate behavioral goal and the suggested method to evaluate goal achievement for each stage of change.

1.3.2   Knowledge of the use and value of the results of the fitness evaluation and exercise test for various populations.

1.3.3   Ability to design and implement a fitness testing/health appraisal program that includes, but is not limited to, staffing needs, physician interaction, documentation, equipment, marketing, and program evaluation.

1.3.4   Ability to recruit, train, and evaluate appropriate staff personnel for performing exercise tests, fitness evaluations, and health appraisals.

GENERAL POPULATION/CORE: MEDICAL AND SURGICAL MANAGEMENT

1.5.1   Ability to identify and describe the principal action, mechanisms of action, and major side effects from each of the following classes of medications: Antianginals, Antihypertensives, Antiarrhythmics, Bronchodilators, Hypoglycemics, Psychotropics, and Vasodilators.

GENERAL POPULATION/CORE: HUMAN BEHAVIOR AND COUNSELING

1.9.1   Knowledge of and ability to apply basic cognitive-behavioral intervention such as shaping, goal setting, motivation, cueing, problem solving, reinforcement strategies, and self-monitoring.

1.9.2   Knowledge of the selection of an appropriate behavioral goal and the suggested method to evaluate goal achievement for each stage of change.

GENERAL POPULATION/CORE: SAFETY, INJURY PREVENTION, AND EMERGENCY PROCEDURES

1.10.1   Ability to identify the process to train the exercise staff in cardiopulmonary resuscitation.

1.10.2   Ability to design and evaluate emergency procedures for a preventive exercise program and an exercise testing facility.

1.10.3   Ability to train staff in safety procedures, risk reduction strategies, and injury care techniques.

1.10.4   Knowledge of the legal implications of documented safety procedures, the use of incident documents, and ongoing safety training.

GENERAL POPULATION/CORE: PROGRAM ADMINISTRATION, QUALITY ASSURANCE AND OUTCOME ASSESSMENT

1.11.1	Ability to manage personnel effectively.
1.11.2	Ability to describe a management plan for the development of staff, continuing education, marketing and promotion, documentation, billing, facility management, and financial planning.
1.11.3	Ability to describe the decision-making process related to budgets, market analysis, program evaluation, facility management, staff allocation, and community development.
1.11.4	Ability to describe the development, evaluation, and revision of policies and procedures for programming and facility management.
1.11.5	Ability to describe how the computer can assist in data analysis, spread-sheet report development, and daily tracking of customer utilization.
1.11.6	Ability to define and describe the total quality management (TQM) and continuous quality improvement (CQI) approaches to management.
1.11.7	Ability to interpret applied research in the areas of exercise testing, exercise programming, and educational programs to maintain a comprehensive and current state-of-the-art program.
1.11.8	Ability to develop a risk factor screening program, including procedures, staff training, feedback, and follow-up.
1.11.9	Knowledge of administration, management and supervision of personnel.
1.11.10	Ability to describe effective interviewing, hiring, and employee termination procedures.
1.11.11	Ability to describe and diagram an organizational chart and show the relationships between a health/fitness director, owner, medical advisor, and staff.
1.11.12	Knowledge of and ability to describe various staff training techniques.
1.11.13	Knowledge of and ability to describe performance reviews and their roll in evaluating staff.
1.11.14	Knowledge of the legal obligations and problems involved in personnel management.
1.11.15	Knowledge of compensation, including wages, bonuses, incentive pro-grams, and benefits.
1.11.16	Knowledge of methods for implementing a sales commission system.
1.11.17	Ability to describe the significance of a benefits program for staff and demonstrate an understanding in researching and selecting benefits.
1.11.18	Ability to write and implement thorough and legal job descriptions.
1.11.19	Knowledge of personnel time management techniques.
1.11.20	Knowledge of administration, management, and development of a budget and of the financial aspects of a fitness center.
1.11.21	Knowledge of the principles of financial management.
1.11.22	Knowledge of basic accounting principles such as accounts payable, accounts receivable, accrual, cash flow, assets, liabilities, and return on investment.
1.11.23	Ability to identify the various forms of a business enterprise such as sole proprietorship, partnership, corporation, and S-corporation.
1.11.24	Knowledge of the procedures involved with developing, evaluating, revis-ing, and updating capital and operating budgets.
1.11.25	Ability to manage expenses with the objective of maintaining a positive cash flow.
1.11.26	Ability to understand and analyze financial statements, including income statements, balance sheets, cash flows, budgets, and pro forma projections.

1.11.27   Knowledge of program-related break-even and cost/benefit analysis.

1.11.28   Knowledge of the importance of short-term and long-term planning.

1.11.29   Knowledge of the principles of marketing and sales.

1.11.30   Ability to identify the steps in the development, implementation, and evaluation of a marketing plan.

1.11.31   Knowledge of the components of a needs assessment/market analysis.

1.11.32   Knowledge of various sales techniques for prospective members.

1.11.33   Knowledge of techniques for advertising, marketing, promotion, and public relations.

1.11.34   Ability to describe the principles of developing and evaluating product and services, and establishing pricing.

1.11.35   Knowledge of the principles of day-to-day operation of a fitness center.

1.11.36   Knowledge of the principles of pricing and purchasing equipment and supplies.

1.11.37   Knowledge of facility layout and design.

1.11.38   Ability to establish and evaluate an equipment preventive maintenance and repair program.

1.11.39   Ability to describe a plan for implementing a housekeeping program.

1.11.40   Ability to identify and explain the operating policies for preventive exercise programs, including data analysis and reporting, confidentiality of records, relationships with health care providers, accident and injury reporting, and continuing education of participants.

1.11.41   Knowledge of the legal concepts of tort, negligence, liability, indemnification, standards of care, health regulations, consent, contract, confidentiality, malpractice, and the legal concerns regarding emergency procedures and informed consent.

1.11.42   Ability to implement capital improvements with minimal disruption of client or business needs.

1.11.43   Ability to coordinate the operations of various departments, including, but not limited to, the front desk, fitness, rehabilitation, maintenance and repair, day care, housekeeping, pool, and management.

1.11.44   Knowledge of management and principles of member service and communication.

1.11.45   Skills in effective techniques for communicating with staff, management, members, health care providers, potential customers, and vendors.

1.11.46   Knowledge of and ability to provide strong customer service.

1.11.47   Ability to develop and implement customer surveys.

1.11.48   Knowledge of the strategies for management conflict.

1.11.49   Knowledge of the principles of health promotion and ability to administer health promotion programs.

1.11.50   Knowledge of health promotion programs (e.g., nutrition and weight management, smoking cessation, stress management, back care, body mechanics, and substance abuse).

1.11.51   Knowledge of the specific and appropriate content and methods for creating a health promotion program.

1.11.52   Knowledge of and ability to access resources for various programs and delivery systems.

1.11.53   Knowledge of the concepts of cost-effectiveness and cost-benefit as they relate to the evaluation of health promotion programming.

1.11.54   Ability to describe the means and amounts by which health promotion programs might increase productivity, reduce employee loss time, reduce health care costs, and improve profitability in the workplace.

Index

Page numbers in *italics* denote figures; those followed by t denote tables; those followed by b denote boxes.

A

AACVPR (American Association of Cardiovascular and Pulmonary Rehabilitation), preparticipation risk stratification for cardiac patients, 19–22, 31, 31b–32b

Absolute intensity, defined, 4

Accolate, (*see* Zafirlukast)

Accupril, (*see* Quinapril)

Accuretic, (*see* Quinapril, and hydrochlorothiazide)

ACE inhibitors, (*see* Angiotensin converting enzyme (ACE) inhibitors)

Acebutolol, 255t, 261t

Aceon, (*see* Perindopril)

ACSM (American College of Sports Medicine)
Certification Resource Center, contact information, 311
certifications of, 309–349 (*see also* ACSM certification)
Committee on Certification and Registry Boards, 310
goals of, for health related physical fitness, 133–134
mission of, 5–7
preparticipation health screening guidelines of, 19–31
risk stratification categories of, 28–29, 28t

ACSM certification, 309–310
as Exercise Specialist, 311, *313*
KSA (knowledge, skills, abilities) requisites for, 332–337
as Health/Fitness Instructor, 311, *312*
KSA (knowledge, skills, abilities) requisites for, 323–331, 346–349
information and application materials for, 311
KSA (knowledge, skills, abilities) requisites for, 314–316
as Personal Trainer, 310–311, *312*
KSA (knowledge, skills, abilities) requisites for, 317–323
as Registered Clinical Exercise Physiologist, 311, *313–314*
KSA (knowledge, skills, abilities) requisites for, 337–346

ACSM Certification Resource Center, contact information, 311

ACSM University Connection Endorsement Program, 310

Activities of daily living (ADLs), 154

Activity Pyramid, 133, *134,* 167

Actos, (*see* Pioglitazone)

Acute mountain sickness, 307t

Adherence to exercise program, 165–167
recommendations for, 167b

Adult Treatment Panel III (ATP III), cholesterol classification of, 45–46

Advair, (*see* Salmeterol, and fluticasone)

Advair Diskus, (*see* Fluticasone, and salmeterol)

Advicor, (*see* Lovastatin, and niacin)

AED (automated external defibrillator), 270

Aerobic fitness, clinical significance of, 118b

Aerobic power, (*see* Maximal oxygen uptake)

AeroBid, (*see* Flunisolide)

Aging, (*see* Elderly people)

AHA (American Heart Association), risk stratification criteria for cardiac patients, 33b–35b

AHA/ACSM, preparticipation screening and risk stratification, 19–36, 33b–35b

AHA/ACSM Health/Fitness Facility Preparticipation Screening Questionnaire, 22, *26*

Albuterol, 259t, 264t, 265t

Alcohol, cardiorespiratory effects of, 265t

Aldactone, (*see* Spironolactone)

Aldalat, (*see* Nifedipine, long-acting)

Aldomet, (*see* Methyldopa)

Aldoril, (*see* Methyldopa, and hydrochlorothiazide)

Alpha adrenergic blockers
cardiorespiratory effects of, 262t
generic and brand names of, 255t

Altace, (*see* Ramipril)

Alternative stretch, 160

Alupent, (*see* Metaproterenol)

Amaryl, (*see* Glimepiride)

Amiloride, 257t, 262t
and hydrochlorothiazide, 258t

Amiodarone, 258t, 263t

Amlodipine, 256t, 261t

Amyl nitrite, 256t, 261t

Angina
scales of assessment, 107
symptoms and clinical significance of, 118b

Angiotensin converting enzyme (ACE) inhibitors
with calcium channel blockers, generic and brand names of, 257t
cardiorespiratory effects of, 262t
with diuretics, generic and brand names of, 257t
generic and brand names of, 256t

Angiotensin II receptor antagonists
cardiorespiratory effects of, 262t

351

Portland Community College